NURSING RESEARCH METHODS

NURSING RESEARCH METHODS

VOLUME II

Qualitative Approaches

Edited by

Peter Griffiths and Jackie Bridges

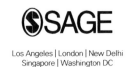

Los Angeles | London | New Delhi
Singapore | Washington DC

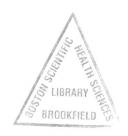

Introduction and editorial arrangement © Peter Griffiths and Jackie Bridges 2010

First published 2010

SAGE Publications Ltd
1 Oliver's Yard
55 City Road
London EC1Y 1SP

SAGE Publications Inc.
2455 Teller Road
Thousand Oaks, California 91320

SAGE Publications India Pvt Ltd
B 1/I 1, Mohan Cooperative Industrial Area
Mathura Road
New Delhi 110 044

SAGE Publications Asia-Pacific Pte Ltd
33 Pekin Street #02-01
Far East Square
Singapore 048763

British Library Cataloguing in Publication Data

A catalogue record for this book is available from the British Library

ISBN: 978-1-84787-946-2 (set of three volumes)

Library of Congress Control Number: 2009921447

Typeset by Star Compugraphics Private Limited, Delhi
Printed on paper from sustainable resources
Printed in Great Britain by the MPG Books Group, Bodmin and King's Lynn

Contents

Volume 2: Qualitative Approaches

Phenomenology

Action Research

Quality in Qualitative Research

Grounded Theory

Myth of Empowerment in Chronic Illness
Barbara Paterson

Introduction

P reviously it was believed that only health professionals should make decisions about disease management. Now people with chronic illness are invited to be partners in decision making. In Canada, as in other countries, health care agencies and governments promise consumers that ill people will have equal say to that of professionals regarding decisions about disease management. The underlying assumption of this promise is that practitioners should invite participation of patients as equal partners.

Much of the current discussion about the need for patient participation in health care decisions is based on a model of empowerment. Empowerment in this context refers to encouraging people to participate as equal partners in decisions about the health care they receive (Opie 1998). Health care professionals who adopt empowering practices respect patients' abilities to make decesions, value their input in such decisions, and are able to relinquish control when a patient rejects their advice (Chapman 1994).

Evidence from research about the self-care decision making of people with diabetes is offered here to suggest that, even when active participation of people with chronic illness is promoted by practitioners, the outcome can be a delegitimization of a patient's ability to participate as an active partner in decisions about care. Our research findings related to self care decision making have been reported elsewhere (Paterson *et al.* 1999, Paterson & Thorne 2000a, 2000b).

Source: *Journal of Advanced Nursing*, 34(5) (2001): 574–581.

Background

The idea that empowerment may be a double edged sword, disguising and sometimes justifying paternalistic practices, has recently received attention from critics of health care (Chapman 1994, Opie 1998). Authors purport that simply changing one's language is not sufficient to effect empowerment; there must also be profound changes in the complex power relations in practitioner–patient interactions (Chapman 1994, Opie 1998, Arksey & Sloper 1999). The primary focus of their critique has been the tendency of practitioners to assume the language of empowerment, including statements that patient participation in treatment decisions is welcome, while at the same time behaving in a manner that implies professional dominance. Although some professionals may support empowerment as a goal of patient participation, their socialization to the 'practitioner as expert' model of health care may be so deeply rooted that they proffer patient participation largely as an extension of their power base, rather than as a collaborative venture (Cahill 1998, Arksey & Sloper 1999). They may perceive patients' attempts to participate in decisions as an invasion of professional territory. For example, participants with cardiac valvular disease reported that although participation was the stated intention of professionals, patients' involvement was frequently restricted to agreeing to comply with the prescribed regime (Jillings 1992).

One of the most significant studies about the contradictory elements of empowerment in health care was conducted by Opie (1998) in New Zealand. The focus of her research was observation of practitioners and families in 45 team reviews and 10 family conferences. Opie determined that although health care professionals believed that they invited and welcomed family participation, they generally positioned themselves as experts, allocating a subordinate, marginalized role to families. A family's input regarding decisions about the patient's plan of care was limited to the agenda established by the health care team. Practitioners often assumed that family members held similar views about the goals and methods of disease management without asking them to validate this assumption.

Similarly, professional dominance is revealed in practitioners' delegitimization of the knowledge and experience of people who have lived with a chronic illness. The experiential insights that people with long-standing chronic illness bring to interactions with professionals can be considered as authoritative knowledge and a source of personal power (Jordan 1993). Authoritative knowledge of people with chronic illness is what they consider legitimate in making self-care decisions and what they mainly weigh in deciding how to manage their disease, even if it contradicts the advice of practitioners (Nyhlin 1990, Mathieu 1993, Kingfisher & Millard 1998). For example, Primomo (1989) discovered that mothers with diabetes tended to evaluate the success of a management plan based on how it affected the family's functioning, not metabolic outcomes. Because, at times, practitioners object to self-care practices that are contrary to professional counsel, people with long-standing chronic illness may choose to hide information about their self-care or at times even lie about it (Paterson & Sloan 1994).

Some professionals, particularly physicians, may devalue the authoritative knowledge of people with chronic illness in favour of more 'objective' data, such as the results of laboratory tests (Fisher 1991). For example, Kingfisher and Millard (1998) determined that clinic staff often ignored or discounted the questions of the women in their study if those questions were perceived to arise from a lay, rather than a biomedical understanding of disease or treatment. Those with chronic pain frequently encounter practitioners who doubt the legitimacy of their illness and label them as hypochondriacs or as difficult (Howell 1994).

Researchers commonly report that although individuals with chronic illness can develop sophisticated awareness of their body's patterns and responses that bear little resemblance to the textbook picture, professionals are sometimes reluctant to acknowledge this expertise as credible (Nyhlin 1990, Paterson & Sloan 1994, Paterson & Thorne 2000a). Paterson and Sloan (1994) found that people with chronic illness were often scolded when they told the doctor of a decision they had made in their self-care management. Such practitioner behaviour emanates from professionals' belief that they know best and that objective evidence, such as physiological indicators or measures of functional integrity, are the only way to determine a person's health status (Molzahn 1991).

Methodology

Our research was guided by the theory of symbolic interactionism (Blumer 1969). Expert self-care managers were viewed as making decisions in accordance with the meaning, derived from their interaction with others, that the situation or event had for them (Annells 1996). For example, we asked participants to record the self-care decisions they made on a daily basis and to reflect on the meaning and significance of these decisions. The investigation was a 2-years longitudinal study of the decision making processes of 22 adults with long-standing (15 years or more) type 1 diabetes. The design was emergent in the tradition of Glaser and Strauss (1967) and followed the procedural and theoretical direction of more recent developments by Thorne *et al.* (1997). An underlying assumption was that the perspective of the insider, or the person with a disease, regarding everyday self-care decisions is best revealed by interpretive research methods.

The research approach entailed simultaneous and ongoing data collection and analysis as well as systematic efforts to check and refine evolving categories of data that determined further literature review, hypothesis development, sample selection and interview questions (Charmaz 1983). For example, when some participants 'shopped around' for practitioners who would facilitate, rather than frustrate, their self-management, the research team conducted a literature review about empowerment and asked participants about what practices would be consistent with empowerment in practitioner–patient relationships. Analysis of the transcripts was guided by traditional constant comparative analytic techniques (Glaser & Strauss 1967).

All 22 participants (14 women and eight men) were Caucasian Canadians who lived in British Columbia, Canada. They ranged in age from 24 to 81 years with a mean of 43 years. They had been diagnosed with diabetes for 15–41 years with a mean of 30 years. Only four had less than high school education; 18 had high school or postsecondary education. Eight participants had one or more diabetes-related complication including nephropathy, retinopathy, atherosclerosis, and neuropathy; 14 had no known diabetes-related complications; 12 lived in urban or suburban areas; the remaining 10 lived in rural areas.

Because a secondary goal of the research was to test and refine the concept of expertise in self-care, we selected participants who were nominated by physicians and those who nominated themselves as expert in self-management of type 1 diabetes. The definition of expert self-management provided to nominators was: the ability to make trustworthy decisions about self-management and to maintain good overall glycaemic control. Eleven people volunteered in response to advertisements in a local newspaper or Canadian Diabetes Association newsletter; they were selected for the study on the basis of self-reports of glycoslylated haemoglobin and self-care decision making ability. Another 11 were nominated by five diabetes internists, physicians who were specialists in the field of diabetes medical care.

The data for the study were derived from an initial interview, audiotaped think-alouds, post-think aloud interviews, and a final focus group interview. In the initial interview, the interviewer asked participants to detail their past and current experiences in diabetes self-management including demographic information such as age and duration of diabetes. All individual interviews occurred in the participants' homes and lasted 90–120 minutes.

Each participant was randomly assigned three periods of 1 week each in the space of a calendar year. During these week-long periods, they were asked to audiotape their self-care decision making using a technique called modified think-aloud or MTA (Fisher & Fonteyn 1995). To permit comparisons between the physician- and self-nominated groups, some participants in each group were given identical MTA schedules. For example, we asked four participants in each group to provide data about self-care decisions during September, immediately following a summer break from work. Think-aloud periods occurred at least 2 months apart to permit sufficient seasonal and other variation to chart the influence of context and other factors on self-management decisions over time. Participants recorded their thoughts, feelings, and decisions made in regard to their diabetes and its management as soon as possible after the decision or situation occurred. For example, one participant recorded, 'a strange sensation in my stomach that might be because I took my insulin too early before I ran', while he was training for a marathon run.

Transcriptions of MTA tapes were used as prompts for questions in an intensive interview, called the post-think-aloud interview (PTAI), that occurred within a week of each MTA data collection period. The purpose of the PTAI was to clarify or extend the participants' statements in the MTA to reveal the complex, multifactorial reasoning of everyday self-care decision making. This entailed repeating participants' statements about a particular self-management decision in the MTA and asking detailed questions about it. For example, an interviewer asked a participant who had experienced hypoglycemia when shopping and waited until she returned home to eat, 'What things about this situation influenced your decision to wait? In what situations might you choose to eat right away? How do you know when a decision to wait is safe and when it isn't?' The PTAI also included questions that were generated in interviews with other participants or the relevant literature. For example, when two men made a decision to eat more at bedtime because they were afraid of nocturnal hypoglycemia, the interviewers explored the experience of nocturnal hypoglycemia with all participants.

A 2-hour focus group interview to share the research findings was held at the conclusion of the study. In each focus group interview, participants in the physician-nominated group were interviewed with others who had been nominated by physicians; those who were self-nominated were interviewed with others who had been nominated themselves. During the focus group, the researcher asked participants to comment about the fit of the findings with their experience in managing their diabetes, any findings they perceived as surprising or confusing, and anything else that they thought was significant about the findings. Participants agreed with the findings as presented but recommended some re-wording (e.g. 'Wait and see' was changed to 'wait and watch' to convey the vigilance that accompanies such a response).

Findings

The findings reported here pertain only to data generated from individual accounts, then validated in the focus group interviews. The data revealed that collaborative partnerships with health care professionals were necessary for participants to actively participate in decision making about their diabetes management. Practitioners who fostered such partnerships were described as 'not necessarily warm and fuzzy' in their approach but as welcoming and respecting the patient's input. One man described a practitioner who had fostered his active participation as 'crusty, no sense of humour, very matter of fact, but willing to really hear me when I say what I think is happening and what needs to happen'. All of the physician-nominated group and only two participants in the self-nominated group had experienced such a partnership. Thes 13 individuals stated that they had met few practitioners whose practices were empowering. They believed that most practitioners 'want to be that way' but that 'empowerment is a great buzz word that is really hard to actually do'. Most practitioners in diabetes care were described as competent but 'more like a professional than a partner'. The participants identified two ways in which practitioners contradicted empowerment: they discounted the experiential knowledge of people who have lived with the disease over time and they did not provide the resources necessary for someone with chronic illness to make informed decisions.

Discounting Experiential Knowledge

Participants concurred that despite the compassionate and competent manner of many health professionals, their response to patients' experiential knowledge often betrayed their essential allegiance to professional dominance. Several indicated that attempts to assume an active role in decisions about their care were met at times with obvious scepticism and, at other times, with anger by health care professionals. For example, many participants told stories of episodes where health care professionals encouraged them to participate in decisions about their care, but then immediately discounted what the patient offered in terms of data. One stated:

> So I went to him (the physician) and I explained how using a grid system for insulin had worked for me. He listened for a second and then said that he didn't believe in that for this and that reason and then he said, 'This is what I use and I think you will find it better'. He was very nice about it. But it was clear that the discussion was over. He was telling me that he didn't want to hear what I thought. He is the doctor and what he says goes. I knew that I needed to shop for another doctor who would be more of a partner with me in this (diabetes management).

Participants perceived such incidents as 'not walking the talk' of empowerment. They stated that until they know that they can be open with a health care professional about their ideas and experiences, they cannot engage in participatory decision making.

Participants stated that practitioners most often communicate their distrust of experiential knowledge in their response to patients' statements about what they believed or desired in their disease management. Three participants indicated that some practitioners respond to such statements by emphasizing the unpredictable nature of diabetes and the complexities of diabetes management that are beyond patients' knowledge and abilities.

He (physician) told me that sure, I could experiment with my insulin if I wanted to. But then he said, 'I hope you don't become unconscious in the night if your blood sugar becomes too low. That will be very hard on your wife.' He knew that I was very afraid of nocturnal hypoglycemia because of that incident in the past. I got the message. He was telling me I should follow what he told me to do. That I would be selfish and irresponsible not to follow his advice to the letter.

Five other participants stated that practitioners convey a distrust of experiential knowledge when they emphasize objective data and dismiss the subjective statements of the person with diabetes. They told of incidents in which practitioners ignored or 'brushed aside' what they told the practitioner because of lack of supportive objective evidence.

I tell her (diabetes educator) about how tired I am, how I just don't have the energy I used to and she says that I am obviously doing well because my A1c (glycosylated haemoglobin) is so good. I am arguing that the new insulin is not for me because I feel terrible and she is saying it's fine because the numbers say it is.

Still others spoke of how practitioners discounted their experiential knowledge by 'quizzing' them about their diabetes knowledge whenever they suggested a change in the prescribed regime.

I get the Spanish Inquisition every time I suggest that we should change what she has ordered. If I don't think it's working or I just want to try something new. She fires questions at me about diabetes or insulin or diet until I don't get the right answer. Then she says that I am not ready to make a decision like that.

Ten participants stated that their experiential knowledge is discounted when practitioners consider only information derived from textbooks as valid and do not heed data that contradict textbook information. As the participants lived with diabetes over time, their patterns of response to situations and treatment changed and their ability to pick up relevant cues about actual or potential diabetes-related problems increased. These cues were often unlike those typically reported in diabetes texts. For example, participants were often able to identify hypo or hyperglycaemia with such subtle signs as 'a slight thickening of the gums', 'the light looking a little brighter than usual', or 'taking a few seconds longer to swing my legs over the bed in the morning'. They perceived textbook signs of hypoglycaemia, such as tremulousness, as 'too late and mostly irrelevant'.

My body has a way of responding that can't be found in any book, The books on diabetes say your blood sugar goes up, not down, with stress. It's the opposite for me when my wife and I fight. If they don't believe me when I tell them that I am different from the books, I know that they don't believe that I know anything.

According to the participants, one of the main ways in which professionals may discount the experiential knowledge of people with chronic illness is when they communicate expectations of compliance. 'They say that they want you to help make decisions about your diabetes but really they only want you to decide to follow what they tell you to do'.

Expectations of compliance were communicated in direct statements ('He told me that I was not to alter the insulin'), by blaming the person for higher than normal blood glucose levels ('He accused me of cheating on my diet'), and by monitoring behaviours, such as expecting the individual to return for frequent appointments ('This doctor wanted to see me every week. He wanted to check up on me to see that I was doing what he told me') and asking to review records of blood glucose levels and insulin ('I could have told her what the patterns were but she needed to see them herself'). Participants agreed that when practitioners focus on compliance, they negate an individual's ability to make decisions and choices that are best for him or her. Several admitted that they lied to practitioners about their self-management strategies because they knew that the professional would disprove of their alterations to a prescribed regime. In fact, these alterations were based on highly sophisticated self-knowledge and experience with the disease and the participants were able to maintain good glycaemic control because of them.

Inadequate Resources for Decision Making

Participants identified a number of resources necessary for them to engage in participatory decision making with practitioners. These included information, time and monetary. Participants stated that the way information is given to persons with chronic illness can affect the willingness and ability to engage in decision making with the practitioner. For example, when practitioners spoke in medical jargon they could not understand, they perceived it as accentuating the power differential between the practitioner and themselves. 'If he can't be bothered to talk so I can understand him, he doesn't really want me to make the decision with him'. Five participants stated that practitioners who do give information irrelevant to their unique situations impair the ability to use that information. A common example was when health care professionals suggested interventions to be used at home without considering the architectural, social or financial constraints that prohibit such a plan.

> So he tells me to get a treadmill and to start using it every day. Or to join a gym. Even though I had been going to him for a year, he didn't remember that I am a student, I have no money, and I live in one room in a friend's house. I was going to say something to him but I – he didn't ask me how

realistic this was for me. He just assumed that this would work because it's what other people do.

One of the resources identified as necessary to participatory decision making is time. Time was described in relation to the duration of their relationship with practitioners, the pace and duration of their visits to the practitioner's office and the duration of waiting time for appointments. Participants stated that lack of time has become a critical issue in recent years as professionals have responded to the ever-increasing demand for chronic illness care. 'Before I could see my doctor in the same day I phone for an appointment. Now there are so many diabetics. He is so swamped, I am lucky if I see him in 3 weeks'.

Participants agreed that changing practitioners on a frequent basis or being referred to specialists who see the ill person only occasionally, constrains the opportunity for participatory decision making. Because they often saw several practitioners, each of whom had a unique and often limited perspective on the diabetes experience, several participants stated that 'no one really has the big picture about what I am all about'. They believed that many practitioners learned to trust their experiential knowledge 'only after they know you and can see that you are serious about your diabetes.' They perceived most short-term relationships with practitioners as 'at best, a beginning point but not sufficient time to know each other well enough to work as a team.' Two commented that some practitioners 'never get to know you, even if you go to them for years. They stay distant because that's their way'.

Participants agreed that participatory decision making is severely constrained whenever practitioners scheduled appointments so that there is little time to ask questions, share ideas or dialogue about available disease management options. They interpreted tight scheduling of appointments as the practitioner being unwilling to include the person with chronic illness as an active participant in health care decisions.

> 'Those people are more concerned with getting you through as fast as possible so they can get onto the next patient, than they are about what's happening to you and what you think.'

One woman who perceived a physician as empowering described him as, 'taking the time, listening to your questions and ideas, not shrugging off what you say because he's scheduled appointments back-to-back and doesn't have the time for you'.

According to participants, practitioners who appeared to lack time frequently convey an allegiance to practitioner 'as the big cheese'. Several stated that practitioners who appear 'too much in a hurry when you are in their office and don't really listen to you' communicate that they are 'not open to a patient's views on things'. They indicated that such practitioners are often unavailable for consultation after hours, do not seem to care about the person's life beyond the disease ('They don't care that you have to live with diabetes in a real world and that there are times when your diabetes isn't the most important part of your life.') and generally offer limited responses to their questions. In their opinion, the accessibility of practitioners to answer questions and to consult about a problem was essential to participatory decision making.

The participants concurred that another constraint to participatory decision making was the costs associated with long waiting times for appointments. They often had to leave work, find child care and pay parking costs in order to attend appointments. If they were required to wait for more than an hour to see the practitioner, they were often reluctant to engage in the time that is required to enact participatory decision making. As one participant stated:

> 'It is often easier simply to let the professional make all the decisions when the (parking) meter is going and you have already waited most of the day'.

Discussion

At first glance, empowerment seems to offer the promise of active participation of people with chronic illness in disease management decisions but the research findings reveal that practitioners' practices often carry subtle but significant messages that contradict the tenets of empowerment (Hess 1996). The paradox that exists concerning empowerment of people with chronic illness is that the stated outcomes are so promising that few practitioners would not agree that it is important. However, the contradictions and challenges that exist in the actualizing of the concept mean that the discourse of empowerment in chronic illness health care may continue to be empty rhetoric (Weissberg 2000).

A central theme in our findings points to why participation in health care decisions is problematic for many people with chronic illness, i.e. the practitioner's positioning as the expert or sole authority. There is a need for further research about the overt and covert ways that practitioners cling to professional dominance and the ways in which practitioners may impede participatory decision making. In contrast to other research that has suggested that people with chronic illness need to develop skills to foster participatory decision making with practitioners, the participants of this research study believed that practitioners should be taught how to enact empowering practices and behaviours. This finding may be a reflection of the 'expert' status of the participants. They perceived that they had already developed the skills of participatory decision making. It is poignant, however, that half the participants had been nominated as successful self-care managers by health care professionals, but even they viewed participatory decision making with practitioners as a rare occurrence.

It is apparent in the research findings that practitioners who view time as a commodity to be juggled in health care present barriers to the enactment of empowerment in health care. For example, in the interest of time management and resource efficiency, health care agencies generally organize the workload of practitioners in such a way that it restricts the amount of time available for individuals with chronic illness to interact with health care professionals. This results in the competing goals of time management and active participation in health care decision making (Golin *et al.* 1996). Time is particularly significant in interactions with clients who have chronic illness because their illness presents complex medical, psychological and social needs that cannot be addressed in the time-efficient medical model of health care in which only the pathology is addressed (Wikblad 1991).

Time with health care professionals is a critical factor in clients being able to assume an active role in decision-making about their care because such a collaborative relationship with health care professionals requires sufficient time to openly explore the client's concerns and ideas (Rheiner 1995). Often clients with chronic illness who visit health care professionals health are required to choose between two or more alternatives of a course of action, each involving significant risk to the individual, without sufficient time or information to do so. If people feel unprepared to make a participatory decision and, in addition, are rushed to arrive at a decision, they will probably rely on practitioners to make the decision independently (Rheiner 1995).

The findings suggest that empowerment is more than simply offering a role in decision making to people with chronic illness. Practitioners can extend invitations to people with chronic illness to engage in participatory decision making, but their behaviours and practices may actually inhibit or negate their intended goal. Interpretations of the research findings must consider the unique nature of the participants as expert self-care managers who demonstrated a commitment to active decision making in regard to their disease management. It is unknown if similar findings would occur in a study that focused on the experiences of people with diabetes who were less experienced in living with the disease or who did not express a desire to be actively involved in the management of the disease.

Conclusions

It is evident in our findings that the discourse of empowerment is not always an actuality in the experience of people with chronic illness. Professionals may talk of empowerment in interactions with people with chronic illness, but then act according to a traditional biomedical model. In that model, the professional is the ultimate decision maker or does not offer the resources that the individual needs to be an active participant in decision making. If health care professionals remain uncritical of the rhetoric of empowerment and are not prepared to identify practices that belie participatory decision making in health care, people with chronic illness may experience unmet expectations and frustration in their interactions with practitioners. As well, uncritical adoption of the discourse of empowerment may lull health care professionals into a false sense of security that all people with chronic illness are able to enter into partnerships with practitioners if only the practitioner extends an invitation to engage in participatory decision making.

References

Arksey H. & Sloper P. (1999) Disputed diagnoses: the case of RSI and childhood cancer. *Social Science & Medicine* **49**, 483–497.

Annells M. (1996) Grounded theory method: philosophical perspectives, paradigm of inquiry, and postmodernism. *Qualitative Health Research* **6**, 379–393.

Blumer H. (1969) *Symxbolic Interactionism.* Prentice-Hall, Englewood Cliffs, NJ.

Cahill J. (1998) Patient participation – a review of the literature *Journal of Clinical Nursing* **7**, 119–128.

Chapman A. (1994) Empowerment. In *Dementia: New Skills for Social Workers* (Chapman A. & Marshall M. eds), Jessica Kinsley. London, pp. 110–124.

Charmaz K. (1983) The grounded theory method: an explication and interpretation. In *Contemporary Field Research* (Emerson R.M. ed.), Waveland, Prospect Heights, IL, pp. 109–126.

Fisher S. (1991) A discourse of the social: medical talk/power talk/oppositional talk? *Discourse & Society* **2**, 157–182.

Fisher A. & Fonteyn M. (1995) An exploration of an innovative methodological approach for examining muses heuristic use in clinical practice - including commentary by J. R. Graves. *Scholarly Inquiry for Nursing Practice* **9**, 263–279.

Glaser B.G. & Strauss A.L. (1967) *The Discovery of Grounded Theory.* Aldine, Chicago, IL.

Golin C.E., DiMatteo M.R. & Gelberg L. (1996) The role of patient participation in the doctor visit: implications for adherence to diabetes care. *Diabetes Care* **19**, 1153–1164.

Hess J.D. (1996) The ethics of compliance: a dialectic. *Advances in Nursing Science* **19**, 18–27.

Howell S.L. (1994) Natural/alternative health care practices used by women with chronic pain: findings from a grounded theory research study. *Nurse Practitioner Forum* **5**, 98–105.

Jillings C.R. (1992) *Back in circulation, or dancing around the circle? Participatory action research in the context of cardiac rehabilitation.* Unpublished Doctoral Dissertation, Union Institute Cincinnati, OH.

Jordan B. (1993) *Birth in Four Cultures: A Cross-cultural Investigation of Childbirth in Yucatan, Holland, Sweden and the United States* 4th edn. Waveland Press, Prospect Heights, IL.

Kingfisher C.P. & Millard A.V. (1998) 'Milk makes me sick but my body needs it': conflict and contradiction in the establishment of authoritarian knowledge. *Medical Anthropology Quarterly* **12**, 447–466.

Mathieu A. (1993) The medicalization of homelessness and the theatre of oppression. *Medical Anthropology Quarterly* **7**, 170–184.

Molzahn A.E. (1991) The reported quality of life of selected home hemodialysis patients. *ANNA Journal* **18**, 173–180, 194.

Nyhlin K.T. (1990) Diabetic patients facing long-term complications: coping with uncertainty. *Journal of Advanced Nursing* **15**, 1021–1029.

Opie A. (1998) 'Nobody's asked me for my view': users' empowerment by multidisciplinary health teams. *Qualitative Health Research* **18**, 188–206.

Paterson B.L. & Sloan J. (1994) A phenomenological study of the decision-making experience of individuals with long-standing diabetes. *Canadian Journal of Diabetes Care* **18**, 10–19.

Paterson B.L. & Thorne. S.E. (2000a) Expert decision making in relation to unanticipated blood glucose levels. *Research in Nursing & Health* **23**, 47–57.

Paterson B.L. & Thorne S. (2000b) The developmental evolution of expertise in diabetes. *Clinical Nursing Research* **9**, 402–419.

Paterson B., Thorne S., Crawford J. & Tarko M. (1999) Living with diabetes as a transformational experience. *Qualitative Health Research* **9**, 786–802.

Primomo J. (1989) *Patterns of chronic illness management, psychosocial development, family and social environment and adaptation among diabetic women.* Unpublished Doctoral Dissertation, University of Washington, Seattle, WA.

Rheiner N.W. (1995) A theoretical framework for research on client compliance with a rehabilitation program. *Rehabilitation Nursing Research* **4**, 90–97.

Roberson M.H.B. (1992) The meaning of compliance: patient perspectives. *Qualitative Health Research* **2**, 7–26.

Thorne S., Kirkham S.R. & MacDonnld-Emes J. (1997) Interpretive description: a non-categorical qualitative alternative for developing nursing knowledge. *Research in Nursing & Health* **20**, 169–177.

Weissberg R. (2000) The vagaries of empowerment. *Society* **37**, 15–21.

Wikblad K.F. (1991) Patient perspectives of diabetes care and education, *Journal of Advanced Nursing* **16**, 837–844.

27

Discovery of Substantive Theory:
A Basic Strategy Underlying
Qualitative Research

Barney G. Glaser and Anselm L. Strauss

In spite of the diversity of problems, approaches and conclusions in the writings of sociologists on qualitative research and analysis, all would seem to support one general position: Qualitative research is a preliminary, exploratory effort to quantitative research since only quantitative research yields rigorously verified findings and hypotheses.[1] The source of this position is that these sociologists appear to take as a guide to being "systematic" the canons of the quantitative analysis on such issues as sampling, coding, reliability, validity, indicators, frequency distributions, conceptual formulization, hypothesis construction and presentation of evidence. Thus these sociologists over-emphasize rigorous testing of hypotheses, and de-emphasize the discovering of what concepts and hypotheses are relevant for the substantive area being researched.

We contend that qualitative research – quite apart from its usefulness as a prelude to quantitative research – should be scrutinized for its usefulness in the discovery of substantive theory.[2] By the discovery of substantive theory we mean the formulation of concepts and their interrelation into a set of hypotheses for a given substantive area – such as patient care, gang behavior, or education – based on research in the area. To view qualitative research as merely preliminary to quantitative research neglects, hence underestimates, several important facts about substantive theory that is based on qualitative research. First, substantive theory is more often than not the end product of

Source: *American Behavioral Scientist*, 8(6) (1965): 5–12.

research within a substantive area beyond which few, if any, research sociologists are motivated to move.[3] Second, it is the basis upon which grounded formal theory is generated.[4] Third, qualitative research is often the most "adequate" and "efficient" method for obtaining the type of information required and for contending with the difficulties of an empirical research situation.[5] Fourth, sociologists (and informed laymen) manage often to profit quite well in their every day work life from substantive theory based on qualitative research.[6]

Together these facts raise doubts as to the applicability of the canons of quantitative research as criteria for judging the credibility of substantive theory based on qualitative research. They suggest rather that criteria of judgment be based on generic elements of qualitative methods for collecting, analyzing and presenting data and for the way in which people read qualitative analyses.

The setting out of these generic elements, to be used both in discovering substantive theory based on qualitative research and in judging its credibility, is the task of this paper. In so doing, we shall regard *qualitative research –* whether utilizing observation, intensive interviews, or any type of document – *as a strategy concerned, with the discovery of substantive theory*, not with feeding quantitative researches. We shall take up the following pertinent matters: 1) the collection and analysis of data, 2) the maximization of substantive theory's credibility by using comparative groups in the research design, 3) the researcher's trust in believing what he knows he knows, 4) the researcher's conveying to others in publication what he knows so that others may judge his theory, and 5) the relation of discovery of substantive theory to its further rigorous testing.

Joint Collection and Analysis of Data

Whether the fieldworker starts out in the confused state of noting everything he sees, because everything may be significant, or whether he starts out with a more defined purpose, observation is quickly accompanied by hypothesizing. When hypothesizing begins, the researcher, even if so disposed, can no longer remain a passive receiver of impressions, but is naturally drawn into actively finding data pertinent to developing and verifying his hypotheses. He looks for that data. He places himself in spaces where his data can be seen "live." He participates in events so that things will pass before his eyes, and so that things will happen to himself which will precipitate further hypothesizing. He may even manipulate events to see what will happen. Although he could manage all these investigatory activities without hypotheses, the hypotheses inevitably arise to guide him.[7]

It is characteristic of fieldwork that multiple hypotheses are pursued simultaneously. Of course, certain events will literally force an important or fascinating hypothesis upon the researcher, so that he spends days or weeks checking out that one hypothesis – especially if its verification is linked with developing social events. Meanwhile other hypotheses are being built into his fieldnotes. Eventually the researcher either actively verifies many of his hypotheses or sufficient verifying events are observed by chance. In either case he no longer packs his notes with evidence pertaining to those particular hypotheses, but goes on to collect data on newer, emerging hypotheses.

The earlier hypotheses may seem unrelated at first, but rather quickly become integrated, to form the basis of a central analytic framework. In fact, fieldworkers have remarked upon the rapid crystallization of that framework, and some have wondered whether later fieldwork does not merely elaborate upon that framework.[8] Whatever the answer, it is certain that experienced researchers quickly develop important concepts, basic categories, and significant hypotheses.[9] Beyond guiding the active search for evidence, these integrated hypotheses immediately provide a central core of theorizing which helps the researcher to develop related hypotheses as well as to prune away those not related. In fact, one hazard of fieldwork is that potentially illuminating perspectives are suppressed in favor of a too rapidly emerging analytic framework.

The analytic framework generally appears on paper in two forms. Analytic comments get written directly into the fieldnotes and are written into occasional memos addressed specifically to matters of analysis. If a research team is involved, the researchers write collective as well as individual memos. Characteristically, researchers withdraw periodically from active field pursuits to reflect upon their observations and write analytic memos. Most field situations force such periods upon the researcher because of the natural lulls in social life. But more important, such respites from active fieldwork are taken by some fieldworkers to avoid collecting huge masses of data without adequate systematic reflection on their research directions and purposes, as guided by their emergent analytic framework.[10]

These reflective periods are immensely important for two additional reasons – other than that the researcher needs occasional relief from observational duty. One reason is, of course, that systematic analysis can better proceed when the researcher thinks uninterruptedly about his observations, interviews and personal field experiences. If a research team is involved, the members can work together better than when scattered about the observational field.

Second, it is necessary to reflect upon what amounts to a process of implicit coding that has been underway since the outset of the research. This reflection by the researcher consists of thinking systematically about the data, in accordance with his basic analytic categories. He need not, however explicitly, code all – or any – of his notes. Fieldworkers actually run through or reread sections of their notes, in order to verify principal hypotheses. They will also run back "in memory" to verify hypotheses. In either case, they do something akin to what ordinarily is termed coding, but do not necessarily raise coding to prominent independent status. Indeed, even when collecting data, researchers will often have an "ah ha!" experience when they recognize that some observed event belongs in a given category. Moreover, strategic memorable events generate new categories and hypotheses, or cast doubt on the efficacy of certain categories and provide negative evidence against previous hypotheses. Those memorable events are either analyzed immediately after they occur, or keep recurring in memory with nagging persistence until systematically analyzed during memo writing periods.

In short, in qualitative work, just as there is no clearcut line between data collection and analysis (except during periods of systematic reflection), there is no sharp division between implicit coding and either data collection or data analysis. There tends to be a continual blurring and intertwining of all three operations from the beginning of the investigation until its near end.

This implicit coding goes on even when researchers do not intend to exploit it purposively, but plan to code explicitly all collected material at the close of fieldwork and then to accomplish the major analysis. However, they may soon realize, *if* substantive theory is their goal, that they have implicitly coded enough material to write their theory already. Therefore, the explicit coding operation can become perceived as a stultifying tedium of little worth, for two reasons.

First, the researchers may find that they are not learning anything new enough about their theory – that is, something that will sufficiently modify the *core* concepts and hypotheses of the theory – to make the explicit procedure seem worthwhile. Of course, explicit coding at the study's close can add further elaboration of details to the substantive theory; but the question is always whether or not the additional effort is worthwhile since there is little chance that the core of the theory will change, and details below the level of generality of the theory seldom add to its wider import and applicability.

Second, little more is likely to be learned by explicit coding after data collection because various segments of the analytic framework get firmed up during chronologically different stages of the fieldwork. Once firmed up, neither more data need be gathered nor analysis rethought for the segment, unless further theoretical work necessitates those additional operations. Experienced fieldworkers know that their fieldnotes not only reflect this continuous firming up, but cannot always be read intelligently by outsiders precisely because at later stages of the research a shorthand reporting occurs which is based upon matters long since firmly known.[11]

The continual intermeshing of data collection and analysis has direct bearing upon how the research is brought to a close. The researcher can always try to mine his data further, and he can always collect more data to check hypotheses or to force new ones. And when writing is done within or near the field, the temptation is especially strong to dash back into the field. This last search for data understandably tends to be either of a specifically confirmatory nature (the researcher moving now with considerable sureness and speed) or of an elaborative nature (the researcher wishing to round out his work by exploring some area that was previously untouched or even unconsidered).[12] This last search can be a strong temptation if personal relations formed in the field are satisfying or if exciting new events are developing there. However, collection and analysis of additional data can be a waste of time because the work merely further elaborates details of the substantive theory; again little of core value is learned.[13]

When the researcher is convinced that his analytic framework forms a systematic substantive theory, that it is a reasonably accurate statement of the matters studied, and that it is couched in a form possible for others to use if they were to go into the same field – then he can publish his results with confidence. He believes in his own knowledgeability and finds no reason to change that belief. He believes not because of an arbitrary judgment but because he has taken very special pains to verify what he thinks he may know every step of the way, from the beginning of his investigation until its publishable conclusion.

Maximizing Credibility through Comparison Groups

In this section we shall present a strategy whereby fieldworkers can facilitate the discovery of a substantive theory, while simultaneously developing confidence in the credibility of that theory. This strategy involves the systematic choice and study of several comparison groups.

Fieldwork in sociology arose from the ethnological tradition of studying one society or group at a time. The sustaining rationale consisted of what one anthropologist or sociologist by himself might be able to observe, plus the conviction that social structure ought to be captured "as a whole." Consequently fieldwork monographs have tended through the years to take the form of single case studies. Even today most fieldworkers study one group at a time and few focus upon more than two or three groups simultaneously.[14] Such comparisons as exist for single case studies are either brought into the monograph (or paper) by footnoting comparable materials and discussing them or by publishing several comparable studies together in one volume.

However, it is feasible in more field studies than have attempted it to *build into the research design a comparison of at least several – and often many – social systems.*[15] The strategy of choosing multiple *comparison groups* is guided by the *logic* of the researcher's emerging analytic framework. Significant categories and hypotheses are first identified in the emerging analysis, during preliminary fieldwork in one or a few groups and while scrutinizing substantive theories and data from other studies. Comparison groups are then located and chosen in accordance with the purposes of providing new data on categories or combinations of them, suggesting new hypotheses, and verifying initial hypotheses in diverse contexts. It is not too difficult to compare as many as forty groups when one considers that they are compared on the basis of a defined set of categories and hypotheses (not compared on the basis of the "whole" group) and that groups within groups are compared (e.g., different and similar wards within different types of hospitals). These groups can be studied one at a time or a number can be studied simultaneously. They can also be studied in quick succession in order to check out major hypotheses before too much theory is built around them.

Multiple comparison groups function in several ways to improve the research and consequent substantive theory. First and foremost the comparisons maximize the credibility of the final theory in two fundamental ways:

A) By precisely detailing the many similarities and differences of the various comparison groups, the analyst knows better, than if he only studied one or a few social systems, under what sets of structural conditions his hypotheses are minimized and maximized, hence to what kinds of social structures his theory is applicable. In increasing the scope and delimiting the generality of his theory, he saves his colleagues work. Ordinarily, readers of fieldwork must figure out the limitations of a published study by making comparisons with their own experience and knowledge of similar groups. By comparison, they figure that the reported material jibes just so far and no further – for given structural reasons. By using multiple comparison groups, much of this burden of delimiting relevant boundaries for the theory is lifted from the reader's shoulders.[16] In short, replication is built into the research.

B) Another way that multiple comparison groups maximize credibility is by helping the researcher to calculate where a given order of events or incidents is most likely to occur or not to occur. This calculus provides an efficient logical guide to groups, for obtaining more data to fill in theoretical gaps and for verifying his hypotheses. This calculus is especially helpful in his efficient search for negative cases that may necessitate reformulation of a hypothesis. Also, the variety lent his study by multiple comparison groups increases the possibility of his being surprised by unanticipated negative cases.

Multiple comparison groups also permit and generate the speedy development of analysis in two principal ways:

A) The constant comparison of many groups rather quickly draws the observer's attention to many similarities and differences among groups that are important for his theory. From these similarities and differences are generated the theoretical categories to be used, their full range of types or continuum, their dimensions, the conditions under which they exist more or less, and their major consequences. In this way, the full generality and meaning of each category is established.[17] Category development is much slower on a single terrain, and the result is a less generalized category imbued with less meaning.

B) In addition, the differences and similarities among groups speedily generate generalized relations among the categories, which of course become the hypotheses soon integrated into the substantive theory. When a negative case is found in a different group, and since a group is an indicator of a set of structural conditions, while reformulating his hypothesis the analyst compares the set of conditions under which it existed to the set under which it is encountered in order to find the particular structural condition(s) making for the change – which condition(s) can then be taken account of in reformulating the hypothesis. This analytic strategy is far different, more powerful, precise, and informative than comparing positive and negative cases within a single structure.[18] In the latter case, one can only compare the *internal* structure of the negative incident to the positive incidents, since both occur under the same structural conditions. That comparison is likely to sound implausible – even tautological – for one ends up saying that an element of an incident caused itself to be different from all other similar incidents. It is more plausible to point to different sets of *external* structural conditions under which positives and negatives exist and, then, suggest differentiating factors in the cases based on comparison of these sets.

Researchers who work with other types of qualitative data can also utilize this efficient method. Using only interviews, for instance, there is no reason why researchers cannot study comparison groups of interviewees, chosen in accordance with emergent analytic frameworks. And historical documents, or other library materials, lend themselves wonderfully to the comparative method. Their use is perhaps even more efficient, since the researcher is saved much time and trouble in his search for comparison groups which are, after all, found concentrated in the library. As in fieldwork, when his analytic framework is far developed, the researcher who uses library materials can always select additional comparison groups to give himself additional confidence in the credibility of his framework. He will also – like the fieldworker who sometimes stumbles upon comparison groups and then makes proper use of them – occasionally profit from such happy accidents which occur when browsing along library shelves.

Trust in One's Own Credible Knowledge

The analytic framework which emerges from the researcher's collection and scrutiny of qualitative data is equivalent to what *he knows systematically about his own data.* Let us discuss why the fieldworker trusts what he knows.

If there is only one fieldworker involved, it is he himself who knows *what* he knows about what he has studied and lived through. They are his perceptions, his personal experiences, and his own hard-won analyses. The fieldworker knows *that* he knows, not only because he's been there in the field and because of his careful verification of hypotheses, but because "in his bones" he feels the worth of his final analysis. He has been living with partial analyses for many months, testing them each step of the way, until he has built his final substantive theory. What is more, if he has participated in the social life of his subjects then he has been living by his analyses, testing them out not only by observation and interview but also in daily livable fact. Hence by the close of his investigation, his conviction about his theory would be hard to shake – as most fieldworkers would attest. This conviction does not mean that his analysis is the only plausible one that might be based on his data, but only that the researcher himself has high confidence in its credibility. What he has confidence in is not a scattered series of analyses, but a systematic ordering of them into an integrated theory.[19] He has, in fact, discovered a substantive theory about delimited arrays of data, through inductive as well as deductive effort, which he is ready to publish.

If a research team is involved, then of course it is their shared knowledge which constitutes the final substantive theory offered to colleagues. Each fieldworker not only knows his own fieldnotes intimately, but has shared his colleagues' observations and experiences by virtue of numerous discussions, "talking out," and memo-writing sessions. The inevitable debates among team members contribute also to the development of a shared analytic framework.

The "real life" character of fieldwork knowledge deserves special under-scoring, especially as many critics think of this and other qualitatively oriented methods as merely preliminary to real (scientific) knowing. A firsthand im-mersion in a sphere of life and action – a social world – different from one's own yields important dividends for the fieldworker. The fieldworker who has observed closely in this social world has had, in a profound sense, to live there. He has not only been sufficiently immersed in the world to know it, but has retained enough detachment to think theoretically about what he has seen and lived through. His informed detachment has allowed him to benefit not only as a sociologist but as a human being who must "make out" in that world. This is true despite the fact that the people there generally do not expect perfect adherence to their ways from the outsider. His detachment has served also to protect him against going more than a little native while yet doing more than a little passing as a native, when the people whom he is studying either have temporarily forgotten his outsider status or have never recognized it. Meanwhile his display of understanding and sympathy for their mode of life permits sufficient trust in him so that he is not cut off from seeing important events, hearing important conversations, and perhaps seeing important docu-ments. If that trust does not develop, his analysis suffers.[20]

The evolving systematic analysis permits the fieldworker quite literally to write prescriptions so that other outsiders might get along in the observed sphere of life and action. That is one benefit of his substantive theory. If he has avoided trouble within the particular social world by following these pre-scriptions, then presumably they accurately represent the world's prominent features; they are workable guides to action and therefore they can, on this account too, be accorded our confidence in their credibility.[21]

In effect this is how shrewd or thoughtful visitors to any social world feel about their knowledge of these worlds. Not infrequently people successfully stake their money, reputations and even lives as well as the fate of others upon their interpretations. *What the fieldworker does is to make this normal strategy of reflective persons into a successful research strategy.* In doing so, of course, a trained, competent researcher is much more systematic in formulating his ideas than is the ordinary visitor; and if a superior researcher, his knowledge is likely to be generalized and systematically integrated into a theory. In addition, he is much more systematic at verifying his ideas than is the ordinary visitor. Such bias as he brings to the field is more likely to be checked upon, while his hypotheses are more likely to arise within the field of observation than to be imported from the outside. In the latter regard, he also differs from researchers who bring such a working baggage of formal theory into the field that they end not by discovering much substantive theory but manage principally to write footnotes to the imported theory. They are not likely, either, to do very well in the pragmatic test of living by their theory while in the field.

Finally, it is worth special mention that those fieldworkers who do *not* really believe in their own hard-won substantive theory are tempted toward a compulsive scientism. Because they do not trust themselves – their own ability to know or reason – they rely additionally upon questionnaires or other "objective" methods of collecting and analyzing quantified data. Used for this purpose these methods do not necessarily lead to greater credibility, but they do permit the insecure researcher to feel greater security in his "results" without genuine consideration of what queries do or do not need this additional "hard" data. It is also true that the insecure fieldworker may know that he is running away from himself, because of a failure of confidence in his ability to render his knowledge credible, but he cannot stop running!

Conveying and Judging Credibility

When the researcher decides to write for publication, then he faces the problem of conveying to colleagues the credibility of his discovered theory so that they can make some sensible judgment about it. The problem of conveying credibility is dividable into two sub-problems, each of which deserves discussion.

The first sub-problem is that of getting readers to understand the theoretical framework. This is generally done by giving an extensive abstract presentation of the framework and its associated theoretical statements, generally at the beginning and/or end of the publication but usually also in segments throughout the publication. This presentation is not particularly difficult since there exists an abstract social science terminology which is quite as applicable to qualitative as to quantitative data as well as a common sociological perspective which furthers the communication.

The related second sub-problem is how to describe the social world studied so vividly that the reader can almost literally see and hear its people – but see and hear in relation to the theoretical framework. To do this, the researcher ordinarily utilizes several of a considerable armamentarium of standard devices.

He can quote directly from interviews or conversations which he has over-heard. He can include dramatic segments of his on-the-spot fieldnotes. He can quote telling phrases dropped by informants. He can summarize events or persons by constructing readable case studies. He can try his hand at describing events and acts; and often at least he will give backdrop descriptions of places and spaces. He will even offer accounts of personal experience to show how events impinged upon himself. Sometimes he will unroll a narrative. Chapter headings can also help to convey sights and sounds.[22]

The first and second sub-problems of conveying credibility through plausible reasoning are reflected in the type of concepts that the researcher chooses for writing his substantive theory. With regard to the first problem, his concepts are analytic – sufficiently generalized to designate the proper-ties of concrete entities (not the concrete entities themselves). With regard to the second problem, his concepts also are sensitizing – yield a "meaningful" picture – abetted by apt illustrations which enable one to grasp the reference in terms of one's own experience.[23] Formulating concepts of this nature, hence tapping the best of two possible worlds, takes considerable study of one's data.[24]

Several aspects of the presentation enter into how the reader, in turn, judges the credibility of the theory that the writer is trying to convey. First of all, if a reader becomes sufficiently caught up in the description so that he feels vicariously that he also had been in the field, then he is more likely to be kindly disposed toward the researcher's theory than if the description seemed flat or unconvincing.

Second, a judgment of credibility will also rest upon assessments con-cerning how the researcher came to his conclusions. The reader will note, for instance, what range of events the researcher saw, whom he interviewed, who talked to him, what kinds of experiences he had, and how he might have appeared to various people whom he studied. That is, the reader will assess the types of data utilized from what is explicitly stated as well as from what can be read between the lines. It is absolutely incumbent upon the reader to make such judgments, partly because the entire publication may be a complete fabrication[25], but more usually because any analysis may require some qualification.

Such qualification we may term "the discounting process." Readers surely discount aspects of many, if not most, analyses which are published (whether resting upon qualitative or quantitative data).[26] This discounting by the reader takes several forms: the theory is *corrected* because of onesided research designs[27], *adjusted* to fit the diverse conditions of different social structures, *invalidated* for other structures through the reader's experience or know-ledge, and deemed *inapplicable* to yet other kinds of structures. It is import-ant to note that when a theory is deemed inapplicable to a social world or social structure, then it cannot be invalidated by their conditions. It is not correct to say that because a theory "does not fit" a structure, then it is invalid.

The invalidation or adjustment of a theory is only legitimate for those social worlds or structures to which it is applicable.

This ongoing discounting process of qualification by the reader allows the researcher to write his theory in general form, because the researcher knows that the reader will make the necessary corrections, adjustments, invalidations and inapplications when thinking about or using the theory. These are qualifications that he could not begin to cover for even a small percentage of one type of reader and, more important, they are qualifications which the researcher must learn to gloss over or to ignore in order to write a substantive theory of some generality.[28] (It is also necessary to leave out qualifications in order to write a theory that is readable, because the rhetoric of qualification is as onerous to read as to write.)

The researcher and his readers thus share a joint responsibility. The researcher ought to provide sufficiently clear statements of theory and description so that readers can carefully assess the credibility of the theoretical framework offered in his publication. A cardinal rule for the researcher is that whenever he himself feels most dubious about an important interpretation – or foresees that readers may well be dubious – then he should specify quite explicitly upon what kinds of data his interpretation rests. The parallel rule for readers is that they should demand explicitness about important interpretations, but if the researcher has not supplied the information then they should assess his interpretations from whatever indirect evidence may be available. These same rules apply to the reading of qualitative materials from libraries and organizational archives, as well as to the writing of those materials.

The Issue of Further Rigor

The presentation of substantive theory, developed through analysis of qualitative data, is often done at a sufficient level of plausibility to satisfy most readers. The theory can be applied and adjusted to many situations with sufficient exactitude to guide thinking, understanding and research. Given certain structural conditions under which sociologists work (such as designing specific action programs, or working in a rather well developed substantive area), then more rigorous testing may be required to raise the level of plausibility of some hypotheses.

Under these conditions, it should be a matter of empirical determination as to how the further testing can best be accomplished – whether through more rigorous or extensive fieldwork itself, or through experiments or survey methods. The two essential points in this decision on method are, first, that the testing be more rigorous than previously (not *which* of all methods is the most rigorous); and, second, that the more rigorous approach be compatible with the research situation in order to yield the most reliable findings. What should not enter into the determination of further testing are the researcher's ideological commitments (with associated career contingencies) to only one method; for instance, that a survey is a more rigorous mode of achieving a high degree of plausibility than field observation, and therefore it is the best and only mode to use in all cases. In the actual research situation, a survey may not be feasible nor worth the time or money, nor yield the type of information needed, and indeed it may even distort the information yielded. An approach to an increased, required level of plausibility should be based, therefore, on the use of the method or methods best suited to the socially structured necessities of the sociologist's research situation.

This cardinal rule for determining which method to use for increasing the plausibility of the substantive theory is broken in another way by researchers who are ideologically committed to quantitative methods. They assume out of context that all research requires a rigorously achieved high level of plausibility and that quantitative research, more rigorous than most qualitative methods, is therefore the *best* method to use in *all* research situations. Thus, whatever qualitative research may be done is seen merely as a preliminary provision of categories to use in the ensuing quantitative research. As noted at the beginning of our paper, this position neglects both the importance of discovering substantive theory based on qualitative research and the fact that this substantive theory is more often than not the end product of research within the substantive area beyond which few, if any, research sociologists are motivated to move.

Substantive theory discovered through qualitative analysis is often the end product of research for a variety of reasons. First, those researchers who do try to move beyond substantive theory by testing it with quantitative data are often told by colleagues and editorial boards that they are simply proving what everyone knows sufficiently well already. They are told their work is trivial and a waste of resources.[29] To "save" their work, they are forced to turn their quantitative work of testing the "already known" hypothesis into an effort at discovering, in their data, new substantive fact and theory. Thus, quantitative data is often used not for rigorous demonstration of theory but as another way to discover more theory, and qualitative data results often in a *de facto* conclusive analysis rather than a preliminary analysis.

Second, it is an old story in social science that contemporary interest switches from certain phenomena once that interest is saturated with substantive theory. This switch usually occurs long before satisfactory quantitative research pertaining to the phenomena has taken place. Meanwhile, informed laymen and social scientists manage to profit quite well by the merely plausible work of discovery published by sociologists who carefully analyse their qualitative data. This ability to profit from substantive theory based on qualitative research forestalls the need for future highly rigorous research among most sociologists and laymen.[30] Since the theory works well enough, it is typically only modified, if even that, not by further demonstrative research on a specific hypothesis but by additional related theory. The researcher's primary effort in working with this related theory is to discover new theory, not to correct or test older theory. Once new theory is discovered and developed, any modification of older theory that then occurs will receive post-hoc recognition.

And third – much the most important reason – a great deal of sociological work, unlike physical science research, never gets to the stage of rigorous demonstration because the social structures which sociologists study are undergoing continuous change. Older structures frequently take on new dimensions before highly rigorous research can be accomplished. The changing of social structures means that a prime sociological task is the exploration – and even literal discovery – of emerging structures. Undue emphasis on being "scientific" is simply not reasonable in light of our need for discovery and exploration amidst very considerable structural changes.

Concluding Remarks

Most writing on sociological method has probably been concerned with how theory can be more rigorously tested. In this paper we have addressed ourselves to the equally important enterprise of how the discovery of substantive theory can be furthered. The formulation of fruitful substantive theory for a substantive area through careful research – as against constructing formal theory for a conceptual area (such as deviance, status congruency, reference groups or hierarchy) – is a major task in sociology. Substantive theory faithful to the empirical situation cannot be formulated, we believe, by merely applying a formal theory to the substantive area. First a substantive theory must be formulated, in order to see which of diverse formal theories are applicable to help further the substantive formulation.[31] And in its turn then substantive theory helps in formulating and reformulating formal theory. Thus substantive theory becomes a strategic link in the formulation and development of formal theory based on data. We have called the latter "grounded" formal theory to contrast it with formal theory based on logical speculation.[32]

Some forty years ago, Thomas and Znaniecki hazarded that one type of qualitative data (autobiographies) might be the most useful kind of data for sociological theory.[33] Anthropologists, however, then and now generally believe that fieldwork data – encompassing observations and interviews as well as case studies and autobiographical accounts – are most useful. And in the recent literature of sociology, there has been some argument on the comparative virtues of various types of qualitative data: for instance, interview *versus* fieldwork data and historical *versus* contemporary data.[34] Regardless of the type of qualitative data preferred, all seem admirably suited for discovery of substantive theory pertaining to the areas and problems with which sociologists are concerned.

Notes

This paper was developed from qualitative research done during a study of terminal care in hospitals, sponsored by NIH Grant NU 00047. We are indebted to Howard S. Becker, Fred Davis, Egon Bittner, Rue Bucher, Virginia Olesen and Stewart Perry for their helpful comments and encouragement during revisions of this paper.

1. See, e.g., A. H. Barton and P. F. Lazarsfeld, "Some Functions of Qualitative Analysis in Social Research," reprinted in Lipset and Smelser, *Sociology: The Progress of a Decade.* Englewood Cliffs: Prentice-Hall 1961, 95–122; B. Berelson, *Content Analysis.* Glencoe: Free Press, 1952, 114–134, esp. 133; S. A. Stouffer, *Social Research to Test Ideas.* New York: Free Press, 1962, 1–10, esp. 10; R. K. Merton, *Social Theory and Social Structure.* Glencoe: Free Press, 1957, 15–16 and chaps. 11 and 111. One author, somewhat ambivalent on this position, seems to agree that discovery in qualitative research is preliminary to rigorous testing, but prefers to establish testing methods applicable to qualitative data using the canons of quantative work (H. S. Becker, "Problems of Inference and Proof in Participant Observation," *Amer. Soc. Rev.,* Dec., 1958, 653). For a critique of this general position sec H. Blumer, "Sociological Analysis and the 'Variable,'" *Amer. Soc. Rev.* 21, 1956, 683–690. Perhaps the latest perspective is the "multiple methodology" approach which sees qualitative analysis as preliminary for some kinds of information (e.g., an enumeration) and the end product for other kinds (e.g., a norm) (M. Zelditch, Jr., "Some Methodological Problems of Field Studies," *Amer. J. Soc.,* March, 1962, 567; and A. Vidich and J. Bensman, "The Validity of Field Data," *Hum. Org.,* 13, 1954, 20–27; and R. N. Adams and J. J. Preiss, *Human Organization Research.* Homewood: Dorsey Press, 1960, 223–4.
2. The richness of qualitative research for the discovery of substantive theory is well known; for detailed explanations of why this is so see Becker, *op. cit.,* 652–3 and 657–8, and H. S. Becker and B. Geer, "The Analysis of Qualitative Field Data," in *Human Organization Research. op. cit.,* 262–3.
3. This fact is discussed above in the section, "The Issue of Further Rigor."
4. This fact is discussed in concluding remarks.
5. Zelditch, *op. cit.,* 575.
6. This fact is brought out in many ways throughout this paper.
7. Becker and Geeer, *op. cit.,* 270–1.
8. B. Geer, "First Days in Field Work," in P. E. Hammond, *Chronicles of Social Research.* New York: Basic Books, Inc., 1964.
9. *Cf.,* B. Paul, "Interview Techniques and Field Relationships," in A. L. Kroeber (ed.), *Anthropology Today.* Chicago: University of Chicago Press, 1953, 430–51.
10. Some inexperienced or compulsive researchers, afraid that they are missing important events, fail to create sufficient breathing space for careful analytic memo writing. The same failing is also characteristic of researchers who work with other kinds of qualitative data.
11. Again, what is true of fieldwork seems equally true of research using other kinds of qualitative data, such as historical materials, in contrast, say, with researchers who use quantified content-analysis methods upon eaches of data.
12. *Cf.,* A. Strauss, L. Schatzman, R. Bucher, D. Ehrlich, and M. Sabshin, *Psychiatric Ideologies and Institutions.* New York: Free Press, 1964, chap. 2. See also H. Becker, B. Geer, E. Hughes and A. Strauss, *Boys in White.* Chicago: University of Chicago Press, 1962, *re* interviews after field observation.
13. Though highly unlikely, there is, of course, the small chance that additional data can "explode" an otherwise finished analytic framework and cause the researcher to spend months or years before he is satisfied enough to publish. This hazard is not confined to work with qualitative data, but is especially characteristic of qualitative work.

14. Two recent field studies which have compared attributes of a specific type of organization, utilizing many such organizations in many nations, are: W. A. Glaser, "American and Foreign Hospitals: Some Sociological Comparisons." in E. Freidson (ed.), *The Hospital in Modern Society*. New York: Free Press, 1963, 37–73; and N. Kaplan, "The Western European Scientific Establishment in Transition," in *Amer. Behav. Sci.*, vi, Dec., 1962, 17–20.

15. The logic of our strategy complies with Nagel's directive for "controlled investigation" in any science: "However, every branch of inquiry aiming at reliable general laws concerning empirical subject matter must employ a procedure that, if it is not strictly controlled experimentation, has the essential logical functions of experiment in inquiry." E. Nagel, *The Structure of Science*. New York: Harcourt, Brace & World, Inc., 1961, 453. We ourselves used this method in a study reported in a forthcoming volume, *Awareness of Dying*.

16. See, i.e., J. Q. Wilson's strictures on D. C. Thompson's. *The Negro Leadership Class*, in *Amer. Soc. Rev.*, 28, Dec., 1963, 1051–52.

17. Consider the full discussion of this point in R. Bendix, "Concepts and Generalizations in Comparative Sociological Studies," *Amer. Soc. Rev.*, 28, Aug., 1963, 532–9.

18. The initial advocates in sociology of a search for negative cases have either focused on them within one structure or omitted explicit focus upon structural conditions. They have, rather, focused upon the search for negative incidents within categories of analysis under which they have amassed a series of positive incidents. Becker and Geer, *op. cit.*, 287–8; A. Lindesmith, *Opiate Addiction*. Bloomingdale: Principia, 1947, chap. 1.

19. This theme is extensively developed throughout H. Zetterberg. *On Theory and Verification In Sociology*. N. J.: Bedminster Press, 1963. It is important that one distinguish between the researcher's conviction in the credibility of his theoretical analysis and his conviction that he understands much about the perspectives and meanings of his subjects. Researchers will readily agree that their own theoretical formulations represent credible interpretations of their data – which could be interpreted differently by others – but it would be hard to shake their conviction that they have correctly understood much about the perspectives and meanings of the people whom they have studied.

20. For a fieldwork account of how tightly closed doors were finally opened after trust was established, see, R. Wax, "Twelve Years Later: An Analysis of Field Experience," *Amer. J. Soc.*, 63, 1957, pp. 133–42.

21. The most vigorous of quantitative researchers may write a methodological article from "heart" with no data collection or coding because he simply knows what he knows. He has lived it and he was successful. People will believe him because they know he has been through it. In writing this article, he is merely doing fieldwork on himself.

22. The researcher's task of conveying credibility is actually much like that of the realistic novelist. The latter generally leaves his analytic framework – his interpretation – much more implicit than does the researcher. Often the novelist's tactics for getting the reader to imagine social reality are more subtle, because he may not only be a more skilled writer but may feel that he can use more license in his presentation. Sometimes too his descriptive task is simpler because his analytic framework is much simpler. Nonetheless, the great novelists have conveyed societal views which readers have long felt to be both complex and real (i.e., credible). We say this not to pit researchers against novelists, but to point out where their respective tasks may be similar and where different.

23. On sensitizing concepts see H. Blumer, "What is Wrong with Social Theory." *Amer. Soc. Rev.*, 19, Feb., 1964, 3–10, quote on page 9.

24. Consider the effort in this direction by H. L. Zetterberg, *Social Theory and Social Practice*. New Jersey: Bedminster Press, 1962, chap. 3. The concepts should also be clearly specified so that they can be readily measured by existing techniques, *if* researchers desire to test quantitatively hypotheses based on them.

25. Note for instance how gullible or unsuspecting readers can believe wholly in purposely fake accounts, such as the papers reprinted in R. Baker (ed.), *Psychology in the Wry.* Princeton: Nostrand, 1963.
26. *Cf.*, B. Berger's review of J. Coleman's quantitative study, *The Adolescent Society*, in *Soc. Prob.*, 10, 1963, 394–400; also J. Q. Wilson, *op. cit.* And whether analysis is quantitative or qualitative, later generations of scholars will discount it by placing it within a larger context of public rhetoric, *cf.*, "Appendix: A Note on Imagery in Urban Sociology," in A. Strauss, *Images of the American City.* Glencoe: Free Press, 1961, 255–58.
27. For instance, when we read that someone has done fieldwork with workers in a factory, we suspect that his interpretive account (as it pertains even to the workers) needs some correction because the administrators have not been similarly studied. What correction is needed may not, of course, be so evident: for instance, some sociologists have studied state mental hospitals from a perspective really borrowed from psychiatry and thus interpreted its structure and functioning from a quasi-psychiatric viewpoint. The needed correction was read in by at least one set of readers, who themselves later studied a mental hospital and came to a rather different conclusion about such institutions (R. Bucher and L. Schatzman, "The Logic of the State Mental Hospital," *Soc. Prob.*, 9, 1962, 337–349). This latter instance suggests that readers are not always merely readers, but can also be or become researchers upon topics about which they have read.
28. Consider the discussion of social laws by E. Nagel, *op. cit.*, 459–66.
29. For a few (or many) diverse comments of concern on the trivial results of "precise" quantitative research, see: on their laboring of the obvious, R. K. Merton, "Problem Finding in Sociology," in R. K. Merton, L. Broom and L. S. Cottrell, Jr. (eds.), *Sociology Today.* New York: Basic Books, 1959, IV–I; on their uselessness for theory construction, H. L. Zetterberg, *On Theory and . . .*, preface, 36, 52, and 67; and on their worth in verifying what is already known, A. Etzioni, "Book Review," *Amer. J. Soc.*, LXVII, Jan., 1962, 466.
30. "While we cannot count on very many research workers being stimulated to conduct crucial tests of middle-range theories, they are likely to be especially stimulated by the concepts that enter into such theories." H. Hyman, "Reflections on the Relations Between Theory and Research." *The Centennial Review*, VII, No. 4, Fall, 1963, 449.
31. Ignoring the task of discovering substantive theory that is relevant to a given substantive area is the result, in most cases, of believing that formal theories can be directly applied to an area, and that these formal theories supply all the necessary concepts and hypotheses. The consequence is often a forcing of data and neglecting of the relevant concepts and hypotheses that may emerge. Allowing substantive concepts and hypotheses to emerge first on their own, enables the analyst to ascertain which of diverse formal theories may be inclusive of his substantive theories, thus enabling him to be more faithful and less forcing of his data (or more objective and less theoretically biased). This means that one cannot merely apply Parsonian categories right off, but must wait to see whether they are linked to the emergent substantive theory concerning the issue in focus.
32. An outstanding example of "grounded" social theory is H. S. Becker, *The Outsiders.* New York: Free Press, 1962.
33. W. I. Thomas and F. Znaniecki, *The Polish Peasant in Europe and America.* New York: Knopf, 1918.
34. See H. S. Becker and B. Geer, "Participant Observation and Interviewing: A Comparison," *Hum. Org.*, XVI, 1957, 28–34; M. Trow, "Comment," *Hum. Org.*, XVI, 1957, 33–35; and Becker and Geer, "Rejoinder," *Hum. Org.*, XVII, 1958, 39–40.

28

Qualitative Data as a Potential Source of Theory in Nursing

Margaret Jacobson

First of all, I'd like to change the title of this paper from that listed on the program "Grounded Theory and its Potential for Adaptation to Nursing" to that of "Qualitative Data as a Potential Source of Theory in Nursing," for the reason that the original title may imply that I plan to take grounded social theory and adapt it as a nursing theory. As nurses, concerned with identifying or building theory in nursing, I propose that we concern ourselves with a more systematic use of our rich sources of qualitative data. I am not primarily concerned with theory development for intellectual exercise, for professionalization or for enhancing nursing in the academe. I am concerned with theory in nursing because I believe that theory has pragmatic value which will ultimately contribute to the improvement of health care.[1]

This does not preclude the use of theory that applies to humans in their processes of growth, development, behavior, socialization, interaction, and so on. The fact that nursing deals with people in their life cycles from preconception to postmortem presumes an interdisciplinary orientation. If we are to generate and develop usable practical theories in nursing they might well be derived, tested, developed and discarded in nursing practice. Some of such theories may stand the tests of time, use, and inquiry.

Glaser and Strauss, sociologists at the University of California at San Francisco have presented their methodology for "discovering" theory from data in the book entitled, **The Discovery of Grounded Theory: Strategies for Qualitative Research**.[2] Grounded theory is theory "discovered" from

Source: *Image*, 4 (1970): 10–14.

data "systematically obtained and analyzed from social research."[3] It is theory generated and inductively developed from data, and it is illustrated by characteristic examples of the data in contrast to logically deduced theory where examples are selected for their confirming value. The writers, themselves, have stated that they perceive their work as a beginning and purposely have not posed clear-cut procedures and definitions.

Probably everyone here knows or has utilized the "Awareness Theory" presented in **Awareness of Dying**.[4] Awareness theory in the substantive area of dying is concerned with the "awareness context," that is, what goes on around the patient who is in the process of dying. There are four types of awareness contexts contained in this theory. These are **closed awareness, suspicion, mutual pretense and open awareness**. This theory is a prime example of a grounded theory which has shown itself to be applicable and practical for nurses and others functioning in the areas of terminal care. It was generated from qualitative data of the type that all of us have been a part of or experienced indirectly in our nursing practice. Because of the impact of the situation and the great need for a guiding theory in this highly sensitive area of dying, many of us have joyfully clasped the "Awareness Theory" to our bosoms. Why has it been so useful? It is a substantive theory of interaction which meets the four requisite properties of grounded theory. These are **Fitness, Understanding, Generality,** and **Control**.[5] It fits the everyday realities of the situation where it is applied for the reason that the data were derived from what actually occurred in a variety of situations of dying. It makes sense and it is understandable by the people involved in the terminal care areas because it is congruent with the realities of the situation. Its concepts have a generality that make for flexibility in the changing conditions of terminal care situations. As to control, nurses and doctors have a great deal of control over the awareness contexts in terminal care.

This theory is a sociological theory of interaction in the substantive area of dying and the method used is comparative analysis. Glaser and Strauss have entitled their use of comparative analysis the "constant comparative" method. The process of selecting data to be treated by the constant comparative method is entitled, "theoretical sampling."[6] Theoretical sampling is defined as the process of data collection for generating theory whereby the analyst jointly collects, codes, and analyzes his data and the decision of what data to collect next and where to collect it is determined by the needs of the developing theory. There is apparently a wide difference between "theoretical sampling" and the rules of inclusion and exclusion of groups as used in research when attempting to control variables. This is evident when one seeks to develop the properties of categories when theory generation rather than theory verification is the goal.

Comparative analysis in itself is not an innovative method. It has long been used by anthropologists as a general method in comparing social groups such as institutions. Glaser and Strauss advocate its use systematically in a wide range of social units of any size and they have demonstrated the use of this method in small groups, such as hospital wards where patients died at different rates. The four states of the constant comparative method are described as a process of continuous development until the analysis is complete. This process is too lengthy for the purposes of this paper, but for the sake of clarity at this point they are (1) the comparison of incidents to formulate a category, (2) the integration of categories and their properties, (3) delimiting the theory, and (4) writing the theory.[7] Briefly, this involves coding each incident into as many categories as possible as categories develop. The coding also identifies the comparison group where the incident occurred. In the first stage incident is compared to incident and in this way similar properties of the categories become evident. In the second stage the process becomes that of comparing incidents with properties of the categories which resulted from stage one. Memos are written through both stages to record the ideas of the developing theory as they occur throughout. As the data accumulate (using theoretical sampling), the categories and their properties become related in many different ways producing a unified whole as the theory emerges. Coding, comparison, categorizing and memo writing are not done as separate tidy tasks, but these are described as part of an ongoing interrelated process. The constant comparative method apparently has its own delimiting features in what could become unwieldy masses of data. The categories become repetitious and new incidents are not coded unless they point to a new aspect which could contribute to the theory. Reducing of the theory occurs by discovering underlying uniformities in the categories or their propertes. This makes it possible to formulate the theory from concepts. In writing the theory, the writer has in his possession coded data, a collection of memos and a theory. The memos provide the content underlying the categories and the categories become the major themes of the theory from which formal propositions can be made. Coding and categorizing as part of the constant comparative method are obviously dependent upon the judgment, skills and sensitivity of the person doing the analysis. The process of integrating the categories and discovering the underlying uniformities from which a theory can be derived is not a simple process. I certainly do not wish to imply that there is a simple formula for deriving theory from qualitative data. The method of comparative analysis is flexible, but it necessitates judgment and discernment as well as experience.

Much of the research by nurses has been concerned with testing established theory applications to various nursing situations, the use of scales for measuring attitudes or opinions, and with the construction of experimental designs. This is appropriate. However, it has been part of our growth pattern that so far most of our nursing research has been in the form of the dissertation for a higher degree. To date we are just reaching the point where we have some postdoctoral research being done, and only recently have we reached a developmental stage where we can anticipate nursing research geared toward theory generation and development. Research and theory are highly interrelated. A logico-deductive type theory needs research to support it. A grounded theory requires research to obtain the data from which the theory is generated or discovered. Both types of theory require research to test the hypotheses they engender.

Nurses have, to my knowledge, always been concerned with the accurate reporting of qualitative data. In fact, some of the old type reporting of nurses was quite objective – to the point of being almost staccato in its lack of embellishments – really, just the facts. Until recent years when nurses have become prepared to conduct their own research investigations, they have habitually functioned as data collectors in the research efforts of others. Major public health studies owe much of their success to the quality of the data collected by nurses. What goes on in the context of patient care is fraught with variables which cannot be controlled or appropriately placed in an experimental design. Oliver Osborne of Michigan State, has made some pertinent observations on this point.

> For nurses there remains the requirement of adequate descriptions of nursing practice. To date, such descriptions have been either too simplistic or prematurely problem oriented. Involved in this has been a tendency to describe nurse interractions only as they illuminate certain constricted theoretical problems . . . There is need for more comprehensive patient care studies. Such studies should be diachronic as well as synchronic. The collection and comparison of such studies will reveal regularities in the patient nurse relationships which will facilitate the development of general and efficient theories of nursing practice. The anthropological ethnography can be used as a prototype for descriptions of such interactions. In anthropology the ethnographic descriptions of social and cultural phenomena have contributed to the development of much anthropological theory within a short period of time.[8]

Nursing has long been concerned with the "whole person," a holistic concept of the individual as a part of his total environment and heritage.[9] This concept is becoming more enunciated as the causes of illness become less attributable to a single causative organism and more related to multiple factors of environmental distresses impinging on individuals and groups.

The sources of qualitative data in nursing are accessible, perhaps more so because nursing is a practice discipline. Nursing is permeated with cumulative data available for systematic analysis with theory as the goal. For a few examples: Nursing has long made use of the case method and care studies have been an inherent part of our teaching, but few teachers have used this method as a source of qualitative data with the thought of theory in mind, and they have not until recently stimulated their students to utilize this type data for seeking concepts and generalizations. I am sure that many of you know a teacher who has collected vast stores of process recordings and who is sensitive to the inherent worth of these materials, yet does not have theory generation in mind. It is interesting to contemplate what diachronic and synchronic accounts of long term illness contexts might hold in potential theory.

Our libraries now hold rich qualitative data in the form of documentary evidence in nursing, as do the archives of our organizations. Documentary evidence need not come from nursing sources, per se. Consider fiction and non-fiction. Most of us can sharpen our skills in the use of library resources. These same skills of selectivity and comparison are needed in the appropriate use of historical documentary materials as they are for materials derived from field and clinical practice areas.

Participant observation as a source of qualitative data in nursing has been criticized because it has been said that the nurse lacks objectivity when acting as a participant and observer simultaneously. This seems very strange to me since so much of anthropological research has been dependent upon the researcher becoming a participating member of the community as do many of the community studies in sociology. Actually to become part of the situation and still retain objectivity is a skill any trained observer has to cultivate. In addition, there are some nursing situations in which it would not be possible to collect data other than as a participant.[10]

Nursing is in need of substantive-type theories applicable in a variety of nursing situations. It is possible to develop such theories directly from the qualitative data of every day nursing contexts. We deal repeatedly with many of the same problems in a variety of settings. Basically many more facts are needed in and of nursing, that is, there is need for more systematic descriptions of what actually occurs in nursing care situations to a cumulative level from which theory might be derived. For example, we say that nurses "promote health." It is conceivable that one could develop a theory of "nurse-type health promotion" derived from the qualitative data of nurses going about the process of intentionally promoting health in various settings. On the other hand, maybe we don't promote health as clearly as we say we do. Examples and non-examples are both required for the formulation of concepts.

In summary, I am saying that nursing is rich in resources of qualitative data as a potential source of nursing theory. I am not precluding the quantifying of qualitative data or theory derived from quantitative data. I am saying that general as well as specific methods and criteria have been developed in the social sciences and nursing which can be very helpful in handling qualitative data for the purposes of theory generation. I am saying that nursing for the reason that it is concerned with human beings is necessarily inter-disciplinary in its orientation but the generation of nursing theory from nursing practice is something that has to be done by nurses; that is, we need to do our own methodology development. Sociological theories are useful, theories of anthropology are useful, as are psychological theories, and nursing theories will, I anticipate, also be useful. It would be interesting and productive if this discussion group would point up some priority areas in nursing practice where appropriate qualitative data might produce applicable theory. If we are convinced that **"Theory begins and ends in practice,"**[11] then it is easier to visualize theory generated from the qualitative data of nursing practice which will fulfill the functions of description, explanation and prediction.

References

1. Theory can contribute to improved health care by guiding practice, predicting outcomes, provoking questions about applicability, and testing generality of application.
2. One of a series of publications developed through a Public Health Service Grant from the Division of Nursing, Bureau of State Services-Community Health. Glaser, Barney G. and Anselm L. Strauss, *The Discovery of Grounded Theory: Strategies for Qualitative Research*. Chicago: Aldine Publishing Co., 1967.
3. Ibid., p. 1.
4. Glaser, Barney G. and Anselm L. Strauss, *Awareness of Dying* Chicago: Aldine Publishing Co., 1965.
5. Ibid., p. 238.
6. The phrases in quotes are those coined by Glaser and Strauss.
7. Ibid., P. 105–115.
8. Osborne, Oliver H., "Anthropology and Nursing: Some Common Traditions and interests," *Nursing Research*, XVIII May–June, 1969, 254.
9. For additional sources on methods and techniques of social anthropology see Gutkind, P. C. W. and G. Sankoff, "Annotated Bibliography on Anthropological Field Work Methods," Chapter 11, pp. 214–271 in *Anthropologist in the Field* by Jongmans, D. G. and P. C. W. Gutkind (eds.) New York: Humanities Press, 1967.
10. For additional discussion of participant observation see Chapter 11 of Oleson, Virginia L., and Elvi W. Whitaker, *The Silent Dialogue*, San Francisco: Jossey Bass Inc., 1968 and Byerly, Elizabeth Lee, "The Nurse Researcher as Participant Observer in a Nursing Setting," *Nursing Research* XVIII, May–June, 1969, p. 230–236.
11. Dickoff, James, Patricia James and Ernestine Weidenback, "Theory in a Practice Discipline," Part 11 "Practice Oriented Research," *Nursing Research* XVIII, November–December, 1968, p. 552.

Bibliography

Beauchamp, George A. Curriculum Theory Wilmette. Illinois: The Kagg Press, 1968.

Byerly, Elizabeth Lee. "The Nurse Researcher as a Participant Observer in a Nursing Setting." *Nursing Research* XVIII, May–June 1969, 230–236.

Dickott, Jones and others. "Theory in a Practice Discipline." Part II. "Practice Oriented Research." *Nursing Research* XVII November–December, 1968, 545–554.

Glaser, Barney G. and Anselm L. Strauss. *The Discovery of Grounded Theory: Strategies for Qualitative Research*. Chicago: Aldine Publishing Co., 1967.

Awareness of Dying. Chicago: Aldine Publishing Company, 1965.

Jongmans, D. G. and P. C. W. Gutkind (eds.) *Anthropologists in the Field*. New York: Humanities Press, 1967.

Kerlinger, Fred N. *Foundations of Behavioral Research*. New York: Hall, Rinehart and Winston, Inc., 1965.

Oleson, Virginia L. and Elvi W. Whitaker. *The Silent Dialogue*. San Francisco: Jossey Bass, Inc., 1968.

Osborne, Oliver H. "Anthropology and Nursing: Some Common Traditions and Interests." *Nursing Research* XVIII May–June 1969, 251–255.

Producing 'Plausible Stories': Interviewing Student Nurses

Kath M. Melia

A t the end of the 1970s, when there was little experience of qualitative research in nursing, I undertook a study of the occupational socialization of student nurses (Melia 1981). The project was in the spirit of Becker et al.'s (1961) study of medical students, drawing on the intellectual legacy of what we have now learned to call the Second Chicago School. Although my research used the ideas that we then called 'symbolic interactionism' and the methodological writings of Glaser and Strauss (1967) on 'grounded theory', it differed from the American work in that there was no participant observation and my data were collected solely by informal interviews. In effect, it was an analysis of student nurses' accounts of their work and training.

At the time, this strategy seemed to be a plausible way of arriving at a picture of the student nurses' world. I saw it as a version of Gold's (1958) observer-as-participant field role: although I had no observational material, I could draw on my own experience and familiarity with the setting to treat the data I gathered as if they were not very different from interview data obtained in the course of participant observation. I analysed the interview transcripts in much the same way as if they had been field notes. As Platt (1983) shows, this is not so far from some of the early practice of qualitative research in inter-war Chicago as it might sound: many of these classic studies owed more to interviews and case reports than tradition allows.

In writing this chapter, I have come to reflect again on the question of the adequacy of interview data for the task of explaining the student nurses' world. I answered the question in the late 1970s, rightly or wrongly, by an appeal to

Source: G. Miller and R. Dingwall, *Context and Method in Qualitative Research* (London: Sage, 1997), pp. 26–36.

the definition of grounded theory offered by Glaser and Strauss (1967: 3) – 'a strategy for handling data in research, providing modes of conceptualization for describing and explaining' – and to the fact that constant comparison allows for drawing on literature and theorizing in the area under study as well as the more obvious comparison of data with data, and data with emerging conceptual categories. In the late 1990s, we might be more sceptical about the adequacy of the informal interview in this kind of research enterprise. There is a climate of methodological angst about the nature of data and the possibilities for analysis. Qualitative analysis texts have become increasingly concerned with the epistemological bases of the methods we adopt, and the range of methods available has expanded well beyond participant observation and the interview to include conversation analysis, narrative and discourse analysis and phenomenology. These developments demand a re-evaluation of the informal interview as a means of gathering data. However, I still think that the analytical procedures associated with grounded theory – constant comparative method and theoretical sensitivity – can take us beyond the interview data themselves to a more conceptual level.

An important problem for such a justification, though, is that the originators of grounded theory, Glaser and Strauss, have recently disagreed between themselves about the nature of the research strategy they promoted in the 1960s. In this chapter, then, I shall review their argument and try to establish where followers of grounded theory might now have been left by it. In conclusion, I propose a pragmatic approach to qualitative methods, which takes account of philosophical and epistemological debates but does not become so preoccupied with them that any form of research can be vetoed on some ground or other.

Method and Methodology

Although it has become fashionable to use the word 'methodology' when it is actually 'method' that is being discussed, the distinction between the two – the 'study of method' and the 'research procedures actually employed' – is a useful one, if only to save the researcher from climbing philosophical heights from which to fall when it comes to the discussion and analysis of data. Much of the current agonizing reflects the challenge of postmodernism and its questions about how we can know anything about the world and what – in that knowing – constitutes data and explanation. At its simplest, postmodernism holds that there are no grand theories, overall explanations or generalized ways of explaining experience and that social life can be better understood as a series of discourses where none is privileged. This position has become entangled with the epistemological justifications that can be put forward for qualitative analysis. If discussions in nursing and health care are anything of a guide to the methods debates in qualitative research, there is cause for some concern. Postmodernism seems to have become something of an excuse for taking what might otherwise be thought of as a rather loose approach to methods.

Atkinson (1995b: 120) has commented on the proliferation of methods texts in qualitative research and the apparent need for some authors to produce taxonomies and neat categories of methods. In his words:

> one may applaud the general intention of clarifying and classifying the array of complementary and contrasting approaches – however it is essentially a text book treatment. As such it can all too easily oversimplify and, ultimately, distort the true picture. This is, moreover, a recurrent problem with many, if not most, listings of qualitative research types. All too often they pull together types and categories that are in different orders of generality.

He goes on to observe that all authors argue for a classification, each produces his or her own list and they are all different. Atkinson's (1995b: 121) main complaint, which I would echo, is that the lists:

> draw together issues and approaches of very different levels of generality. Some represent theoretical schools or traditions that have some affinities with qualitative research (symbolic interactionism, ethnomethodology, phenomenology); some are labels for general approaches to research (ethnography) or strategies of research design and analysis (grounded theory); yet others are of extreme generality and have no claim to be research methods at all (constructionism, deconstructionism, feminism, critical theory).

Atkinson (1995b: 123) concludes that 'the goals of research will not be served by a slavish adherence to the historical accidents and arbitrary boundaries that separate methodological traditions and particular research methods.' We should not, he says, 'turn the pedagogical half truths of textbook knowledge into prescriptions for research practice'.

Attempts to bring methodological perspectives into some order need not have the unfortunate consequences that Atkinson outlines. Denzin (1989b: 7), for instance, makes a heroic attempt to pull a good deal together under the term *interpretive interactionism*. With this title he is, in his own words, trying:

> to make the world of problematic lived experience of ordinary people directly available to the reader. The interactionist interprets these worlds. The research methods of this approach include open-ended, creative interviewing; document analysis; semiotics; life-history; life-story; personal experience and self-story construction; participant observation; and thick description.

According to Denzin, the term 'interpretive interactionism' signifies an attempt to join traditional symbolic interactionist thought with participant observation and ethnography; semiotics and fieldwork; postmodern ethnographic research; naturalistic studies; creative interviewing; the case-study method; hermeneutic phenomenology; cultural studies and feminist critiques of positivism. This seems to be an impossible task, but it purs interactionist thought centre stage while allowing space for current methods debates. If symbolic interactionism has been overrun by postmodernists, Denzin's compass and his caution may offer us a way through this fad. Writing with Lincoln at the end of their edited collection on qualitative research, he notes that 'what is passe today may be in vogue a decade from now. Just as the postmodern, for example reacts to the modern, some day there may well be a neomodern phase that extols Malinowski and the Chicago school and finds the current post-structural, postmodern moment abhorrent' (Denzin and Lincoln 1994: 575).

Interestingly, in the introduction to *Interpretive Interactionism*, Denzin states that an aim of the book is to continue C. Wright Mills's project of the 'sociological imagination', to allow the examination of private troubles of individuals to be connected to public issues and public responses. However, we might also remember another passage from Mills (1959: 215) where he discusses intellectual craft:

> To the individual social scientist who feels himself a part of the classic tradition, social science is the practice of a craft. A man at work on problems of substance, he is among those who are quickly made impatient and weary by elaborate discussions of method-and-theory-in-general; so much of which interrupts his proper studies.

Mills continues by saying it is much better 'to have one account by a working student about how he is going about his work than a dozen "codifications of procedure" by specialists who as often as not have never done much work of consequence'.

It is clearly oversimplifying the case to argue that philosophy and method should be kept apart. It is, however, helpful if what researchers 'do' – method, and the methodological justification for that doing, epistemology – are treated as rather separate entities, if only to avoid the epistemological justification being mistaken for the method itself. Most philosophies can be taken to an ultimate conclusion where research becomes impossible. If the world is only discourse and narrative without structure or context, how can we make sense of, for instance, interview data?

Interviews as Text: Interviews as Data

The basic challenge that all methodological discussion must face is the question: 'how does all this help in the analysis of data and the production of explanation?' What is the connection between the resultant explanation of the data and the epistemological starting point described by the analyst? How close is the methodological rhetoric to the method of doing of the research? If we had not been told in a methodological preamble, would we know that what follows is postmodern, discourse analysis, grounded theory or whatever? The link between what a researcher does and the philosophical position set out to justify the method is often problematic.

In the light of current debates, returning to the work on the student nurses' world has been a curious experience. The growing interest in the analysis of text, and the reluctance to allow interview data to be analysed beyond the textual level, challenges those of us who relied on interviews to produce qualitative data that would shed some light on a substantive topic. The data for the study comprised 40 tape-recorded interviews with student nurses. The interviews were fully transcribed and the transcripts treated as raw data. I used the approach described by Glaser and Strauss (1967) in *The Discovery of Grounded Theory*. Arguably, Glaser and Strauss were the most influential writers in the qualitative methods field in the 1970s and, through the work of Strauss and Corbin (1987), into the 1980s. As qualitative methods have spread, this pre-eminence has, perhaps, faded a little with the rise of ethno-methodology, phenomenology and discourse analysis. However, despite the incongruity, grounded theory is often still yoked to these other positions.

In the late 1970s, when I was working on the student nurse study, grounded theory was assumed to rest on the general tenets of Blumer's version of symbolic interactionism derived from the work of G.H. Mead. Coupled with some awareness of Berger and Luckmann's (1966) version of Schutz and the early work of Garfinkel (1967), these formed the epistemological under-pinnings of the project. I started with the premise that life – that of the student nurse in this case – can be understood by asking questions about it so that the person experiencing that life can convey his or her understanding of it by his or her own descriptions and insights. The researcher can then, taking an interactionist approach, seek to communicate the view of the informant and to place it within a more general, second-order framework. This involves allowing the inclusion of interpretation which goes beyond the raw data, draw-ing upon cognate work and thinking to see the specific case as an instance of a more general social process or institution. This generalization provides an additional dimension to the informant's specific account, which, in turn, also exemplifies or modifies the general account.

The analysis of nursing as a profession was one example. Drawing on previous studies of work, occupations and organizations, the students' accounts were crafted into a discussion of nursing as an occupation and the problems posed for many of its members by the professionalizing aspirations of an influential segment. This took issue with the self-serving accounts that had been written by that segment, while enlarging our general understanding of the differentiation that may occur within professions.

Analysing interviews presents a critical methodological challenge. Are the data to be regarded as straight accounts of the interviewees' experiences or stories about that experience told as an exercise in self-presentation by the interviewee? Here lurks the temptation to abandon the enterprise on the grounds that it is impossible to determine the status of the data. However, if we allow all possible objections to cause us to doubt the status and utility of the data, the chances are that we would not undertake research at all. Notwithstanding the philosophical debates from Wittgenstein to the post-moderns, if we are going to tell a story, we have to be less epistemologically squeamish and get on with it.

Grounding Analysis

A greater worry for me is the way in which the originators of grounded theory have fallen out about what it really is. In Glaser's (1992) book, *Emergence vs Forcing: Basics of Grounded Theory Analysis*, he reproduces a letter to Strauss: 'I request that you pull the book [*Basics of Qualitative Research*]. It distorts and misconceives grounded theory, while engaging in a gross neglect of 90% of its important ideas.' He continues, in equally strong terms, with: 'You wrote a whole different method so why call it "grounded theory"? It indicates that you never have grasped what we did, not studied it to try to carefully extend it' (Glaser 1992: 2).[1] If there is room for dispute between the founders, it is not surprising that qualitative methods debates become so complicated. Glaser and Strauss now clearly have different views about the essential nature of the analytical strategy which they co-originated: indeed, if we were to accept Glaser's version, they may have had different understandings from the outset![2]

Working in the UK means that one is reliant upon the books and papers produced by the originators of grounded theory. Much of the work claiming to adopt this approach, whatever it is, emanates from California (cf. Cheni and Swanson 1986) and many of the researchers involved are, or have been, students of Strauss. Those using grounded theory tend to cite Glaser and Strauss (1967), possibly Glaser (1978) and then skip to Strauss and Corbin (1990). Glaser's major contribution to the method in *Theoretical Sensitivities* (1978) is well known in the UK. However, my unsystematic enquiries suggest that few are aware of Glaser's latest work and that there is an increasing tendency to rely on Strauss and Corbin (1990) as the main source. Grounded theory seems to be becoming synonymous with the use of the Strauss and Corbin text. At worst, this can amount to little more than a nod in the general direction of grounded theory and then a progression to a generalized qualitative analysis.

The original version of grounded theory stressed the idea that theory emerged from, and was grounded in, data. Careful analysis of data items using the constant comparative method would lead to the emergence of conceptual categories that would describe and explain the phenomenon under study. Several explanatory or conceptual categories would be integrated around a core category and so the theory would emerge. The idea was to follow up conceptually fruitful avenues and allow emergent concepts to dictate the direction and nature of the data collection. Glaser and Strauss described this as a process of 'theoretical sensitivity', whereby data collection and analysis went on side by side until a core category emerged and was 'saturated'.

Glaser, however, is now questioning the extent to which concepts emerge or data are forced into them. He ultimately comes to the view that: 'Anselm's methodology is one of full conceptual description and mine is grounded theory. They are very different, the first focusing on forcing and the second on emergence. The first keeping all the problems of forcing data, the second giving them up in favour of emergence, discovery, and inductive theory generation' (Glaser 1992:122). In Glaser's view, Strauss is not advancing theory, but producing something he calls *full conceptual description*. This seems to be more formulaic in style than the original version of grounded theory, with a greater use of certain prior concepts which are expected to recur in different settings.

Strauss's (1987) and Strauss and Corbin's (1990) more recent writings have certainly had a procedural emphasis which Glaser (1992: 5) sees as betraying their original vision:

> What is written in Strauss' book is out of the blue, a present piece with no historical reference on the idea level, and an almost new method borrowing an older name – Grounded Theory – and funny thing, it produces simply what qualitative researchers had been doing for sixty years or more: forced, full conceptual description.

In full conceptual description, Glaser asserts, there is a preconceived and verificational approach to qualitative data analysis. In his own expressive terms he says:

> If you torture the data enough it will give up! This is the underlying approach in the forcing preconceptions of full conceptual description. The data is not allowed to speak for itself, as in grounded theory, and to be heard from infrequently it has to scream. Forcing by preconception constantly derails it from relevance. (Glaser 1992: 123)

It is certainly notable that one of the main ideas in both *The Discovery of Grounded Theory* (1967) and *Theoretical Sensitivity* (1978), namely that of 'saturation' – the compilation of data until a conceptual category becomes credible – does not figure in Strauss and Corbin (1990). This was an important element of my use of interview data: the student nurses repeated some very clear story lines again and again. The category which turned out to be the core – 'fitting in' – was well saturated. Almost every student had a tale to tell where the moral was that the student goal was to become a registered nurse and that they would do just about whatever it took in college and on the ward to achieve that aim.

While *Basics of Qualitative Research* (Strauss and Corbin 1990) has been of some help in teaching and laying out some of the ideas discussed in great detail in Strauss's 1987 book, I have a nagging doubt that the procedures are getting in the way: the technical tail is beginning to wag the theoretical dog. On the matter of procedures, it also has to be said that, on first reading, *Theoretical Sensitivity* (Glaser 1978), and its 18 coding families, took some getting used to and produced some of the same feelings of overload experienced on reading Glaser's latest work. The saving grace then, and now with *Emergence vs Forcing*, is the simplicity of the central idea of the constant comparative method. Glaser (1992: 43) argues that Strauss's methods are now unnecessarily laborious and tedious:

> Strauss's method of labelling and then grouping is totally unnecessary, laborious and is a waste of time. Using constant comparison method gets the analyst to the desired conceptual power, quickly, with ease and joy. Categories emerge upon comparison and properties emerge upon more comparison. And that is all there is to it.

Who could resist that?

It has been argued that grounded theory is not that different from long-accepted good practice in sociology. Bechhofer (1974: 77–78), while applauding Glaser and Strauss's call for the generation of theory, wrote in a discussion of theoretical sampling that: 'the search for contrasting empirical situations is suggested by good experimental practices, and the search for conceptually related, but empirically different situations is very much good scientific practice.' If this is the case, and I have some sympathy with Bechhofer's position, it may not matter so much if there are the two versions of grounded theory in circulation. Indeed, if what Glaser and Strauss were doing was what many good sociologists had done for years, perhaps, as Bechhofer has suggested in a recent personal communication, it is not too surprising that subsequent attempts to make grounded theory appear to be more and more special have led to a split between the two. In the 1967 *Discovery* book, both authors stressed the point that researchers should feel free to develop the method. That this freedom has in the fullness of time included themselves is a matter of record.

This is echoed by Strauss and Corbin (1994: 283) in their recent contribution to a major qualitative methods tome (Denzin and Lincoln 1994), which is, in effect, their reply to Glaser:

> Recently an astute sociologist asked us to say something about the outer limits of research that we would or could continue to call 'grounded theory'. The feature of this methodology that we consider so central that their abandonment would signify a great departure are the grounding of theory upon data through data-theory interplay, the making of constant

comparisons, the asking of theoretical oriented questions, theoretical coding, and the development of theory. Yet, no inventor has permanent possession of the invention – certainly not even of its name – and furthermore we would not wish to do so. No doubt we will always prefer the later versions of grounded theory that are closest to or elaborate on our own, but a child once launched is very much subject to a combination of its origins and the evolving contingencies of life. Can it be otherwise with a methodology?

Whether or not the current debate would have influenced the way in which I analysed my interviews is a moot point. The account was grounded in the data supplied by the students, yet moved to an analytical level beyond the raw data themselves. The point at issue seems to be more whether the data jumped or were pushed – emergence *v.* forcing – rather than whether informal interviews are up to the job.

I am not sure how Glaser would describe my work (Melia 1987). The 1967 book contains some near mystical passages, but I suspect that that was its charm and ultimately the reason for its success. Strauss's continued interest in writing on qualitative methods can simply be seen as part of the trend noted by Atkinson. Again, we have to ask whether it is the methods text itself that is a problem for qualitative research: if researchers were less hung up on debating methods might we do rather better in getting the story out? Methods texts and epistemological discussions are interesting, but do they lead to any difference in the product? The debate between the fathers of grounded theory gives some substance to the arguments about justification of methods. If the results of Strauss's work provide useful insights and explanations while his methods discussions have become more and more laboured – certainly in Glaser's view and at times in mine – does it matter? Are we, perhaps, looking at two different issues: one being the way in which methods are written up in the increasingly self-conscious 'methods text' genre; the other being the research itself. It is tempting to ask whether, if Glaser had undertaken the substantive work that Strauss published, the results would actually have been very different.

Where Does This Leave Us with the Interview?

The starting point for me in this chapter was the student nurse interviews (Melia 1987), and the question remains that of the legitimacy of using them to move to a discussion of the organization of nursing practice and the nursing profession more generally. The original justification lay in grounded theory and an accepted practice in the analysis of qualitative data. More recent phenomenological discussions, with their talk of 'lived worlds' and meanings lying in wait to be uncovered, prompt me to wonder if telling my plausible story was rather naive or maybe not such a bad idea after all.

Informal interview data are yielded by a series of questions and general lines of enquiry embedded in a seemingly natural conversation with the interviewee. The data can be seen, then, as an account of the interviewee's opinions and views, arrived at as a result of the interaction with the researcher. The effect of this interaction cannot be denied, whether on the pragmatic ground that the interviewee's talk is produced by the interviewer's questions or on the theoretical ground that symbolic interactionism rests on the assumption of the intersubjective construction of social reality. We can view the interview as a presentation of self by the interviewee with the data as a representation that has no further credibility. Or we can see the interview as a means of gaining insight into a world beyond the story that the interviewee tells, a means of getting a handle on a more complex set of ideas than the ones that the interviewee is ostensibly talking about. This is not to say that the interviewer moves into the territory of the paranormal and can somehow see through the data to things otherwise concealed. However, it does mean that a researcher with an interest in, and open mind about, a particular topic can, with practised care, take an analysis beyond its face value. In the case of the student nurses, this moved on from their accounts to become a discussion of nursing as a segmented occupational group with different approaches to the question of profession: a move from interviews about the student nurses' worldview of nursing to a discussion of nursing as a profession. If we were to take a seriously postmodern view, I suppose that we would never know the answer to these bigger questions.

'Is the interview an account, a story about a world described or does it provide an index of a world beyond the story? Moreover, does the nature of the analytical route taken through the data – be it discourse analysis, narrative, constant comparative method or full conceptual description – produce an answer to this question of the status of the interview data? Will the answers be different? And, if so, why so and how so? It may be counter-productive to get further and further into a philosophically interesting mire which keeps us from the plausible story. If the world in which we exist manages to get along with its business by means of, for the most part, a commonsense, if cautious, approach to daily experiences, this might be the best, possibly the only, strategy open to the social scientist hoping to understand that world. Ultimately, it becomes perverse to say that life cannot be understood by the same means that it is lived. Data are what we see, hear or read: no more but certainly no less. Even a phenomenologist cannot transcend these major conditions. The challenge is to convert these sense data into an explanation of the situation, an explanation which Becker (1958) points out, in his classic piece on 'inference and proof', has to convince others. Or, as Strong (1979: 250) put it, 'the best we can hope for in this world, even if we study practical reasoning, is a plausible story.'

There is a tendency to treat methods as belief systems and to light up one, see all its attractions and adopt its rhetoric. As with any new faith, proselytizing stage is probably the most unhelpful as it usually takes the form of rubbishing other belief systems. In the 1970s, a generalized attacking positivism was employed to legitimize qualitative methods, which, atleast in a philosophical sense, still rest themselves on a positivist foundation. As the methods debates have become more philosophical, or at least epistemological they have become less useful for the doing of research. Whatever high-flown rhetoric is adopted about uncovered meanings and understandings of discourse and narratives, what is required for a discussion of empirical work is some means of translating data from the field – interviews, observations, documents – into an explanation of the topic in hand which can be conveyed to others and understood by others. All the social processes are epistemological considerations that went into problematizing the data gathering and interpretation exist in the understanding of the research output.

This chapter has raised questions about the limits of the interview in light of the recent methods debates, in particular the Glaser and Strauss disputed. The epistemological and philosophical distinctions associated with different approaches to data collection and analysis may have more relevance for methods texts than they do for research practices. If we can collect data with which to tell a plausible story, perhaps we should settle for that. Phenomenology and postmodernism have challenged interactionism, but if the upshot is methodological paralysis it may be better to take a more anarchic, or at least pragmatic, approach to methods and do what is plausible. Mouzelis (1995: 54) has deplored what he terms a 'strategy of dedifferentiation' where there is a 'free and indiscriminate mixture of concepts and ideas derived from philosophy, literature, sociology, psychoanalysis and elsewhere'. He calls for a means of relating one discipline to another, allowing insights from one discipline to be usefully incorporated into another. 'It is precisely this free for all strategy of dedifferentiation, and the abolition of distinctions and boundaries, that has led to the present incredible situation where anything goes, and where complex macro phenomena are reductively explained in terms of signs, texts, the unconscious or what have you' (Mouzelis 1995: 54). He goes on to say:

> It is not surprising that postmodern theorising is marked by a relativism that tries to persuade us that any theoretical construction, however bizarre or crude, is just as true or false as any other. It is also not surprising that postmodernist theory tends to adopt a style where lack of depth and of substantive analysis is concealed by a quasi poetical language glorying in the obscure, the ambivalent, in plays on words and similar gimmicks. (1995: 54–55)

With all that in mind, going off to interview people and coming back to tell Strong's 'plausible story' probably is, as he said, 'the best we can hope for'.

Notes

1. The harsh words are tempered by the signature, 'your pal Barney': indeed, a rather angry book is peppered throughout with friendly comments on the value of Anselm Strauss's work as a qualitative sociologist.
2. Stern (1994: 212) Says that: 'students of Glaser and Strauss in the 1960s and 1970s knew that the two had quite different modus operandi, but Glaser only found out when Strauss and Corbin's *Basics of Qualitative Research* came out in 1990.'

References

Atkinson, P. (1995b) 'Some perils of paradigms', *Qualitative Health Research*, 5: 117–124.

Bechhofer, F. (1974) 'Current approaches to empirical research: some central ideas', in J. Rex (ed.), *Approaches to Sociology*. London: Routledge and Kegan Paul.

Becker, H.S. (1958) 'Problems of inference and proof in participant observation', *American Sociological Review*, 23: 652–660.

Becker, H.S., Geer, B., Hughes, E.C. and Strauss, A.L. (1961) *Boys in White*. Chicago: University of Chicago Press.

Berger, P.L. and Luckmann, T. (1966) *The Social Construction of Reality: a Treatise in the Sociology of Knowledge*. New York: Doubleday.

Chenitz, W.C. and Swanson, J.M. (1986) *From Practice to Grounded Theory*. Menlo Park, CA: Addison-Wesley.

Denzin, N. (1989b) *Interpretive Interactionism*. London: Sage.

Denzin, N. and Lincoln, Y. (eds) (1994) *Handbook of Qualitative Research*. London: Sage.

Garfinkel, H. (1967) *Studies in Ethnomethodology*. Englewood Cliffs, NJ: Prentice Hall.

Glaser, B. (1978) *Theoretical Sensitivity: Advances in the Methodology of Grounded Theory Analysis*. Mill Valley, CA: The Sociology Press.

Glaser, B. (1992) *Emergency vs Forcing: Basics of Grounded Theory Analysis*. Mill Valley, CA: The Sociology Press.

Glaser, B. and Strauss A. (1967) *The Discovery of Grounded Theory*. Chicago: Aldine.

Gold, R.L. (1958) 'Roles in sociological field observations', *Social Forces*, 36: 217–223.

Melia, K.M. (1981) 'Student nurses' accounts of their work and training: a qualitative analysis'. PhD thesis, University of Edinburgh.

Melia, K.M. (1987) *Learning and Working: the Occupational Socialization of Nurses*. London: Tavistock.

Mills, C.W. (1959) *The Sociological Imagination*. New York: Oxford University Press.

Mouzelis, N. (1995) *Sociological Theory: What Went Wrong?* London: Routledge.

Platt, J. (1983) 'The development of the participant observation method', *Journal of the History of the Behavioural Sciences*, 19: 379–393.

Strauss, A. and Corbin, J. (1990) *Basics of Qualitative Research: Grounded Theory Procedures and Techniques*. Newbury Park, CA: Sage.

Strauss, A. and Corbin J. (1994) 'Grounded theory methodology: an overview', in N. Denzin and Y. Lincoln (eds), *Handbook of Qualitative Research*. London: Sage. pp. 273–285.

Strong, P.M. (1979) *The Ceremonial Order of the Clinic*. London: Routledge.

30

Grounded Theory in the 21st Century: Applications for Advancing Social Justice Studies

Kathy Charmaz

G rounded theory methods of the 20th century offer rich possibilities for advancing qualitative research in the 21st century. Social justice inquiry is one area among many in which researchers can fruitfully apply grounded theory methods that Barney G. Glaser and Anselm L. Strauss (1967) created. In keeping with the theme for the current *Handbook* of advancing constructive social critique and change through qualitative research, this chapter opens discussion about applying grounded theory methods to the substantive area(s) of social justice. Inquiry in this area assumes focusing on and furthering equitable distribution of resources, fairness, and eradication of oppression (Feagin, 1999).[1]

The term "grounded theory" refers both to a method of inquiry and to the product of inquiry. However, researchers commonly use the term to mean a specific mode of analysis (see Charmaz, 2003a). Essentially, grounded theory methods are a set of flexible analytic guidelines that enable researchers to focus their data collection and to build inductive middle-range theories through successive levels of data analysis and conceptual development. A major strength of grounded theory methods is that they provide tools for analyzing processes, and these tools hold much potential for studying social justice issues. A grounded theory approach encourages researchers to remain close to their studied worlds and to develop an integrated set of theoretical

Source: *The Sage Handbook of Qualitative Research*, 3 (2005): 507–535.

concepts from their empirical materials that not only synthesize and interpret them but also show processual relationships.

Grounded theory methods consist of simultaneous data collection and analysis, with each informing and focusing the other throughout the research process.[2] As grounded theorists, we begin our analyses early to help us focus further data collection.[3] In turn, we use these focused data to refine our emerging analyses. Grounded theory entails developing increasingly abstract ideas about research participants' meanings, actions, and worlds and seeking specific data to fill out, refine, and check the emerging conceptual categories. Our work results in an analytic interpretation of participants' worlds and of the processes constituting how these worlds are constructed. Thus, we can use the processual emphasis in grounded theory to analyze relationships between human agency and social structure that pose theoretical and practical concerns in social justice studies. Grounded theorists portray their understandings of research participants' actions and meanings, offer abstract interpretations of empirical relationships, and create conditional statements about the implications of their analyses.

Applying grounded theory methods to the substantive area of social justice produces reciprocal benefits. The critical stance in social justice in combination with the analytic focus of grounded theory broadens and sharpens the scope of inquiry. Such efforts locate subjective and collective experience in larger structures and increase understanding of how these structures work (see also Clarke, 2003, 2005; Maines, 2001, 2003). Grounded theory can supply analytic tools to move social justice studies beyond description, while keeping them anchored in their respective empirical worlds.[4] Not only are justice and injustice abstract concepts, but they are, moreover, *enacted processes*, made real through actions performed again and again. Grounded theorists can offer integrated theoretical statements about the conditions under which injustice or justice develops, changes, or continues. How might we move in this direction? Which traditions provide starting points?

Constructivist Re-Visions of Grounded Theory

To develop a grounded theory for the 21st century that advances social justice inquiry, we must build upon its constructionist elements rather than objectivist learnings. In the past, most major statements of grounded theory methods minimized what numerous critics (see, for example, Atkinson, Coffey, & Delamont, 2003; Bryant. 2002, 2003; Coffey, Holbrook, & Atkinson, 1996; Silverman, 2000) find lacking: interpretive, constructionist inquiry. Answering this criticism means building on the Chicago school roots in grounded theory consistent with my constructivist statement in the second edition of this handbook (Charmaz, 2000a).[5] Currently, the Chicago school antecedents of grounded theory are growing faint and risk being lost. Contemporary grounded theorists may not realize how this tradition influences their work or may not act from its premises at all. Thus, we need to review, renew, and revitalize links to the Chicago school as grounded theory develops in the 21st century.

Building on the Chicago heritage supports the development of grounded theory in directions that can serve inquiry in the area of social justice. Both grounded theory methods and social justice inquiry fit pragmatist emphases on process, change, and probabilistic outcomes.[6] The pragmatist conception of emergence recognizes that the reality of the present differs from the past from which it develops (Strauss, 1964). Novel aspects of experience give rise to new interpretations and actions. This view of emergence can sensitize social justice researchers to study change in new ways, and grounded theory methods can give them the tools for studying it. Thus, we must revisit and reclaim Chicago school pragmatist and fieldwork traditions and develop their implications for social justice and democratic process.[7] To do so, we must move further into a constructionist social science and make the positivist roots of grounded theory problematic.

For many researchers, grounded theory methods provided a template for doing qualitative research stamped with positivist approval. Glaser's (see, especially, Glaser, 1978, 1992) strong foundation in mid-20th-century positivism gave grounded theory its original objectivist cast with its emphases in logic, analytic procedures, comparative methods, and conceptual development and assumptions of an external but discernible world, unbiased observer, and discovered theory. Strauss's versions of grounded theory emphasized meaning, action, and process, consistent with his intellectual roots in pragmatism and symbolic interactionism. These roots seem shrunken in his methodological treatises with Juliet Corbin (Strauss & Corbin, 1990, 1998) but grow robust in other works (see, for example, Corbin & Strauss, 1988; Strauss, 1993). Like Glaser, Strauss and Corbin also advanced positivistic procedures, although different ones. They introduced new technical procedures and made verification an explicit goal, thus bringing grounded theory closer to positivist ideals.[8] In divergent ways, Strauss and Corbin's works as well as Glaser's treatises draw upon objectivist assumptions founded in positivism.

Since then, a growing number of scholars have aimed to move grounded theory in new directions away from its positivist past. I share their goal and aim to build on the constructivist elements in grounded theory and to reaffirm its Chicago school antecedents. To date, scholars have questioned the epistemologies of both Glaser's and Strauss and Corbin's versions of grounded theory. We challenge earlier assumptions about objectivity, the world as an external reality, relations between the viewer and viewed, the nature of data, and authors' representations of research participants. Instead, we view positivist givens as social constructions to question and alter. Thus, when we adopt any positivist principle or procedure, we attempt to do so knowingly and to make our rationales explicit. In the second edition of this handbook (Charmaz, 2000a), I argued for building on the pragmatist underpinnings in grounded theory and developing it as a social constructionist method. Clive Seale (1999) contends that we can retain grounded theory methods without adhering to a naïve realist epistemology. Antony Bryant (2002, 2003) calls for re-grounding grounded theory in an epistemology that takes recent methodological developments into account, and Adele E. Clarke (2003, 2005) aims to integrate postmodern sensibilities with grounded theory and to provide new analytic tools for discerning and conceptualizing subtle empirical relationships. These moves by grounded theorists reflect shifts in approaches to qualitative research.[9]

A constructivist grounded theory (Charmaz, 1990, 2000a, 2003b; Charmaz & Mitchell, 2001) adopts grounded theory guidelines as tools but does not subscribe to the objectivist, positivist assumptions in its earlier formulations. A constructivist approach emphasizes the studied phenomenon rather than the methods of studying it. Constructivist grounded theorists take a reflexive stance on modes of knowing and representing studied life. That means giving close attention to empirical realities and our collected renderings of them – *and* locating oneself in these realities. It does not assume that data simply await discovery in an external world or that methodological procedures will correct limited views of the studied world. Nor does it assume that impartial observers enter the research scene without an interpretive frame of reference. Instead, what observers see and hear depends upon their prior interpretive frames, biographies, and interests as well as the research context, their relationships with research participants, concrete field experiences, and modes of generating and recording empirical materials. No qualitative method rests on pure induction – the questions we ask of the empirical world frame what we know of it. In short, we share in constructing what we define as data. Similarly, our conceptual categories arise through our interpretations *of* data rather than emanating *from* them or from our methodological practices (cf. Glaser, 2002). Thus, our theoretical analyses are interpretive renderings of a reality, not objective reportings of it.

Whether informed by Glaser (1978, 1992, 1998, 2002) or Strauss and Corbin (1990, 1998), many researchers adopted positivist grounded theory as a template. The constructivist position recasts this template by challenging its objectivist underpinnings. We can use a constructivist template to inform social justice research in the 21st century. Clearly, much research in the area of social justice is objectivist and flows from standard positivist methodologies. A constructivist grounded theory offers another alternative: a systematic approach to social justice inquiry that fosters integrating subjective experience with social conditions in our analyses.

An interest in social justice means attentiveness to ideas and actions concerning fairness, equity, equality, democratic process, status, hierarchy, and individual and collective rights and obligations. It signifies thinking about being human and about creating good societies and a better world. It prompts reassessment of our roles as national and world citizens. It means exploring tensions between complicity and consciousness, choice and constraint, indifference and compassion, inclusion and exclusion, poverty and privilege, and barriers and opportunities. It also means taking a critical stance toward actions, organizations, and social institutions. Social justice studies require looking at both realities and ideals. Thus, contested meanings of "shoulds" and "oughts" come into play. Unlike positivists of the past, social justice researchers openly bring their shoulds and oughts into the discourse of inquiry.

Reexamining Grounded Theory of the Past

In the 20th century, grounded theory methods offered guidelines and legitimacy for conducting research. Glaser and Strauss (1967) established qualitative research as valuable in its own right and argued that it proceeds from a different logic than quantitative research. Although researchers did not always understand grounded theory methods and seldom followed them beyond a step or two, they widely cited and acclaimed these methods because they legitimized and codified a previously implicit process. Grounded theory methods offered explicit strategies, procedural rigor, and seeming objectivity. As Karen Locke (1996) notes, many researchers still use grounded theory methods for "a rhetoric of justification as opposed to a rhetoric of explication" (p. 244; see also Charmaz, 1983; Silverman, 2000).

All analyses come from particular standpoints, including those emerging in the research process. Grounded theory studies emerge from wrestling with data, making comparisons, developing categories, engaging in theoretical sampling, and integrating an analysis. But *how* we conduct all these activities does not occur in a social vacuum. Rather, the entire research process is interactive; in this sense, we bring past interactions and current interests into our research, and we interact with our empirical materials and emerging ideas as well as, perhaps, granting agencies, institutional review boards, and community agencies and groups, along with research participants and colleagues. Neither data nor ideas are mere objects that we passively observe and compile (see also Holstein & Gubrium, 1995).

Glaser (2002) treats data as something separate from the researcher and implies that they are untouched by the competent researcher's interpretations. If, perchance, researchers somehow interpret their data, then according to Glaser, these data are "rendered objective" by looking at many cases. Looking at many cases strengthens a researcher's grasp of the empirical world and helps in discerning variation in the studied phenomenon. However, researchers may elevate their own assumptions and interpretations to "objective" status if they do not make them explicit.

No analysis is neutral – despite research analysts' claims of neutrality. We do not come to our studies uninitiated (see also Denzin, 1994; Morse, 1999; Schwandt, 1994, 2000). What we know shapes, but does not necessarily determine, what we "find." Moreover, *each* stage of inquiry is constructed through social processes. If we treat these processes as unproblematic, we may not recognize how they are constructed. Social justice researchers likely understand their starting assumptions; other researchers may not – including grounded theorists.[10] As social scientists, we *define* what we record as data, yet how we define data outlines how we represent them in our works. Such definitional decisions – whether implicit or explicit – reflect moral choices that, in turn, spawn subsequent moral decisions and actions.[11]

Rather than abandoning the traditional positivist quest for empirical detail, I argue that we advance it – *without the cloak of neutrality and passivity enshrouding mid-century positivism*. Gathering rich empirical materials is the first step. Recording these data systematically prompts us to pursue leads that we might otherwise ignore or not realize. Through making systematic recordings, we also gain comparative materials to pinpoint contextual conditions and to explore links between levels of analysis. By seeking empirical answers to emerging theoretical questions, we learn about the worlds we enter and can increase the cogency of our subsequent analyses. Hence, data need to be informed by our theoretical sensitivity. Data alone are insufficient; they must be telling and must answer theoretical questions.

Without theoretical scrutiny, direction, and development, data culminate in mundane descriptions (see also Silverman, 2000). The value of the product then becomes debatable, and critics treat earlier studies as reified representations of the limits of the method itself rather than how it was used (Charmaz, 2000a). Burawoy (1991) categorizes the products of grounded theory as empirical generalizations. Moreover, he claims that the method does not consider power in micro contexts and that "it represses the broader macro forces that both limit change and create domination in the micro sphere" (p. 282). I disagree. Simply because earlier authors did not address power or macro forces does not mean that grounded theory methods cannot. In contrast to Burawoy's claims, I argue that we should use grounded theory methods in precisely these areas to gain fresh insights in social justice inquiry.

Critics of grounded theory commonly miss four crucial points: (a) theorizing is an activity; (b) grounded theory methods provide a way to proceed with this activity; (c) the research problem and the researcher's unfolding interests shape the *content* of this activity, not the method; and (d) the products of theorizing reflect how researchers acted on these points. As Dan E. Miller (2000) argues, the ironic issue is that researcher's have done so little grounded theory, despite their claims to use it. Its potential for developing theory remains untapped, as does its potential for studying power and inequality.

Social justice studies require data that diverse audiences agree represent the empirical world and that researchers have given a fair assessment. I do not mean that we reify, objectify, and universalize these data. Instead, I mean that we must start by gathering thorough empirical materials precisely because social justice research may provoke controversy and contested conclusions. Thus, we need to identify clear boundaries and limits of our data. Locating the data strengthens the foundation for making theoretical insights and for providing evidence for evaluative claims. Critics can then evaluate an author's argument on its merits. The better they can see direct connections between the evidence and points in the argument, the more this argument will persuade them. The lingering hegemony of positivism still makes controversial research suspect, as Fine, Weis, Weseen, and Wong (2000) observe. Therefore, the data for such studies must be unassailable.

A strong empirical foundation is the first step in achieving credibility – for both social justice researchers and grounded theorists. Despite reliance on data-driven interpretations, the rush to "theorize" – or perhaps to publish – has led some grounded theorists to an unfortunate neglect of thorough data collection, which has persisted since Lofland and Lofland (1984) first noted it. Glaser (1992, 2002) discounts quests for accurate data and dismisses full description as distinguishing conventional qualitative data analysis from grounded theory. However, leading studies with implications for social justice and policy have had solid empirical foundations (see, for example, Duneire, 1992; Glaser & Strauss, 1965; Goffman, 1961; Mitchell, 2002; Snow & Anderson, 1993). Grounded theory studies that lack empirical vitality cannot support a rationale for major social change – or even minor policy recommendations. The stronger the social justice arguments derived from a study, particularly controversial ones, the greater the need for a robust empirical foundation with compelling evidence.

Using Grounded Theory to Study Social Justice Issues

Initial Reflections

Both the steps and the logic of grounded theory can advance social justice research. Grounded theorists insist that researchers define what is happening in the setting (Glaser, 1978; Glaser & Strauss, 1967). Sensitivity to social justice issues fosters defining latent processes as well as explicit actions. Grounded theory tools for studying action – collective as well as individual action – can make social justice analysis more precise and predictive. By focusing the data gathering, a researcher can seek new information to examine questions concerning equality, fairness, rights, and legitimacy.[12] The grounded theory openness to empirical leads spurs the researcher to pursue emergent questions and thus shifts the direction of inquiry.

A social justice researcher can use grounded theory to anchor agendas for future action, practice, and policies in the *analysis* by making explicit connections between the theorized antecedents, current conditions, and consequences of major processes. Social justice research, particularly participatory action research (Kemmis & McTaggart, 2000), proceeds from researchers' and participants' joint efforts and commitments to change practices. Because it arises in settings and situations in which people have taken a reflexive stance on their practices, they already have tools to conduct systematic research on their practices in relation to subjective experience, social actions, and social structures. Hence, adopting constructivist grounded theory would foster their efforts to articulate clear links between practices and each level and, thus, to strengthen their arguments for change.

Other researchers need to weigh whether, when, how, and to what extent to bring research participants into the process. Although well intended, doing so may create a series of knotty problems in concrete situations.[13] Janice Morse (1998) finds that the consequences of bringing participants into research decisions include keeping the analytic level low, overstating the views of participants who clamored for more space in the narrative, and compromising the analysis. Moreover, Morse (1998) notes that qualitative analyses differ from participants' descriptive accounts and may reveal paradoxes and processes of which participants are unaware.

Adopting grounded theory strategies in social justice research results in putting ideas and perspectives to empirical tests. Any extant concept must earn its way into the analysis (Glaser, 1978). Thus, we cannot import a set of concepts such as hegemony and domination and paste them on the realities in the field. Instead, we can treat them as sensitizing concepts, to be explored in the field settings (Blumer, 1969; van den Hoonaard, 1997). Then we can define if, when, how, to what extent, and under which conditions these concepts become relevant to the study (Charmaz, 2000b). We need to treat concepts as problematic and look for their characteristics as lived and understood, not as given in textbooks. Contemporary anthropologists, for example, remain alert to issues of cultural imperialism. Most sociologists attend to agency, power, status, and hierarchy.

Grounded theory studies can show how inequalities are played out at interactional and organizational levels. True, race, class, and gender – and age and disability – are everywhere. But how do members of various groups define them?[14] How and when do these status variables affect action in the scene? Researchers must define how, when, and to what extent participants *construct* and *enact* power, privilege, and inequality. Robert Prus (1996) makes a similar point in his book *Symbolic Interaction and Ethnographic Research*. Race, class, gender, age, and disability are social constructions with contested definitions that are continually reconstituted (see, for example, Olesen, Chapter 10, this volume). Using them as static variables, as though they have uncontested definitions that explain data and social processes *before* or *without* looking, undermines their potential power. Taking their meanings as given also undermines using grounded theory to develop fresh insights and ideas. Adopting my alternative tack involves juxtaposing participants' definitions against academic or sociological notions. In turn, researchers themselves must be reflexive about how they represent participants' constructions and enactments.

What new dimensions will social justice foci bring to research? Societal and global concerns are fundamental to a critical perspective. Thus, these studies situate the studied phenomenon in relation to larger units. How and where does it fit? For example, a study of sales interactions could look not only at the immediate interaction and how salespeople handle it but also at the organizational context and perhaps the corporate world, and its global reach, in which these interactions occur. Like many qualitative researchers, grounded theorists often separate the studied interactions from their situated contexts. Thus, a social justice focus brings in more structure and, in turn, a grounded theory treatment of that structure results in a dynamic, processual analysis of its enactment. Similarly, social justice research often takes into account the historical evolution of the current situation, and a grounded theory analysis of this evolution can yield new insights and, perhaps, alternative understandings. For that matter, researchers can develop grounded theories from analyses of pertinent historical materials in their realm of inquiry (see, for example, Clarke, 1998; Star, 1989).

Critical inquiry attends to contradictions between myths and realities, rhetoric and practice, and ends and means. Grounded theorists have the tools to discern and analyze contradictions revealed in the empirical world. We can examine what people *say* and compare it to what they *do* (Deutscher, Pestello, & Pestello, 1993). Focusing on words or deeds are ways of representing people; however, observed contradictions between the two may indicate crucial priorities and practices. To date, grounded theorists have emphasized the *overt* – usually overt statements – more than the tacit, the liminal, and the implicit. With critical inquiry, we can put our data to new tests and create new connections in our theories.

Social Justice Emphases: Resources, Hierarchies, and Policies and Practices

A social justice focus can sensitize us to look at both large collectivities and individual experiences in new ways. Several emphases stand out: *resources, hierarchies*, and *policies and practices*. First, present, partial, or absent resources – whether economic, social, or personal – influence interactions and outcomes. Such resources include information, control over meanings, access to networks, and determination of outcomes. Thus, information and power are crucial resources. As Martha Nussbaum (1999) argues, needs for resources vary among people, vary at different times, and vary according to capabilities. Elders with disabling conditions need more resources than other people do or than they themselves needed in earlier years. What are the resources in the empirical worlds we study? What do they mean to actors in the field? Which resources, if any, are taken for granted? By whom? Who controls the resources? Who needs them? According to which and whose criteria of need? To what extent do varied capabilities enter the discussion? Are resources available? If so, to whom? How, if at all, are resources shared, hoarded, concealed, or distributed?

How did the current situation arise? What are the implications of having control over resources and of handling them, as observed in the setting(s)?

Second, any social entity has hierarchies – often several. What are they? How did they evolve? At what costs and benefits to involved actors? Which purported and actual purposes do these hierarchies serve? Who benefits from them? Under which conditions? How are the hierarchies related to power and oppression? How, if at all, do definitions of race, class, gender, and age cluster in specific hierarchies and/or at particular hierarchical levels? Which moral justifications support the observed hierarchies? Who promulgates these justifications? How do they circulate? How do these hierarchies affect social actions at macro, meso, and micro social levels? How and when do the hierarchies change?

Third, the consequences of social policies and practices are made real in collective and individual life. Here we have the convergence of structure and process. What are the rules – both tacit and explicit? Who writes or enforces them? How? Whose interests do the rules reflect? From whose standpoint? Do the rules and routine practices negatively affect certain groups or categories of individuals? If so, are they aware of them? What are the implications of their relative awareness or lack of it? To what extent and when do various participants support the rules and the policies and practices that flow from them? When are they contested? When do they meet resistance? Who resists, and which risks might resistance pose?

By asking these questions, I aim to stimulate thinking and to suggest diverse ways that critical inquiry and grounded theory research may join. The potential of advancing such endeavors already has been indicated by symbolic interactionists who point the way to demonstrating micro consequences of structural inequalities (L. Anderson & Snow, 2000; Scheff, 2003; Schwalbe et al., 2000). Combining critical inquiry and grounded theory furthers these efforts.

Working with Grounded Theory

Studying the Data

The following interview stories provide the backdrop for introducing how grounded theory guidelines can illuminate social justice concerns. My research is social psychological; however, grounded theory methods hold untapped potential for innovative studies at the organizational, societal, and global levels of analysis. The examples below offer a glimpse of the kinds of initial comparisons I make.[15] I began studying the experience of chronic illness with interests in meanings of self and time. Such social psychological topics can reveal hidden effects of inequality and difference on the self and social life that emerge in research participants' many stories of their experiences.

Both grounded theory and critical inquiry are inherently comparative methods. In earlier renderings, I treated the excerpt of Christine Danforth below as a story of suffering and Marty Gordon's initial tale as a shocking significant event that marked a turning point in her life. The first step of grounded theory analysis is to study the data. Grounded theorists ask: What is happening? and What are people doing? A fresh look at the accounts below can suggest new leads to pursue and raise new questions.

At the time of the following statement, Christine was a 43-year-old single woman who had systemic lupus erythematosus, Sjögren's syndrome, diabetes, and serious back injuries. I had first met her 7 years earlier, when her multiple disabilities were less visible, although intrusive and worrisome. Since then, her health had declined, and she had had several long stretches of living on meager disability payments. Christine described her recent episode:

> I got the sores that are in my mouth, got in my throat and closed my throat up, so I couldn't eat or drink. And then my potassium dropped down to 2.0. I was on the verge of cardiac arrest.... That time when I went in they gave me 72 bottles of pure potassium, burned all my veins out.
>
> I asked, "What does that mean, that it burned your veins out?"
>
> She said, "It hurts really bad; it's just because it's to so strong and they can't dilute it with anything. They said usually what they do is they dilute with something like a numbing effect, but because I was 2.0, which is right on cardiac arrest that they couldn't do it, they had to get it in fast."
>
> I asked, "Did you realize that you were that sick?" She said, "Well, I called the doctor several times saying, 'I can't swallow.' I had to walk around and drool on a rag. They finally made an appointment, and I got there and I waited about a half hour. The lady said that there was an emergency and said that I'd have to come back tomorrow. And I said, 'I can't.' I said, 'As soon as I stand up, I'm going to pass out' And she said, 'Well there's nothing we can do.'... And then this other nurse came in just as I got up and passed out, so then they took me to emergency.... And it took them 12 hours to – they knew when I went in there to admit me, but it took them 12 hours to get me into a room. I sat on a gurney. And they just kept fluid in me until they got me to a room.
>
> Later in the interview, Christine explained,
>
> [When the sores] go to my throat, it makes it really hard to eat or drink, which makes you dehydrated. After that first time... when I called her it had been 3 days since I'd are or drank anything... and by the time I got an appointment, it was, I believe, six or seven days, without food or water.

Imagine Christine walking slowly and determinedly up the short sidewalk to my house. See her bent knees and lowered head, as she takes deliberate steps. Christine looks weary and sad, her face as laden with care as her body is burdened by pain and pounds. Always large, she is heavier than I have ever seen her, startlingly so.

Christine has a limited education; she can hardly read. Think of her trying to make her case for immediate treatment – without an advocate. Christine can voice righteous indignation, despite the fatigue and pain that saps her spirit and drains her energy. She can barely get through her stressful workday, yet she must work as many hours as possible because she earns so little. The low pay means that Christine suffers directly from cutbacks at the agency where she works. Her apartment provides respite, but few comforts. It has no heat – she cannot afford it. Christine does not eat well. Nutritious food is an unobtainable luxury; cooking is too strenuous, and cleanup is beyond imagination. She tells me that her apartment is filled with pictures and ceramic statues of cats as well as stacks of things to sort. Maneuverable space has shrunk to aisles cutting through the piles. Christine seldom cleans house – no energy for that. I've never been to her apartment; it embarrasses her too much to have visitors. Christine would love to adopt a kitten but cats are not permitted. Her eyes glaze with tears when my skittish cat allows her to pet him.

Christine has become more immobile and now uses a motorized scooter, which she says has saved her from total disability. But since using the scooter and approaching midlife, she also has gained one hundred pounds and needs a better vehicle to transport the scooter. Christine has little social life by now; her friends from high school and her bowling days have busy family and work lives. When she first became ill, Christine had some nasty encounters with several of those friends who accused her of feigning illness. She feels her isolation keenly, although all she can handle after work is resting on the couch. Her relationship with her elderly mother has never been close; she disapproves of her brother, who has moved back in with their mother and is taking drugs. One continuing light in Christine's life is her recently married niece, who just had a baby.

The years have grown gray with hardships and troubles. Christine has few resources – economic, social, or personal. Yet she perseveres in her struggle to remain independent and employed. She believes that if she lost this job, she would never get another one. Her recent weight gain adds one more reason for the shame she feels about her body.

Christine suffers from chronic illness and its spiraling consequences. Her physical distress, her anger and frustration about her life, her sadness, shame, and uncertainty all cause her to suffer. Christine talks some about pain and much about how difficult disability and lack of money make her life. She has not mentioned the word "suffering." Like many other chronically ill people, Christine resists describing herself in a way that might undermine her worth and elicit moral judgments. Yet she has tales to tell of her turmoil and troubles. (Charmaz, 1999, pp. 362–363)

The following interview account of Marty Gordon's situation contrasts with Christine's story. Marty received care from the same health facility as Christine and also had a life-threatening condition that confounded ordinary treatment and management. However, Marty's relationship to staff there and the content and quality of her life differed dramatically from Christine's.

When I first met Marty Gordon in 1988, she was a 59-year-old woman with a diagnosis of rapidly progressing pulmonary fibrosis. A hospitalization for extensive tests led to the diagnosis of Marty's condition. She had moved to a new area after her husband, Gary, retired as a school superintendent, and she herself retired early from her teaching and grant-writing post at a high school.

Marty said that she and Gary were "very, very close." They had had no children, although Gary had a son by an earlier marriage and she, a beloved niece.

Pure retirement lasted about 3 months before they became bored. Subsequently, Marty became a part-time real estate agent and Gary worked in sales at a local winery. Not only did working bring new interests into their lives, but it also helped pay their hefty health insurance costs. They had not realized that their retirement benefits would not cover a health insurance plan. They both found much pleasure in their new lives and in their luxurious home high in the hills overlooking the city. Marty seemed to remain almost as busy as she was before retiring. While working full-time, she had entertained her husband's professional associates, had run a catering business, and had created special meals to keep Gary's diabetes and heart condition under control. She had taken much pride – and still did – in keeping up her perfectly appointed house and in keeping her weight down through regular exercise. For years, she had arisen at 5 each morning to swim an hour before going to work, then stopped at church afterward to say her rosaries.

When I first met Marty, she told the following tale about her first hospitalization:

> The doctor came in to tell me, "Uh, it didn't look good and that this was a – could be a rapidly" – and it appeared that mine was really going rapidly and that it might be about six weeks. Whoa! That blew my mind. It really did.... Right after that – I'm a Catholic – right after that, a poor little volunteer lady came in and said, "Mrs. Gordon?" And the doctor had said, "Mrs. Gordon?" "Yeah, OK." And then he told me. She said, "I'm from St. Mary's Church." I said, "Jesus, Mary, and Joseph, they've got the funeral already." And it really just – then I began to see humor in it, but I was scared....
>
> This was the point when – [I decided], "If this is going to happen OK, but I'm not going to let it happen." ... And I think probably that was the turning point when I said I wouldn't accept it. You know, I will not accept that uhm, death sentence, or whatever you want to call it. (Charmaz, 1991, p. 215)

However, from that point on, Marty had Gary promise her that she would die first. She needed him to take care of her when she could no longer care for herself; moreover, she could not bear the thought of living without him. During the next 5 years, Marty made considerable gains, despite frequent pain, fatigue, and shortness of breath. One Sunday evening, when Gary came home from a wine-pouring and Marty saw his ashen face, she insisted, "We're going to emergency." He had had a second heart attack, followed by a quadruple bypass surgery. Marty said, "He sure is a lot better now. And, of course, *I was very angry with him.* I said to him, 'You can never leave me. *I tell you, I'll sue you!*' [She explained to me.] Because we've had a deal for a long time." When telling me about her own health, she recounted this conversation with her surgeon:

I come in for an appointment and I had just played 18 holes of golf, and so he said, "I think we misdiagnosed you." And I said, "Well, why do you think that?" And he said, "You're just going over, you're surpassing everything." So I said, "Well, that doesn't necessarily mean a diagnosis is wrong." I said, "Are you going to give me credit for anything?" And he said, "Well, what do you mean?" I said, "You have to have a medical answer, you can't have an answer that I worked very hard, on my whole body and my mind, to get, you know, the integral part of myself, and that maybe that might be helping? And the fact that I don't touch fats and I don't do this and I do exercise? *That's not helping, huh?*" So he said, "Well, I guess so." And I said, "Well, do you want to take out my lungs again and see?" I said, "You took them out [already]." So he acknowledged, he said, "Yeah, it's just that it's so unusual." And maybe not accepting something, you know, denial is one thing, but not *excepting* is another thing.

Marty strove to be the exception to her dismal prognosis – she insisted on being an exception. She made great efforts to keep herself and her husband alive, functioning, and enjoying life. By confronting her doctor and challenging *his* definition of her, Marty rejected his narrow, medicalized definition of her. She implied that he was *denying her wellness*. Thus, she enacted a dramatic reversal of the conventional scenario of a doctor accusing the patient of denying her illness. Marty fought feelings of self-pity and sometimes talked about suffering and self-pity interchangeably. When she reflected on how she kept going, she said:

I do, do really think that, if you sit down, and I mean, literally sit down, because it's hard to get up, you do start feeling sorry for yourself. And I'm saying, "Oh, God if I could only get up without hurting." And I've begun to feel, once in a while, I get this little sorry for myself thing, that if I could have a day without pain, I wonder what I'd do? *Probably nothing.* Because I wouldn't push myself and I'd get less done.

I asked, "How so?"

Marty replied, "My whole thing is faith and attitude. You've just got to have it. I feel so sorry for people who give in. But maybe that's why … you've got to have some people die. [Otherwise they'd] be hanging around forever."

Marty had fortitude – and attitude. Marty intended to live – by will and grit. Dying? The prospect of dying undermined her belief in individual control and thus conflicted with her self-concept.

Integrating Grounded Theory with Social Justice Research

What do these stories indicate? What might they suggest about social justice? How do grounded theory methods foster making sense of them? Both women have serious debilitating conditions with multiple harrowing episodes that make their lives uncertain. Both are courageous and forthright, are aware of their conditions, and aim to remain productive and autonomous.

Coding is the first step in taking an analytic stance toward the data. The initial coding phase in grounded theory forces the researcher to define the action in the data statement. In the figures illustrating coding (Figures 1–3), my

Recognizing illness spiral Recounting symptom progression Approaching crisis	I got the sores that are in my mouth, got in my throat and closed my throat up, so I couldn't eat or drink. And then my potassium dropped down to 2.0. I was on the verge of cardiac arrest…. That time when I went in they gave me 72 bottles of pure potassium, burned all my veins out.
	I asked, "What does that mean, that it burned your veins out?"
Suffering the effects of treatment Receiving rapid treatment Forfeiting comfort for speed	She said, "It hurts really bad; it's just because it's so strong and they can't dilute it with anything. They said usually what they do is they dilute with something like a numbing effect, but because I was 2.0, which is right on cardiac arrest that they couldn't do it, they had to get it in fast."
	I asked, "Did you realize that you were that sick?
	She said,

Seeking help
Remaining persistent
Explaining symptoms
Encountering bureaucratic
   dismissal
Experiencing turning point
Explaining severity
Receiving second refusal
Collapsing
Prolonging the ordeal – fitting
   into organizational time
	"Well, I called the doctor several times saying, 'I can't swallow.' I had to walk around and drool on a rag. They finally made an appointment, and I got there and I waited about a half hour. The lady said that there was an emergency and said that I'd have to come back tomorrow. And I said, 'I can't.' I said, 'As soon as I stand up, I'm going to pass out.' And she said, 'Well there's nothing we can do'…. And then this other nurse came in just as I got up and passed out, so then they took me to emergency…. And it took them 12 hours to – they knew when I went in there to admit me, but it took them 12 hours to get me into a room. I sat on a gurney. And they just kept fluid in me until they got me to a room.

	Later in the interview, Christine explained:
Explaining symptoms Awareness of complications Enduring the wait Suffering induced by organization	[When the sores] go to my throat, it makes it really hard to eat or drink, which makes you dehydrated. After that first time … when I called her it had been three days since I'd ate or drank anything … and by the time I got an appointment, it was, I believe, six or seven days, without food or water.

Figure 1: Initial coding – Christine Danforth

Receiving bad news Facing death Suffering diagnostic shock Identifying religion Recounting the identifying moment Finding humor Feeling frightened	The doctor came in to tell me, "Uh, it didn't look good and that this was a – could be a rapidly" – and it appeared that mine was really going rapidly and that it might be about six weeks. Whoa! That blew my mind. It really did…. Right after that – I'm a Catholic – right after that, a poor little volunteer lady came in and said, "Mrs. Gordon?" And the doctor had said, "Mrs. Gordon?" "Yeah, OK." And then he told me. She said, I'm from St. Mary's Church." I said, "Jesus, Mary, and Joseph, they've got the funeral already." And it really just – then I began to see humor in it, but I was scared….

Accepting the present, but not
   the prognosis
Insisting on controlling the illness
Turning point –
   Refusing the death sentence
	This was the point when – [I decided], "If this is going to happen OK, but I'm not going to let it happen." … And I think probably that was the turning point when I said I wouldn't accept it. You know, I will not accept that uhm, death sentence, or whatever you want to call it.

Figure 2: Initial coding – Marty Gordon

	Christine Danforth	*Marty Gordon*
Awareness of illness	Predicting symptom intensification Recognizing illness spiral Lack of control over escalating symptoms Experiencing stigma	Learning and experimenting Becoming an expert Realizing the potential stigma
Developing a stance toward illness	Remaining persistent Monitoring progression of symptoms Seeking help	Suffering initial diagnostic shock Feeling frightened Taking control Refusing death sentence Making deals Challenging physician's view Attacking physician's assumptions Discrediting physician's opinion Rejecting medical model Working on body and mind Following strict regimen Swaying physician's view Believing in her own perceptions Seeing self as an exception
Material resources	Fighting to keep the job Having a health plan Struggling to handle basic expenses Eking out a life – Juggling to pay the rent; Relying on an old car	Working part-time for extras Having a health plan Having solid retirement income Enjoying comfortable lifestyle with travel and amenities
Personal resources	Persevering despite multiple obstacles Defending self Recognizing injustice Abiding sense of shame about educational deficits and poverty Hating her appearance Trying to endure life Feeling excluded from organizational worlds	Preserving autonomy Forging partnerships with professionals Trusting herself Having good education Assuming the right to control her life Believing in individual power Finding strength through faith Possessing a sense of entitlement Aiming to enjoy life Having decades of experience with organizations and professionals
Social resources	Living in a hostile world Taking delight in her niece Retreating from cruel accusations Suffering loneliness Realizing the fragility of her existence Foreseeing no future help	Taking refuge in a close marriage Having strong support, multiple involvements Maintaining powerful images of positive and negative role models Knowing she could obtain help, if needed
Strategies for managing life	Minimizing visibility of deficits Avoiding disclosure of illness Limiting activities	Obtaining husband's promise Avoiding disclosure of illness Controlling self-pity Remaining active Maintaining religious faith

Figure 3: Comparing life situations

codes reflect standard grounded theory practice. The codes are active, immediate, and short. They focus on defining action, explicating implicit assumptions, and seeing processes. By engaging in line-by-line coding, the researcher makes a close study of the data and lays the foundation for synthesizing it.

Coding gives a researcher analytic scaffolding on which to build. Because researchers study their empirical materials closely, they can define both new leads from them and gaps in them. Each piece of data – whether an interview, a field note, a case study, a personal account, or a document – can inform earlier data. Thus, should a researcher discover a lead through developing a code in one interview, he or she can go back through earlier interviews and take a fresh look as to whether this code sheds light on earlier data. Researchers can give their data multiple readings and renderings. Interests in social justice, for example, would lead a researcher to note points of struggle and conflict and to look for how participants defined and acted in such moments.

Grounded theory is a comparative method in which the researcher compares data with data, data with categories, and category with category. Comparing these two women's lives illuminates their several similarities and striking contrasts between their personal, social, and material resources. I offer these comparisons here for heuristic purposes only, to clarify points of convergence and divergence. Both women shared a keen interest in retaining autonomy, and both were aware that illness and disability raised the specter of difference, disconnection, and degradation. Nonetheless, Marty Gordon enjoyed much greater economic security, choices, privileges, and opportunities throughout her life than did Christine Danforth, Marty's quick wit, articulate voice, organizational skills, and diligence constituted a strong set of capabilities that served her well in dealing with failing health.

Poverty and lack of skills had always constrained Christine's life and curtailed her choices. They also diminished her feelings of self-worth and moral status, that is, the extent of virtue or vice attributed to a person by others and self (Charmaz, in press). Then illness shrunk her limited autonomy, and her moral status plummeted further. Christine lived under a cloud of nagging desperation. The anger she felt earlier about being disabled, deprived, and disconnected had dissipated into a lingering sadness and shame. Clearly, Christine has far fewer resources than Marty. She also has had fewer opportunities to develop capabilities throughout her life that could help her to manage her current situation.

Marty struggled periodically with daily routines, but she exerted control over her life and her world. Her struggles resided at another level; she fought against becoming inactive and sinking into self-pity. She treated both her body and her mind as objects to work on and to improve, as projects. Marty worked with physicians, if they agreed on her terms. Although she had grown weaker and had pronounced breathing problems, she believed living at all testified to her success.

For long years, Marty kept her illness contained, or at least mostly out of view. Her proactive stance toward her body and her high level of involvements sustained her moral status. Whatever social diminishment of moral status she experienced derived more from age than from suffering.

The kinds of insights that grounded theory methods can net social justice research vary according to level, scope, and objectives of the study. Through comparing the stories above, we gain some sense of structural and organizational sources of suffering and their differential effects on individuals. The comparisons suggest how research participants' relative resources and capabilities became apparent through studying inductive data.

The comparisons also lead to ideas about structure. Most policy research emphasizes *access* to health care. Comparing these two interviews indicates differential treatment *within* a health care organization. In addition, the comparisons raise questions about rhetoric and realities of receiving care. Marty Gordon credited her "faith and attitude" for managing her illness; however, her lifestyle, income, supportive relationships, and quick wit also helped to buffer her losses. But might not her attitude and advantages be dialectic and mutually reinforcing? Could not her advantages have also fostered her faith and attitude? Each person brings a past to the present. When invoking a similar logic, the residues of the past – limited family support, poor education, undiagnosed learning problems, and lack of skills – complicated and magnified Christine Danforth's troubles with chronic illness and in negotiating care. The structure of Christine's life led to her increasing isolation and decreasing moral status. Might not her anger and sadness have followed? From Marty and Christine's stories, we can discern hidden advantages of high social class status as well as hidden injuries of low status (Sennett & Cobb, 1973).

Last, coding practices can help us to see *our* assumptions, as well as those of our research participants. Rather than raising our codes to a level of objectivity, we can raise questions about how and why we developed certain codes.[16] Another way to break open our assumptions is to ask colleagues and, perhaps, research participants themselves to engage in the coding. When they bring divergent experience to the coding, their responses to the data may call for scrutiny of our own.

Reclaiming Chicago School Traditions

Marty Gordon and Christine Danforth's situations and statements above indicate the construction of their views and actions. Note that at certain points, they each struggle with obdurate social structures that take on tangible meaning in their stories of crucial interactions. To make further sense of situations and stories like these and to interpret the social justice issues with them, I have called for reclaiming Chicago school underpinnings in grounded theory. These underpinnings will move grounded theory more completely into constructionist social science. What are these underpinnings? What does reclaiming them entail? On which assumptions does Chicago school sociology rest? Why are they significant for both the development of grounded theory methods and social justice inquiry?

In brief, the Chicago school assumes human agency, attends to language and interpretation, views social processes as open-ended and emergent, studies action, and addresses temporality. This school emphasizes the significance of language for selfhood and social life and understands that human worlds consist of meaningful objects. In this view, subjective meanings emerge from experience, and they change as experience changes (Reynolds, 2003a).

Thus, the Chicago school assumes dynamic, reciprocal relationships between interpretation and action, and it views social life as people fitting together diverse forms of conduct (Blumer, 1979, p. 22).[17] Because social life is interactive and emergent, a certain amount of indeterminacy characterizes it (Strauss & Fisher, 1979a, 1979b). How might we use Chicago school sociology now to inform contemporary grounded theory studies and social justice inquiry? Where might it lead us? What moral direction might it give?

Both pragmatist philosophy and Chicago school ethnography foster openness to the world and curiosity about it. The Meadian concept of role-taking assumes empathetic understanding of research participants and their worlds. To achieve this understanding, we must know how people define their situations and act on them. Social justice researchers can turn this point into a potent tool for discovering if, when, and to what extent people's meanings and actions contradict their economic or political interests – and whether and to what extent they are aware of such contradictions (see, for example, Kleinman, 1996). Thus, seeking these definitions and actions can make critical inquiry more complex and powerful. Knowing them can alert the researcher to points of actual or potential conflict and change – or compliance. Similarly, learning what things mean to people makes what they do with them comprehensible – at least from their world-view. Conversely, how people act toward things in their worlds indicates their relative significance. Such considerations prompt the researcher to construct an inductive analysis rather than, say, impose structural concepts on the scene.

Although Chicago school sociology has been viewed as microscopic, it also holds implications for the meso and macro levels that social justice researchers aim to engage. A refocused grounded theory would aid and refine connections with these levels. Horowitz (2001) shows how extending Mead's (1934) notion of "generalized other" takes his social psychology of the self to larger social entities and addresses expanding democratic participation of previously excluded groups. Her argument is two-pronged: (a) the development of a critical self is prerequisite for democracy and (b) groups that achieve self-regulation gain empowerment.

The naturalistic inquiry inherent in Chicago school tradition means studying what people in specific social worlds do over time and gaining intimate familiarity with the topic (Blumer, 1969; Lofland & Lofland, 1984, 1995). Hence, to reclaim the Chicago tradition, we must first: *Establish intimate familiarity with the setting(s) and the events occurring within it – as well as with the research participants.*[18] This point may seem obvious; however, much qualitative research, including grounded theory studies, skate the surface rather than plumb the depths of studied life.

An emphasis on action and process leads to considerations of time. The pragmatist treatment of social constructions of past, present, and future could direct social justice researchers to look at timing, pacing, and temporal rhythms. These concerns could alert us to new forms of control and organization.

In addition, understanding timing and sequencing can shed light on the success or failure of collective action. Thus, attending to temporality affords us new knowledge of the worlds we study.

Chicago fieldwork traditions have long emphasized situated analyses embedded in social, economic, and occasionally political contexts, as evident in urban ethnographies (see, for example, E. Anderson, 2003; Horowitz, 1983; Suttles, 1968; Venkatesh, 2000). Numerous grounded theory studies have not taken account of the context in which the studied research problem or process exists. Combining Chicago intellectual traditions with social justice sensitivities would correct tendencies toward decontextualized – and, by extension, objectified – grounded theory analyses.

Looking at data with a Chicago school lens entails focusing on meaning and process at both the subjective and social levels. Like many other people with chronic illness, the women above are aware of the pejorative moral meanings of illness and suffering and sensed the diminished status of those who suffer. When I asked Marty Gordon how her condition affected her job, she said, "I never let it show there. *Never*. Never give cause for anybody either to be sorry for you or want to get rid of you." Although Christine Danforth hated her job, she viewed it as her lifeline and feared losing it. After telling me about receiving written ultimatums from her supervisor, she said:

> Nobody else is going to hire me... An able body can't get one [job], how am I going to get one? So if I'm dyslexic, you know, those people don't even know what it is, let alone how to deal with it. I wouldn't be able to get a job as a receptionist because I can't read and write like most people, so I'm there for life.

Christine Danforth's employers knew the names of her medical diagnoses, but they did not understand her symptoms and their effects in daily life. Christine's story took an ironic twist. She worked for an advocacy agency that served people with disabilities. Several staff members who challenged her work and worth had serious physical disabilities themselves. Christine also discovered that her supervisors had imposed rules on her that they allowed other staff to ignore. Thus, the situation forced Christine to deal with multiple moral contradictions. She suffered the consequences of presumably enlightened disability advocates reproducing negative societal judgments of her moral worth. Tales of such injustice inform stories of suffering.

These examples suggest the second step to reclaiming the Chicago tradition: *Focus on meanings and processes*. This step includes addressing subjective, situational, and social levels. By piecing together many research participants' statements, I developed a moral hierarchy of suffering. Suffering here is much more than pain; it defines self and situation – and ultimately does so in moral terms that support inequities. Suffering takes into account stigma and social definitions of human worth. Hence, suffering includes the lived experience of stigma, reduced autonomy, and loss of control of the defining images of self.

As a result, suffering magnifies difference, forces social disconnection, elicits shame, and increases as inequalities mount.[19]

Meanings of suffering, however, vary and are processual. As researchers, we must find the range of meanings and learn how people form them. Figure 4 shows how suffering takes on moral status and assumes hierarchical form. In addition, it suggests how suffering intersects with institutional traditions and structural conditions that enforce difference. In keeping with a grounded theory perspective, any attributes taken as status variables must earn their way into the analysis rather than be assumed. Note that I added resources and capabilities as potential markers of difference as their significance became clear in the data.[20] Figure 4 implies how larger social justice issues can emerge in open-ended, inductive research. In this case, these issues concern access, equitable treatment, and inherent human worth in health care.

HIERARCHY of MORAL STATUS in SUFFERING

HIGH MORAL STATUS – VALIDATED MORAL CLAIMS

MEDICAL EMERGENCY

INVOLUNTARY ONSET

BLAMELESSNESS FOR CONDITION

"APPROPRIATE" APPEARANCE AND DEMEANOR

SUSTAINED MORAL STATUS – ACCEPTED MORAL CLAIMS

CHRONIC ILLNESS

NEGOTIATED DEMANDS

PRESENT OR PAST POWER & RECIPROCITIES

Diminished Moral Status – Questionable Moral Claims

CHRONIC TROUBLE

BLAME FOR CONDITION AND COMPLICATIONS

"INAPPROPRIATE/REPUGNANT" APPEARANCE AND/OR DEMEANOR

PERSONAL VALUE

Worth less

Worth less

Worth Less

WORTHLESS

Institutional Traditions   **Structural Conditions**

Difference – class, race, gender, age, sexual preference, resources, capabilities

---

Figure 4: Hierarchy of moral status in suffering

Source: Adapted and expanded from Charmaz (1999), "Stories of Suffering: Subjects' Stories and Research Narratives," *Qualitative Health Research*, 9, 362–382.

The figure reflects an abstract statement of how individual experience and social structure come together in emergent action. The figure derives from inductive and comparative analyses of meaning and action, consistent with Chicago school sociology. When we compare individual accounts, we can see that Marty Gordon and Christine Danforth develop their stance toward illness from different starting places and different experiences, yet they both are active in forming their definitions. The Chicago school concept of human nature has long contrasted with much of structural social science. We not only assume human agency but also study it and its consequences. People are active, creative beings who *act*, not merely behave. They attempt to solve problems in their lives and worlds. As researchers, we need to learn how, when, and why participants act. Thus, the third step in reclaiming Chicago traditions follows: *Engage in a close study of action.* The Chicago emphasis on process becomes evident here. What do research participants see as routine? What do they define as problems? In Marty Gordon's case, the problems disrupted her life and could kill her. She had good reason for wanting to oversee her care. At one point, she described her conversation with Monica, her lung specialist, about ending treatment with prednisone:

> I've had a couple of setbacks.... The first time I went off it [prednisone], my breathing capacity cut right in half, so she said, "No." And I make deals with her.... So I'm going to Ireland and she said, "Okay, I want you to double it now, go back up while you're traveling, and then we'll talk about it. But no deals, and don't be stupid." So when I came back I said. "Let's try it again."

But when Marty came back from Ireland, she had complications. She described what happened while she was playing golf:

> I wound up in emergency Easter Sunday because I thought ... I pulled a muscle...But they thought it was a pulmonary embolism.... They said, "Well, with your condition we have to take an X ray, a lung X ray." And he [physician] said, "Oh, I don't like what I see here." And I said, "Look, you're not the doctor that looks at that all the time, don't get nervous, it's been there." So he said, "No, there's a lot more scar tissue than your other X ray." And I said, "Yeah, well that's par for the course, from what I under-stand." And he said, "But there's a hole there I don't like to see." I said, "Look, it's a pulled muscle. *Give me the Motrin.*" [At the time of this inter-view, Motrin was a prescription drug.] And finally he said, "... Maybe it is a pulled muscle." So she [Monica, her lung specialist] called me the next day and she said, "Okay, let's slow down on this going down on the prednisone, too many side things are happening, so we're going slower." And I think it will work.... I'm still playing golf and still working.

Marty Gordon's recounted conversations attest to her efforts to remain autonomous. She insisted on being the leading actor in her life and on shaping its quality. From the beginning, she had remained active in her care and unabashed in her willingness to challenge her physicians and to work with them – on her terms.

Agency does not occur in isolation; it always arises within a social context already shaped by language, meaning, and modes of interaction. This point leads us to the next step in reclaiming the Chicago tradition: *Discover and detail the social context within which action occurs.* A dual focus on action and context can permit social justice researchers to make nuanced explanations of behavior. What people think, feel, and do must be analyzed within the relevant social contexts, which, in turn, people construct through action and interaction. Individuals take into account the actions of those around them as they themselves act. Interaction depends on fitting lines of action together, to use Herbert Blumer's term (Blumer, 1969, 1979). We sense how Marty Gordon and Monica fit lines of actions together to quell her symptoms. Marty crafted an enduring professional partnership with Monica that has eased her way through an increasingly less accessible health care organization for more than 10 years. Knowing that others are or will be involved shapes how people respond to their situations. The more participants create a shared focus and establish a joint goal, the more they will build a shared past and projected future. Marty and Monica shared the goal of keeping Marty alive and of reducing her symptoms while minimizing medication side effects. They built a history of more than a decade, and to this day they project a shared future.

The women in these two stories grapple with the issues that confront them and thus affect the social context in which they live. Marty had a voice and made herself heard; Christine tried but met resistance. She lacked advocates, social skills, and a shared professional discourse to enlist providers as allies, which commonly occurs when class and culture divide providers and patients. The construction of social context may be more discernible in Marty's statements than in other kinds of interviews. In Christine's attempt to obtain care, she related the sequence and timing of events. We see that she received care only because she became a medical emergency, and we learn how earlier refusals and delays increased her misery.

These interview statements contain words and phrases that tell and hint of meaning. Marty Gordon talks about "making deals," "working hard," "not excepting," "wallowing," and "pushing myself." Christine Danforth contrasts herself with an "able body" and recounts how the sequence of events affected her actions. The fifth step in reclaiming the Chicago school tradition follows this dictum: *Pay attention to language.* Language shapes meaning and influences action. In turn, actions and experiences shape meanings. Marty's interview excerpts suggest how she uses words to make her meanings real and tries to make her meanings stick in interaction. Chicago school sociology assumes reciprocal and dynamic relations between interpretation and action. We interpret what happens around and to us and shape our actions accordingly, particularly when something interrupts our routines and causes us to rethink our situations.

In addition to the points outlined above, Chicago school scholars have generated other concepts that can fruitfully inform initial directions in social justice research and can sensitize the researcher's empirical observations. Among these concepts are Glaser and Strauss's (1965) concept of awareness contexts, Scott and Lyman's (1968) idea of accounts, Mills's (1990) notion of vocabularies of motive, Goffman's (1959) metaphor of the theater, and Hochschild's (1983) depiction of emotion work and feeling rules. Establishing who knows what, and when they know it, can provide a crucial focus for studying interaction in social justice research. Both the powerful and the powerless may be forced to give accounts that justify or excuse their actions. People describe their motives in vocabularies in situated social, cultural, historical, and economic contexts. Viewing life as theater can alert social justice researchers to main actors, minor characters and audiences, acts and scenes, roles and scripts, and front-stage impressions and backstage realities. Different kinds of emotion work and feeling rules reflect the settings in which they arise. Expressed emotions and stifled feelings stem from rules and enacted hierarchies of power and advantage that less privileged actors may unwittingly support and reproduce (see, for example, Lively, 2001).

Rethinking Our Language

Just as we must attend to how our research participants' language shapes meaning, we must attend to our own language and make *it* problematic. I mention a few key terms that we qualitative researchers assume and adopt. These terms have served as guiding metaphors or, more comprehensively, as organizing concepts for entire studies. Perhaps ironically, Chicago school sociologists and their followers have promulgated most of these terms. Researchers have made them part of their taken-for-granted lexicon and, I believe, imposed them too readily on our studied phenomena. The logic of both the earlier Chicago school and grounded theory means developing our concepts *from* our analyses of empirical realities, rather than applying concepts *to* them. If we adopt extant concepts, they must earn their way into the analysis through their usefulness (Glaser, 1978). Then we can extend and strengthen them (see, for example, Mamo, 1999; Timmermans, 1994).

Two major concepts carry images of tactical manipulations by a calculating social actor: strategies and negotiations. Despite what we social scientists say, much of human behavior does not reflect explicit *strategies*. Subsuming ordinary actions under the rubric of "strategies" implies explicit tactical schemes when, in fact, an actor's intentions may not have been so clear to him or her, much less to this actor's audience. Rather than strategies, much of what people do reflects their taken-for-granted habitual actions. These actions become routine and scarcely recognized unless disrupted by change or challenge. Note that in the long lists of codes comparing Christine Danforth's and Marty Gordon's situations, I list many actions but few strategies.

When looking for taken-for-granted actions in our research, John Dewey's (1922) central ideas about habit, if not the term itself, can prove helpful to attend to participants' assumptions and taken-for-granted practices, which may not always be in their own interests. Like Snow's (2001) point that much of life is routine and proceeds without explicit interpretation, Dewey (1922) views habits as patterned predispositions that enable individuals to respond to their situations with economy of thought and action: People can act while focusing attention elsewhere (see also Clark, 2000; Cutchin, 2000). Thus, habits include those taken-for-granted modes of thinking, feeling, and acting that people invoke without reflection (Dewey, 1922; Hewitt, 1994). The habits of a lifetime enabled Marty Gordon to maintain hope and to manage her illness. Christine's habits let her eke by but also increased her isolation and physical problems.

Like the concept of strategies, negotiation also imparts a strategic character to interaction. Negotiation is an apt term to describe Marty Gordon's "deals" and disputes with her practitioners. At least from her view, contests did emerge, and bargaining could bring them to effective closure. Then interaction could proceed from the negotiated agreement. Marty brought not only her resolve to her negotiations, but also years of skills and fearlessness in dealing with professionals, a partnership with her primary physician, a network of supportive others, and the ability to pay for nutritious food, conveniences, and a good health plan. Little negotiation may proceed when a person has few such resources and great suffering, as Christine Danforth's story suggests.

Although the concept of negotiations may apply in Marty Gordon's case, we have stretched its applicability, as if it reflected most interactions. It does not. Much of social life proceeds as people either unconsciously adapt their response to another person or interpret what the other person says, means, or does and then they subsequently respond to it (Blumer, 1979). Interaction can alter views, temper emotions, modify intentions, and change actions – all without negotiation. The strategic quality of negotiation may be limited or absent during much sociability. People can be persuasive without attempting to negotiate. Negotiation assumes actors who are explicitly aware of the content and structure of the ensuing interaction. Negotiation also assumes that participants' interactional goals conflict or need realignment if future mutual endeavors are to occur. For that matter, the term assumes that all participants have sufficient power to make their voices heard, if not also to affect outcomes. Judith Howard (2003) states, "The term 'negotiation' implies that the interacting parties have equal opportunities to control the social identities presented, that they come to the bargaining table with equal resources and together develop a joint definition of the situation" (p. 10). Nonetheless, much negotiation ensues when the parties involved do not have equal resources, and much foment may occur about enforcing definitions of social identities, despite unequal positions. For negotiations to occur, each party must be involved with the other to complete joint actions that matter to both, likely for different reasons.

The problems of applying these concepts and of importing their meanings and metaphors on our data extend beyond the concepts above. These problems also occur with applying the concepts of "career," "work," or "trajectory," which we could examine with the same logic. However, the current social scientific emphasis on stories merits scrutiny here.

Metaphors of Stories and Meanings of Silences

The term "story" might once have been a metaphor for varied qualitative data such as interview statements, field note descriptions, or documents. However, we cease to use the term "story" as metaphor and have come view it as concrete reality, rather than a construction we place on these data. With several exceptions (e.g., Charmaz, 2002, in press; Frank, 1997), social scientists have treated the notion of "story" as unproblematic. We have questioned whose story we tell, how we tell it, and how we represent those who tell us their stories, but not the idea of a story itself or whether our materials fit the term "story." The reliance on qualitative interviews in grounded theory studies (Creswell, 1997), as well as in other qualitative approaches, such as narrative analysis, furthered this focus on stories. In addition, the topics themselves of intensive interviews foster producing a story.

Limiting data collection to interviews, as is common in grounded theory research, delimits the theory we can develop. In social justice studies, we must be cautious about which narrative frame we impose on our research, and when and how we do it. The frame itself can prove consequential. The story frame assumes a linear logic and boundaries of temporality that we might over- or underdraw.[21]

Part of my argument about stories concerns silences. In earlier works (Charmaz, 2002, in press), I have emphasized silences at the individual level of analysis; they are also significant at the organizational, social worlds, and societal levels. Clarke (2003, 2005) provides a new grounded theory tool, situational mapping, for showing action and inaction, voices and silences, at varied levels of analysis. She observes that silences reveal absent organizational alignments. Thus, mapping those silences, in their relation to active alignments, can render invisible social structure visible. Invisible aspects of social structure and process are precisely what critical inquiry needs to tackle.[22]

Silences pose significant meanings and telling data in any research that deals with moral choices, ethical dilemmas, and just social policies. Silence signifies absence and sometimes reflects a lack of awareness or inability to express thoughts and feelings. However, silence speaks to power arrangements. It also can mean attempts to control information, to avoid redirecting actions, and, at times, to impart tacit messages. The "right" to speak may mirror hierarchies of power: *Only those who have power dare to speak.* All others are silenced (see, for example, Freire, 1970). Then, too, the powerless may retreat into silence as a last refuge. At one point, Christine Danforth felt that her life was out of control. She described being silenced by devastating events and by an aggressive psychiatrist, and she stopped talking. In all these ways, silence is part of language, meaning, *and* action.

Making stories problematic and attending to silences offers new possibilities for understanding social life for both social justice and grounded theory research. What people in power do not say is often more telling than what they do say. We must note those who choose to remain silent, as well as those who have been silenced. Treating both stories and silences with a critical eye and comparing them with actions and inaction provides empirical underpinnings for any emerging grounded theory. Subsequently, the constructed theory will gain usefulness in its explanatory and predictive power.

Establishing Evaluation Criteria

Using grounded theory for social justice studies requires revisiting the criteria for evaluating them. Glaser and Strauss's (1967; Glaser, 1978) criteria for assessing grounded theory studies include fit, workability, relevance, and modifiability. Thus, the theory must fit the empirical world it purports to analyze, provide a workable understanding and explanation of this world, address problems and processes in it, and allow for variation and change that make the core theory useful over time. The criterion of modifiability allows for refinements of the theory that simultaneously make it more precise and enduring.

Providing cogent explanations stating how the study meets high standards will advance social justice inquiry and reduce unmerited dismissals of it. However, few grounded theorists provide a model. They seldom offer explicit discussions about how their studies *meet* the above or other criteria, although they often provide statements on the logic of their decisions (cf. S. I. Miller & Fredericks, 1999). In the past, some grounded theorists have claimed achieving a theoretical grounding with limited empirical material. Increasingly, researchers justify the type, relative depth, and extent of their data collection and analysis on *one* criterion: saturation of categories. They issue a claim of saturation and end their data collection (Flick, 1998; Morse, 1995; Silverman, 2000). But what does saturation mean? To whom? Janice Morse (1995), who initiated the critique of saturation, accepts defining it as "data adequacy" and adds that it is "operationalized as collecting data until no new information is obtained" (p. 147). Often, researchers invoke the criterion of saturation to justify small samples – very small samples with thin data. Such justifications diminish the credibility of grounded theory. Any social justice study that makes questionable claims of saturation risks being seen as suspect.

Claims of saturation often reflect rationalization more than reason, and these claims raise questions. What stands as a category?[23] Is it conceptual? Is it useful? Developed? By whose criteria? All these questions add up to the big question: *What stands as adequate research?* Expanded criteria that include the Chicago school's rigorous study of context and action makes any grounded theory study more credible and advances the claims of social justice researchers. Then we can augment our criteria by going beyond "saturation" and ask if our empirical detail also achieves Christians's (2000) and Denzin's (1989) criterion of "interpretive sufficiency," which takes into account cultural complexity and multiple interpretations of life.

To reopen explicit discussion of criteria for grounded theory studies, and particularly those in social justice research, I offer the following criteria.

Criteria for Grounded Theory Studies in Social Justice Inquiry

Credibility

- Has the researcher achieved intimate familiarity with the setting or topic?
- Are the data sufficient to merit the researcher's claims? Consider the range, number, and depth of observations contained in the data.
- Has the researcher made systematic comparisons between observations and between categories?
- Do the categories cover a wide range of empirical observations?
- Are there strong logical links between the gathered data and the researcher's argument and analysis?
- Has the researcher provided enough evidence for his or her claims to allow the reader to form an independent assessment – and *agree* with the researcher's claims?

Originality

- Are the categories fresh? Do they offer new insights?
- Does the analysis provide a new conceptual rendering of the data?
- What is the social and theoretical significance of the work?
- How does the work challenge, extend, or refine current ideas, concepts, and practices?

Resonance

- Do the categories portray the fullness of the studied experience?
- Has the researcher revealed liminal and taken-for-granted meanings?
- Has the researcher drawn links between larger collectivities and individual lives, when the data so indicate?
- Do the analytic interpretations make sense to members and offer them deeper insights about their lives and worlds?

Usefulness

- Does the analysis offer interpretations that people can use in their everyday worlds?
- Do the analytic categories speak to generic processes?
- Have these generic processes been examined for hidden social justice implications?

- Can the analysis spark further research in other substantive areas?
- How does the work contribute to making a better society?

A strong combination of originality and credibility increases resonance, usefulness, and the subsequent value of the contribution. The criteria above account for the empirical study and development of the theory. They say little about how the researcher writes the narrative or what makes it compelling. Other criteria speak to the aesthetics of the writing. Our written works derive from aesthetic principles and rhetorical devices – in addition to theoretical statements and scientific rationales. The act of writing is intuitive, inventive, and interpretive, not merely a reporting of acts and facts, or, in the case of grounded theory, causes, conditions, categories, and consequences. Writing leads to further discoveries and deeper insights; it furthers inquiry. Rather than claiming silent authorship hidden behind a scientific facade, grounded theorists – as well as proponents of social justice – should claim audible voices in their writings (see Charmaz & Mitchell, 1996; Mitchell & Charmaz, 1996). For grounded theorists, an audible voice brings the writer's self into the words while illuminating intersubjective worlds. Such evocative writing sparks the reader's imagined involvement in the scenes portrayed and those beyond. In this sense, Laurel Richardson's (2000) criteria for the evocative texts of "creative analytic practice ethnography" also apply here. These criteria consist of the narrative's substantive contribution, aesthetic merit, reflexivity, impact, and expression of a reality (p. 937).

A grounded theory born from reasoned reflections and principled convictions that conveys a reality makes a substantive contribution. Add aesthetic merit and analytic impact, and then its influence may spread to larger audiences. Through reclaiming Chicago traditions, conducting inquiry to make a difference in the world, and creating evocative narratives, we will not be silenced. We will have stories to tell and theories to proclaim.

Summary and Conclusions

A turn toward qualitative social justice studies promotes combining critical inquiry and grounded theory in novel and productive ways. An interpretive, constructivist ground theory supports this turn by building on its Chicago school antecedents. Grounded theory can sharpen the analytic edge of social justice studies. Simultaneously, the critical inquiry inherent in social justice research can enlarge the focus and deepen the significance of grounded theory analyses. Combining the two approaches enhances the power of each.

A grounded theory informed by critical inquiry demands going deeper into the phenomenon itself and its situated location in the world than perhaps most grounded theory studies have in the past. This approach does not mean departing from grounded theory guidelines. It does not mean investigative reporting.

Grounded theory details process and context – and goes into the social world and setting far beyond one investigative story. Grounded theory contains tools to study how processes become institutionalized practices. Such attention to the processes that constitute structure can keep grounded theory from dissolving into fragmented small studies.

With the exception of those studies that rely on historical documents, grounded theory studies typically give little scrutiny to the past and sometimes blur inequalities with other experiences or overlook them entirely. Studying social justice issues means paying greater attention to inequality and its social and historical contexts. Too much of qualitative research today minimizes current *social* context, much less historical evolution. Relying on interview studies on focused topics may preclude attention to context – particularly when our research participants take the context of their lives for granted and do not speak of it. Hence, the mode of inquiry itself limits what researchers may learn. Clearly, interviewing is the method of choice for certain topics, but empirical qualitative research suffers if it becomes synonymous with interview studies.

Like snapshots, interviews provide a picture taken during a moment in time. Interviewers gain a view of research participants' concerns as they present them, rather than as events unfold. Multiple visits over time combined with the intimacy of intensive interviewing do provide a deeper view of life than one-shot structured or informational interviews can provide. However, anyone's retelling of events may differ markedly from an ethnographer's recording of them. In addition, as noted above, what people say may not be what they do (Deutscher et al., 1993). At that, what an interviewer asks and hears or an ethnographer records depends in part on the overall context, the immediate situation, *and* his or her training and theoretical proclivities.

At its best, grounded theory provides methods to explicate an empirical process in ways that prompt seeing beyond it. By sticking closely to the leads and explicating the relevant process, the researcher can go deeper into meaning and action than given in words. Thus, the focused inquiry of grounded theory, with its progressive inductive analysis, moves the work theoretically and covers more empirical observations than other approaches. In this way, a focused grounded theory portrays a picture of the whole.

Author's Note

I thank Adele E. Clarke, Norman K. Denzin, Udo Kelle, Anne Marie McLauglin, and Janice Morse for their comments on an earlier version of this chapter. I also appreciate having the views of the following members of the Sonoma State University Faculty Writing Program: Karin Enstam, Scott Miller, Tom Rosin, Josephine Schallehn, and Thaine Stearns. I presented brief excerpts from earlier drafts in a keynote address, "Reclaiming Traditions and Re-forming Trends in Qualitative Research," at the Qualitative Research Conference, Carleton University, Ottawa, Canada, May 22, 2003, and in a presentation, "Suffering and the Self: Meanings of Loss in Chronic Illness," at the Sociology Department, University of California, Los Angeles, January 9, 2004.

Notes

1. Such emphases often start with pressing social problems, collective concerns, and impassioned voices. In contrast, Rawls's (1971) emphasis on fairness begins from a distanced position of theorizing individual rights and risks from the standpoint of the rational actor under hypothetical conditions. Conceptions of social justice must take into account both collective goods and individual rights and must recognize that definitions both of rationality and of "rational" actors are situated in time, space, and culture – and both can change. To foster justice, Nussbaum (2000, p. 234) argues that promoting a collective good must not subordinate the ends of some individuals over others. She observes that women suffer when a collective good is promoted without taking into account the internal power and opportunity hierarchies within a group.

2. For descriptions of grounded theory guidelines, see Charmaz (2000a, 2003b), Glaser (1978, 1992), and Strauss and Corbin (1990, 1998).

3. I use the term "data" throughout for two reasons: It symbolizes (a) a fund of empirical materials that we systematically collect and assemble to acquire knowledge about a topic and (b) an acknowledgment that qualitative resources hold equal significance for studying empirical reality as quantitative measures, although they differ in kind.

4. In this way, integrating a critical stance offers a corrective to narrow and limited studies conducted as grounded theory studies. Neither a narrow focus nor limited empirical material is part of the method itself. We cannot blur how earlier researchers have used grounded theory with the guidelines in the method. Although social justice inquiry suggests substantive fields, it also assumes questions and concerns about power, privilege, and hierarchy that some grounded theorists may not yet have entertained.

5. Chicago school sociology shaped an enduring tradition of qualitative research in sociology, of which grounded theory remains a part. What stands as "the" Chicago school varies depending on who defines it (Abbott, 1999; L. H. Lofland 1980). In my view, the Chicago school theoretical heritage goes back to the early years of the 20th century, in the works, for example, of Charles Horton Cooley (1902), John Dewey (1922), George Herbert Mead (1932, 1934), and Charles S. Peirce (Hartshorne & Weiss, 1931–1935). In research practice, the Chicago school sparked study of the city and spawned urban ethnographies (see, for example, Park & Burgess, 1925; Shaw, 1930; Thomas & Znaniecki, 1927; Thrasher, 1927). Chicago sociologists often held naïve and partial views but many sensed the injustices arising in the social problems of the city, and Abbott (1999) notes that Albion Small attacked capitalism. Nonetheless, some Chicago school sociologists reinforced inequities in their own bailiwicks (Deegan, 1995). Mid-century ethnographers and qualitative researchers built on their Chicago school intellectual heritage and created what scholars have called a second Chicago school (G. A. Fine, 1995). For recent renderings of the Chicago school, see Abbott (1999), G. A. Fine (1995), Musolf (2003), and Reynolds (2003a, 2003b). Chicago school sociology emphasizes the contextual backdrop of observed scenes and their situated nature in time, place, and relationships. Despite the partial emergence of grounded theory from both theoretical and methodological Chicago school roots, Glaser (2002) disavows the pragmatist, constructionist elements in grounded theory.

6. Symbolic interactionism provides an open-ended theoretical perspective from which grounded theory researchers can start. This perspective is neither inherently prescriptive nor microsociological. Barbara Ballis Lal (2001) not only suggests the contemporary

usefulness of early Chicago school symbolic interactionist ideas for studying race and ethnicity but also notes their implications for current political action and social policy. David Maines (2001) demonstrates that symbolic interactionist emphases on agency, action, and negotiated order have long had macrosociological import. He shows that the discipline of sociology has incorrectly – and ironically – compartmentalized symbolic interactionism while increasingly becoming more interactionist in its assumptions and directions.

7. In particular, the Chicago school provides antecedents for attending to social reform, as in Jane Addams's (1919) work at Hull-House and Mead and Dewey's interests in democratic process. The field research founded in Chicago school sociology has been called into question at various historical junctures from Marxist and postmodernist perspectives (see, for example, Burawoy, Blum, et al., 1991; Burawoy, Gamson, et al., 2002; Clough, 1992; Denzin, 1992; Wacquant, 2002). Criticisms of Chicago school sociology have suggested that grounded theory represents the most codified and realist statement of Chicago school methodology (Van Maanen, 1988).

8. Strauss and Corbin's (1990, 1998) emphasis on technical procedures has been met with chagrin by a number of researchers (Glaser, 1992; Melia, 1996; Stern, 1994). In his 1987 handbook *Qualitative Analysis for Social Scientists*, Strauss mentions axial coding and verification, which depart from earlier versions of grounded theory, and he and Juliet Corbin (1990, 1998) develop them in their coauthored texts.

9. My critique mirrors a much larger trend. Lincoln and Guba (2000) find that the movement away from positivism pervades the social sciences. They state that the turn toward interpretive, postmodern, and critical theorizing makes most studies vulnerable to criticism (p. 163).

10. Grounded theory provides tools that researchers can – and do – use from any philosophical perspective – or political agenda. Studies of worker involvement, for example, may start from addressing employees' concerns or management's aim to increase corporate profits.

11. Tedlock (2000) states, "Ethnographers' lives are embedded within their field experiences in such a way that all their interactions involve moral choices" (p. 455). Ethnography may represent one end of a continuum. Nevertheless, does not grounded theory research also involve moral choices?

12. Feminist research suggests ways to proceed. DeVault (1999) and Olesen (2000) provide excellent overviews of and debates in feminist research.

13. Issues of exploitation arise when participants work without pay or recognition. Feminist researchers often recommend having participants read drafts of materials, yet even reading drafts may be too much when research participants are struggling with losses, although they may have requested to see the researcher's writings in progress. When research participants express interest, I share early drafts, but I try to reduce participants' potential feelings of obligation to finish reading them. Morse (1998) agrees with sharing results but not the conduct of inquiry.

14. Schwalbe et al: (2000) and Harris (2001) make important moves in this analytic direction.

15. The first two interview excerpts appear in earlier published accounts. I include them so that readers interested in seeing how I used them in social psychological accounts may obtain them. Subsequent interview statements have not been published. The data are part of an evolving study of 170 interviews of chronically ill persons. A subset of research participants that includes these two women have been interviewed multiple times.

16. Further specifics of grounded theory guidelines are available in Charmaz (2000a, 2003b, Charmaz & Mitchell, 2001), Glaser (1978, 1992, 2001), Strauss, (1987), and Strauss and Corbin (1990, 1998).

17. I realize that presenting the Chicago school as a unified perspective is something of a historical gloss because differences are discernible between the early pragmatists as well as among the sociologists who followed them. Furthermore, a strong quantitative tradition developed at the University of Chicago (see Bulmer, 1984).

18. See Lofland and Lofland (1984, 1995) for an emphasis on describing the research setting. Lincoln and Guba (1985) offer a sound rationale for naturalistic inquiry as well as good ideas for conducting it. When the data consist of extant texts such as documents, films, or texts, then the researcher may need in seek multiple empirical sources.

19. See Scheff (2003) for a discussion of relationships between shame and society.

20. Grounded theory methods can inform traditional quantitative research, although these approaches seldom have been used together. Hypotheses can be drawn from Figure 20.4, such as that the greater the definitions of an individual's difference, the more rapid his or her tumble down the moral hierarchy of suffering. Quantitative researchers could pursue such hypotheses.

21. And as I have pointed out with individual accounts (Charmaz, 2002), raw experience may fit neither narrative logic nor the comprehensible content of a story.

22. Clarke's (2003, 2004) concept of implicated actors can be particularly useful to analyze voices and silences in social justice discourses.

23. See Dey (1999) for an extensive discussion on constructing categories in the early grounded theory works.

References

Abbott, A. (1999). *Department & discipline: Chicago sociology at one hundred.* Chicago: University of Chicago Press.

Addams, J. (1919). *Twenty years at Hull-House.* New York: Macmillan.

Anderson, E. (2003). Jelly's place: An ethnographic memoir. *Symbolic Interaction, 26,* 217–237.

Anderson, L., & Snow, D. A. (2001). Inequality and the self: Exploring connections from an interactionist perspective. *Symbolic Interaction, 24,* 396–406.

Atkinson, P., Coffey, A., & Delamont, S. (2003). *Key themes in qualitative research: Continuities and changes.* New York: Rowman and Littlefield.

Blumer, H. (1969). *Symbolic interactionism.* Englewood Cliffs, NJ: Prentice-Hall.

Blumer, H. (1979). Comments on "George Herbert Mead and the Chicago tradition of sociology." *Symbolic Interaction, 2*(2), 21–22.

Bryant, A. (2002). Regrounding grounded theory. *The Journal of Information Technology Theory and Application, 4,* 25–42.

Bryant, A. (2003). A constructive/ist response to Glaser. *Forum Qualitative Sozialforschung/ Forum: Qualitative Social Research, 4,* Retrieved from www.qualitative-research.net/fqs-texte/1–03/1-bryant-e-htm

Bulmer, M. (1984). *The Chicago school of sociology: Institutionalization, diversity, and the rise of sociology.* Chicago: University of Chicago Press.

Burawoy, M (1991). Reconstructing social theories. In M. Burawoy, J. Gamson, J. Schiffman, A. Burton, A. A. Ferguson, L. Salzinger, L., et al. (Eds.), *Ethnography unbound: Power and resistance in the modern metropolis* (pp. 8–28). Berkeley: University of California Press.

Burawoy, M., Blum, J. A., George, S., Gill, Z., Gowan, T., Haney, L., et al. (2000). *Global ethnography: Forces, connections, and imaginations in a postmodern world.* Berkeley: University of California Press.

Burawoy, M., Gamson, J., Schiffman, J., Burton, A., Ferguson, A. A., Salzinger, L., et al. (1991). *Ethnography unbound: Power and resistance in the modern metropolis.* Berkeley: University of California Press.

Charmaz, K. (1983). The grounded theory method: An explication and interpretation. In R. M. Emerson (Ed.), *Contemporary field research* (pp. 109–126). Boston: Little, Brown.

Charmaz, K. (1990). Discovering chronic illness: Using grounded theory. *Social Science and Medicine, 30,* 1161–1172.

Charmaz, K. (1991). *Good days, bad days: The self in chronic illness and time.* New Brunswick, NJ: Rutgers University Press.

Charmaz, K. (1999). Stories of suffering: Subjects' Stories and research narratives. *Qualitative Health Research, 9,* 362–382.

Charmaz, K. (2000a). Constructivist and objectivist grounded theory. In N. K. Denzin & Y. S. Lincoln (Eds.), *Handbook of qualitative research* (2nd ed., pp. 509–535). Thousand Oaks, CA: Sage.

Charmaz, K. (2000b). Looking backward, moving forward: Expanding sociological horizons in the twenty-first century. *Sociological Perspectives, 43,* 527–549.

Charmaz, K. (2002). Stories and silences: Disclosures and self in chronic illness. *Qualitative Inquiry, 8,* 302–328.

Charmaz, K. (2003a). Grounded theory. In M. Lewis-Beck, A. E. Bryman, & T. F. Liao (Eds.), *The Sage encyclopedia of social science research methods* (pp. 440–444). Thousand Oaks, CA: Sage.

Charmaz, K. (2003b). Grounded theory. In J. A. Smith (Ed.), *Qualitative psychology: A practical guide to research methods* (pp. 81–110). London: Sage.

Charmaz, K. (in press). Stories and silences: Disclosures and self in chronic illness. In D. Brashers & D. Goldstein (Eds.), *Health communication.* New York: Lawrence Erlbaum.

Charmaz, K., & Mitchell, R. G. (1996). The myth of silent authorship: Self, substance, and style in ethnographic writing. *Symbolic Interaction, 19*(4), 285–302.

Charmaz, K., & Mitchell, R. G. (2001). Grounded theory in ethnography. In P. Atkinson, A. Coffey, S. Delamont, J. Lofland, & L. H. Lofland (Eds.), *Handbook of ethnography* (pp. 160–174). London: Sage.

Christians, C. G. (2000). Ethics and politics in qualitative research. In N. K. Denzin & Y. S. Lincoln (Eds.), *Handbook of qualitative research* (2nd ed., pp. 133–155). Thousand Oaks, CA: Sage.

Clark, F. A. (2000). The concepts of habit and routine: A preliminary theoretical synthesis. *The Occupational Therapy Journal of Research, 20,* 123S–138S.

Clarke, A. E. (1998). *Disciplining reproduction: Modernity, American life sciences and the "problem of sex."* Berkeley: University of California Press.

Clarke, A. E. (2003). Situational analyses: Grounded theory mapping after the postmodern turn. *Symbolic Interaction, 26,* 553–576.

Clarke, A. E. (2004). *Situational analysis: Grounded theory after the postmodern turn.* Thousand Oaks, CA: Sage.

Clough, P. T. (1992). *The end(s) of ethnography: From realism to social criticism.* Newbury Park, CA: Sage.

Coffey, A., Holbrook, P., & Atkinson, P. (1996). Qualitative data analysis: Technologies and representations. *Sociological Research Online, 1*(1). Retrieved from www.socresonline.org.uk/1/1/4.html

Cooley, C. H. (1902). *Human nature and the social order.* New York: Scribner's.

Corbin, J. M., & Strauss, A. (1988). *Unending care and work.* San Francisco: Jossey-Bass.

Creswell, J. W. (1997). *Qualitative inquiry and research design.* Thousand Oaks, CA: Sage.

Cutchin, M. P. (2000). Retention of rural physicians: Place integration and the triumph of habit. *The Occupational Therapy Journal of Research, 20,* 106S–111S.

Deegan, M. J. (1995). The second sex and the Chicago school: Women's accounts, know-ledge, and work, 1945–1960. In G. A. Fine (Ed.), *A second Chicago school?* (pp. 322–364). Chicago: University of Chicago Press.

Denzin, N. K. (1989). *Interpretive biography.* Newbury Park, CA: Sage.

Denzin, N. K. (1992). *Symbolic interactionism and cultural studies: The politics of interpretation.* Oxford, UK: Basil Blackwell.

Denzin, N. K. (1994). The art and politics of interpretation. In N. K. Denzin & Y. S. Lincoln (Eds.), *Handbook of qualitative research* (pp. 500–515). Thousand Oaks, CA: Sage.

Deutscher, I., Pestello, R., & Pestello, H. F. (1993). *Sentiments and acts.* New York: Aldine de Gruyter.

DeVault, M. L. (1999). *Liberating method: Feminism and social research.* Philadelphia: Temple University Press.

Dewey, J. (1922). *Human nature and conduct.* New York: Modern Library.

Dey, I. (1999). *Grounding grounded theory.* San Diego: Academic Press.

Duneire, M. (1992). *Slim's table: Race, respectability, and masculinity.* Chicago: University of Chicago Press.

Feagin, J. R. (1999). Social justice and sociology: Agendas for the twenty-first century. *American Sociological Review, 66,* 1–20.

Fine, G. A. (Ed.). (1995). *A second Chicago school? The development of a postwar American sociology.* Chicago: University of Chicago Press.

Fine, M., Weis, L., Weseen. S., & Wong, L. (2000). For whom? Qualitative research, representations, and social responsibilities. In N. K. Denzin & Y. S. Lincoln (Eds.), *Handbook of qualitative research* (2nd ed., pp. 107–131). Thousand Oaks. CA: Sage.

Flick, U. (1998). *An introduction to qualitative research.* Thousand Oaks, CA: Sage.

Frank, A. W. (1997). Enacting illness stories: When, what, and why. In H. L. Nelson (Ed.), *Stories and their limits: Narrative approaches to bioethics* (pp. 31–49). New York: Routledge.

Freire, P. (1970). *The pedagogy of the oppressed* (M. B. Ramos, Trans.). New York: Herder and Herder.

Glaser, B. G. (1978). *Theoretical sensitivity.* Mill Valley, CA: Sociology Press.

Glaser, B. G. (1992). *Basics of grounded theory analysis.* Mill Valley, CA: Sociology Press.

Glaser, B. G. (1998). *Doing grounded theory: Issues and discussions.* Mill Valley, CA: Sociology Press.

Glaser, B. G. (2001). *Conceptualization contrasted with description.* Mill Valley, CA: Sociology Press.

Glaser, B. G. (2002). Constructivist grounded theory? *Forum Qualitative Sozialforschung/ Forum: Qualitative Social Research, 3*(3). Retrieved from www.qualitative-research. net/fqs-texte/3–02/3–02glasere-htm

Glaser, B. G., & Strauss, A. L. (1965). *Awareness of dying.* Chicago: Aldine.

Glaser, B. G., & Strauss, A. L. (1967). *The discovery of grounded theory.* Chicago: Aldine.

Goffman, E. (1959). *The presentation of self in everyday life.* Garden City, NY: Doubleday.

Goffman, E. (1961). *Asylums.* Garden City, NY: Doubleday.

Harris, S. R. (2001). What can interactionism contribute to the study of inequality? The case of marriage and beyond. *Symbolic Interaction, 24,* 455–480.

Hartshorne, C., & Weiss, P. (Eds.). (1931–1935). *Collected papers of Charles Saunders Peirce* (Vols. 1–6). Cambridge, MA: Harvard University Press.

Hewitt, J. P. (1994). *Self and society: A symbolic Interactionist social psychology* (6th ed.). Boston: Allyn & Bacon.

Hochschild, A. (1983). *The managed heart: Commercialization of human feeling.* Berkeley: University of California Press.

Holstein, J. A., & Gubrium, J. F. (1995). *The active interview.* Thousand Oaks, CA: Sage.

Horowitz, R. (1983). *Honor and the American dream: Culture and identity in a Chicano community.* New Brunswick, NJ: Rutgers University Press.

Horowitz, R. (2001). Inequalities, democracy, and fieldwork in the Chicago schools of yesterday and today. *Symbolic Interaction, 24,* 481–504.

Howard, J. A. (2003). Tensions of social Justice, *Sociological Perspectives, 46,* 1–20.

Kemmis, S., & McTaggart, R. (2000). Participatory action research. In N. K. Denzin & Y. S. Lincoln (Eds.), *Handbook of qualitative research* (2nd ed., pp. 567–605). Thousand Oaks. CA: Sage.

Kleinman, S. (1996). *Opposing ambitions: Gender and identity in an alternative organization.* Chicago: University of Chicago Press.

Lal, B. B. (2001). Individual agency and collective determinism: Changing perspectives on race and ethnicities in cities, the Chicago school 1918–1958. In J. Mucha, D. Kaesler, & W. Winclawski (Eds.), *Mirrors and windows: Essays in the history of sociology* (pp. 183–196). Torun: International Sociological Association.

Lincoln, Y. S., & Guba, E. G. (1985). *Naturalistic inquiry.* Beverly Hills, CA: Sage.

Lincoln, Y. S., & Guba, E. G. (2000). Paradigmatic controversies, contradictions, and emerging confluences. In N. K. Denzin & Y. S. Lincoln (Eds.), *Handbook of Qualitative Research* (2nd ed., pp. 163–188). Thousand Oaks. CA: Sage.

Lively, K. (2001). Occupational claims to professionalism: The case of paralegals. *Symbolic Interaction, 24,* 343–365.

Locke, K. (1996). Rewriting *The Discovery of Grounded Theory* after 25 years? *Journal of Management Inquiry, 5,* 239–245.

Lofland, J., & Lofland, L. H. (1984). *Analyzing social settings* (2nd ed.). Belmont, CA: Wadsworth.

Lofland, J., & Lofland, L. H. (1995). *Analyzing social settings* (3rd ed.). Belmont, CA: Wadsworth.

Lofland, L. H. (1980). Reminiscences of classic Chicago. *Urban Life, 9,* 251–281.

Maines, D. R. (2001). *The faultline of consciousness: A view of interactionism in sociology.* New York: Aldine de Gruyter.

Maines, D. R. (2003). Interactionism's place. *Symbolic Interaction, 26,* 5–18.

Mamo, L. (1999). Death and dying: Confluences of emotion and awareness. *Sociology of Health and Illness, 21,* 13–26.

Mead, G. H. (1932). *Philosophy of the present.* LaSalle, IL: Open Court.

Mead, G. H. (1934). *Mind, self and society.* Chicago: University of Chicago Press.

Melia, K. M. (1996). Rediscovering Glaser. *Qualitative Health Research, 6,* 368–378.

Miller, D. E. (2000). Mathematical dimensions of qualitative research. *Symbolic Interaction, 23,* 399–402.

Miller, S. I., & Fredericks, M. (1999). How does grounded theory explain? *Qualitative Health Research, 9,* 538–551.

Mills, C.W. (1990). Situated actions and vocabularies of motive. In D. Brissett & C. Edgley (Eds.), *Life as theatre* (2nd ed., pp. 207–218). New York: Aldine de Gruyter.

Mitchell, R. G., Jr. (2002). *Dancing to Armageddon: Survivalism and chaos in modern times.* Chicago: University of Chicago Press.

Mitchell, R. G., & Charmaz, K. (1996). Telling tales, writing stories. *Journal of Contemporary Ethnography, 25,* 144–166.

Morse, J. M. (1995). The significance of saturation. *Qualitative Health Research, 5,* 147–149.

Morse, J. M. (1998). Validity by committee. *Qualitative Health Research, 8,* 443–445.

Morse, J. M. (1999). The armchair walkthrough. *Qualitative Health Research, 9,* 435–436.

Musolf, G. R. (2003). The Chicago school. In L. T. Reynolds & N. J. Herman-Kinney (Eds.), *Handbook of symbolic interactionism* (pp. 91–117). Walnut Creek, CA: AltaMira.

Nussbaum, M. C. (1999). *Sex and social justice.* New York: Oxford University Press.

Nussbaum, M. C. (2000). Women's capabilities and social justice, *Journal of Human Development, 1,* 219–247.

Olesen, V. L. (2000). Feminisms and qualitative research at and into the millennium. In N. K. Denzin & Y. S. Lincoln (Eds.), *Handbook of qualitative research* (2nd ed., pp. 215–255). Thousand Oaks, CA: Sage.

Park, R. E., & Burgess, E. W. (1925). *The city.* Chicago: University of Chicago Press.

Prus, R. (1996). *Symbolic interaction and ethnographic research: Intersubjectivity and the study of human lived experience.* Albany: State University of New York Press.

Rawls, J. (1971). *A theory of justice.* Cambridge, MA: Belknap Press of Harvard University Press.

Reynolds, L. T. (2003a). Early representatives. In L. T. Reynolds & N. J. Herman-Kinney (Eds.), *Handbook of symbolic interactionism* (pp. 59–81). Walnut Creek, CA: AltaMira.

Reynolds, L. T. (2003b). Intellectual precursors. In L. T. Reynolds & N. J. Herman-Kinney (Eds.), *Handbook of symbolic interactionism* (pp. 39–58). Walnut Creek, CA: AltaMira.

Richardson, L. (2000). Writing: A method of inquiry. In N. K. Denzin & Y. S. Lincoln (Eds.), *Handbook of qualitative research* (2nd ed., pp. 923–948). Thousand Oaks, CA: Sage.

Scheff, T. J. (2003). Shame in self and society. *Symbolic Interaction, 26,* 239–262.

Schwalbe, M. S., Goodwin, S., Holden, D., Schrock, D., Thompson, S., & Wolkomir, M. (2000). Generic processes in the reproduction of inequality: An interactionist analysis. *Social Forces, 79,* 419–452.

Schwandt, T. A. (1994). Constructivist, interpretivist approaches to human inquiry. In N. K. Denzin & Y. S. Lincoln (Eds.), *Handbook of qualitative research* (pp. 118–137). Thousand Oaks, CA: Sage.

Schwandt, T. A. (2000). Three epistemological stances for qualitative inquiry: Interpretivism, hermeneutics, and social constructionism. In N. K. Denzin & Y. S. Lincoln (Eds.), *Handbook of qualitative research* (2nd ed., pp. 189–213). Thousand Oaks, CA: Sage.

Scott, M., & Lyman, S. M. (1968). Accounts. *American Sociological Review, 33,* 46–62.

Seale, C. (1999). *The quality of qualitative research.* London: Sage.

Sennett, R., & Cobb, J. (1973). *The hidden injuries of class.* New York: Vintage.

Shaw, C. (1930). *The jack-roller.* Chicago: University of Chicago Press.

Silverman, D. (2000). *Doing qualitative research: A practical handbook.* London: Sage.

Snow, D. (2001). Extending and broadening Blumer's conceptualization of symbolic interactionism. *Symbolic Interaction, 24,* 367–377.

Snow, D., & Anderson, L. (1993). *Down on their luck: A study of homeless street people.* Berkeley: University of California Press.

Star, S. L. (1989). *Regions of the mind: Brain research and the quest for scientific certainty.* Stanford, CA: Stanford University Press.

Stern, P. N. (1994). Eroding grounded theory. In J. Morse (Ed.), *Critical issues in qualitative research methods* (pp. 212–223). Thousand Oaks, CA: Sage.

Strauss, A. L (Ed.). (1964). *George Herbert Mead on social psychology.* Chicago: University of Chicago Press.

Strauss, A. L. (1987). *Qualitative analysis for social scientists.* New York: Cambridge University Press.

Strauss, A. L. (1993). *Continual permutations of action.* New York: Aldine de Gruyter.

Strauss, A., & Corbin, J. (1990). *Basics of qualitative research: Grounded theory procedures and techniques.* Newbury Park, CA: Sage.

Strauss, A., & Corbin, J. (1998). *Basics of qualitative research: Grounded theory procedures and techniques* (2nd ed.). Thousand Oaks, CA: Sage.

Strauss, A., & Fisher, B. (1979a). George Herbert Mead and the Chicago tradition of sociology, Part 1. *Symbolic Interaction, 2*(1), 9–26.

Strauss, A., & Fisher, B. (1979b). George Herbert Mead and the Chicago tradition of sociology, Part 2. *Symbolic Interaction, 2*(2), 9–19.

Suttles, G. (1968). *Social order of the slum.* Chicago: University of Chicago Press.

Tedlock, B. (2000). Ethnography and ethnographic representation. In N. K. Denzin & Y. S. Lincoln (Eds.), *Handbook of qualitative research* (2nd ed., pp. 455–486). Thousand Oaks, CA: Sage.

Thomas, W. I. & Znaniecki, F. (1927). *The Polish peasant in America.* New York: Knopf.

Thrasher, F. (1927). *The gang.* Chicago: University of Chicago Press.

Timmermans, S. (1994). Dying of awareness: The theory of awareness contexts revisited. *Sociology of Health and Illness, 17,* 322–339.

van den Hoonaard, W. C. (1997). *Working with sensitizing concepts: Analytical field research.* Thousand Oaks, CA: Sage.

Van Maanen, J. (1988). *Tales of the field.* Chicago: University of Chicago Press.

Venkatesh, S. (2000). *American project: The rise and fall of a modern ghetto.* Cambridge, MA: Harvard University Press.

Wacquant, L. (2002). Scrutinizing the street: Poverty, morality, and the pitfalls of urban ethnography. *American Journal of Sociology, 107,* 1468–1534.

Ethnography

31

Doing Occupational Demarcation: The "Boundary-Work" of Nurse Managers in a District General Hospital

Davina Allen

" . . . these processes may be understood as micro-political strategies through which work identities and occupational margins are negotiated."

T his article analyzes how nurse managers attempted to accomplish the formal boundaries of clinical nursing work in a large UK district general hospital. As a site where occupational jurisdictions are claimed and sustained, the management arena has been hitherto neglected in interactionist studies of hospital settings. The sociological eye has focused primarily on the ways in which staff in the clinical domain negotiate their occupational roles, and the formal organizational plan is typically treated as a background against which the daily constitution of work boundaries takes place. Yet, as proponents of the negotiated-order perspective have pointed out, the formal organizational structure is itself a negotiated order, even if it becomes more-or-less stable at particular points in time and/or for specific analytic purposes. In this article, I explore the ways in which nurse managers charged, inter alia, with the formalization of nursing jurisdiction, attempted to do occupational demarcation. The strategies they employed are treated herein as examples of "boundary-work" (Gieryn 1983, 1999). My aim is to examine the detail of these micro-political processes and to consider their contribution to the interactional accomplishment of the division of labor between nursing, medical, and support staff. I shall be using ethnographic data from a wider study (Allen 1996) into the ways in which hospital-based nurses routinely produced their work boundaries.

Source: *Journal of Contemporary Ethnography,* 29(3) (2000): 326–356.

The Division of Labor – Agency and Structure

Most interactionist studies of hospital workplace settings undertaken over the past thirty years owe an enormous intellectual debt to Strauss and colleagues' work on negotiated orders (Strauss 1978; Strauss, Fagerhaugh, and Suczet 1985; Strauss et al. 1963, 1964). Introduced into the literature as a way of conceptualizing the ordered flux found in their study of two North American psychiatric hospitals, the negotiated-order perspective attempted to address the question of how social order was maintained in the face of change. Critical of the emphasis given to formal structures and regulations which characterized the then dominant paradigm in organizational studies, Strauss et al. (1963) proposed an alternative approach in which the social order was (re)conceptualized as in-process, reconstituted continually.

In underlining the dynamic nature of social organizations, negotiated-order theorists were attempting to create an analytic space for human agency as a counterbalance to the excessive determinism of the orthodox view. Contrary to the claims of its critics (Benson 1977a, 1977b, 1978; Day and Day 1977,1978; Dingwall and Strong 1997), however, the approach did not assume that social life was *indefinitely* negotiable. Strauss (1978) developed the concepts of "negotiation context" and "structural context" to sensitize researchers to those factors which shape social action. The former refers to immediate features of a social setting which enter into negotiations and directly influence their form and course; the latter relates to the circumstances which transcend the immediate negotiation context. Many of the studies undertaken within this tradition have focused on the interaction of personal processes and social structures.

> Negotiated orders refer to those arenas through which structural constraint, in the form of rules, policies, laws, normative proscription, and ideology are defined, interpreted, and incorporated into the daily activities of organizational members. (Maines and Charlton 1985, 303)

Nevertheless, negotiated-order theorists insist that while "structures" exhibit stability at a particular point in time and/or for certain analytic purposes, ultimately they too are negotiated orders (Glaser and Strauss 1964; Maines 1977). Maines (1977, 244) cites the example of the tax structure of the United States which, on the one hand, constitutes the framework in which negotiations about tax deductions take place but which, on the other, was itself the focus of negotiation between various competing interests at the point of legislative reform. The division of labor may also be considered in an analogous way. At one level, as Freidson has pointed out:

> it seems accurate to see the division of labor as a process of social interaction in the course of which the participants are continuously engaged in attempting to define, establish, maintain and renew the tasks they perform and the relationship with others which their tasks presuppose. (Freidson 1976, 311)

At another level, however, as Freidson (1976) himself stresses, these negotiative processes are not entirely free. Social interaction may be constrained, for example, by the relative power of the participants or the material features of the negotiation context. Moreover, however central social interaction is to the division of labor, it is also the case that abstract conceptions of roles and responsibilities *are* made – in formal organizational policy and, in the case of certain occupations, in state legislature – and while they may not determine work boundaries in a straightforward way, they certainly help to fashion their contours. Although more-or-less fixed for certain purposes, these "official" divisions of labor are themselves negotiated orders: occupational jurisdictions have to be claimed and sustained in public, legal, and workplace arenas and the particular context in which negotiations take place shapes the form that they assume (Abbott 1988).

The Social Production of Hospital Work

Although its proponents emphasize that the negotiated-order perspective can be applied to all kinds of organizations, it has been most extensively employed in research on hospital settings. The interpenetration of the structural and the social on the health care division of labor has been a central concern of much of this work.

A dominant theme in this literature is how formal divisions of labor are mediated in daily practice by features of the work setting. For example, a number of studies have shown how nurses are able to exert influence over doctors in relation to clinical decision making (Hughes 1988; Svensson 1996; Porter 1991). Work boundaries may also be fashioned by the hospital's temporal organization (Zerubavel 1979). As the only occupational group in the hospital providing 24-hour care, nurses frequently find themselves crossing occupational boundaries (Evers 1982; Millman 1976; Roth and Douglas 1983; Taylor 1970; Zerubavel 1979). Work pressures are another mediator of formal jurisdictions in the hospital context (Sudnow 1967; Hughes 1980; Roth and Douglas 1983). Sudnow (1967) and Hughes (1980) describe how the development of informal practices between casualty and ambulance staff led to ambulance crews being accorded the power to declare a patient "dead" although, legally, this should have been performed by a doctor.

Others have run the lines of emphasis in the opposite direction, highlighting the constraining effects of the hospital structure on the daily practice of health workers and the conflicts to which this gives rise (Anspach 1987, 1993; Chambliss 1997; Rosenthal et al. 1980). Anspach (1987, 1993) describes how the division of labor between nursing and medical staff in the neonatal intensive care setting leads to different perceptions of infant prognosis. Chambliss (1997) draws attention to the moral and ethical dilemmas which are created for nursing staff as a result of their position of subordination in relation to both doctors and hospital administrators. He argues that what appear as ethical arguments are, in actuality, thinly disguised turf battles.

Another theme in the ethnographic literature on hospital settings relates to the micro-political processes via which occupational boundaries are negotiated at the point of service delivery (Guillemin and Holmstrom 1986; Mesler 1989, 1991; Porter 1991; Svensson 1996). Mesler (1989, 1991) has explored the strategies clinical pharmacists employed in attempting to expand their role. He argues that by deploying "tact and diplomacy," "role-taking," and "tactical socialization" (1989), they were able to enlarge their jurisdiction in ways which were acceptable to nursing and medicine. Others have pointed to the importance of the workplace as the site of occupational "identity work" (Brown 1989; Emerson and Pollner 1976). Emerson and Pollner (1976) argue that by designating certain tasks as "shit work," mental health workers were able to distance themselves from those activities which threatened their occupational identity, thereby marking the legitimate boundaries of their practice.

There is, then, a rich body of literature which has examined the interrelationship of structure and agency in the social constitution of the hospital division of labor. Although we now have a much better understanding of the factors which shape work boundaries at the point of service delivery, relatively little is known about the ways in which the formal division of labor is produced by those charged with the formulation of organizational polices and plans. Indeed, despite the claim of negotiated-order theorists that all social orders are in some sense negotiated orders, in most of the hospital workplace studies arising from this tradition, the formal plan of work is consistently treated as a stable "background" feature against which shop floor negotiations take place. Thus, while the negotiated-order perspective clearly provided an important corrective to the overemphasis on formal organizational structures which characterized traditional approaches to the field, the balance of sociological attention may now have shifted too far the other way, thereby inverting the original error (Dingwall and Strong 1997). The corollary is that we have only a partial understanding of the ways in which division(s) of labor are socially constituted, and our conceptualization of the relationship between the formal and social organization of hospital work remains tentative.

The Changing Boundary between Nurses, Doctors and Support Workers: Policy Context

One possible reason for the absence of studies of formal organizational plans as negotiated orders is lack of opportunity. As negotiated-order theorists point out, organizations are not in a permanent state of flux; they can become more or less stable at particular points in time. It is during conditions of change, uncertainty and ambiguity, disagreement, ideological diversity, and newness and inexperience that negotiations are most likely to arise. In the UK in the early 1990s a number of developments in medical and nursing education (General Medical Council 1993; Department of Health and Social Security 1987; United Kingdom Central Council for Nursing, Midwifery and Health Visiting 1987) and health policy (Department of Health 1989) converged to provide the impetus for jurisdictional shifts at two of nursing's key occupational boundaries: at the interface with medicine on one hand, and with support staff, on the other. Rekindling deep-seated historical tensions between professional and service versions of nursing, these policy changes provided a natural laboratory for the study of the micro-political processes via which occupational jurisdictions are socially constituted.

First there was Project 2000. This was the United Kingdom Central Council For Nursing, Midwifery and Health's (UKCC) plan for the reform of nursing education, structure, and practice.[1] At one level, an explicit professionalizing strategy, at another, an attempt to overcome the fragmentation and technical orientation of health provision, its proponents argued that it had the potential to overcome some of the occupation's most persistent problems: low status, poor retention, and the lack of a clearly defined area of expertise with a scientific basis for practice (Beardshaw and Robinson 1990). The Project 2000 reforms were wide-ranging. Nurse education was relocated from hospital-based schools of nursing to institutes of higher education, and emphasis was given to education rather than training. A single portal of entry was established by abolishing the SEN (State Enrolled) grade of nurse.[2] There was a shift in the curriculum from an emphasis on disease to health and the introduction of a "New Nursing" (Beardshaw and Robinson 1990) ideology which advocated a holistic, rather than a task-oriented, approach to care.[3] Crucially, for the purposes of this article, learners' contribution to service provision was reduced from 60 percent to 20 percent. Nurses in training had always been an important source of labor on hospital wards; there was now a need to find ways of replacing their contribution.

Project 2000 was an explicitly elitist program of reform and its acceptance by the government was initially puzzling to some observers. Similar proposals had previously been constrained by economic realities (Dingwall, Kafferty, and Webster 1988), and the general thrust of government policy at the time was directed at curbing professional power in the public sector. As Rafferty (1992, 1996) has pointed out, however, historically the success of nurse-driven policy changes can be traced to their synchronization with wider organizational and policy concerns and, in the case of Project 2000, there appeared to be several possible reasons for the government's willingness to embrace its recommendations. First, there was the specter of the "demographic timebomb." During the late 1980s policy making was dominated by the prospect of having to recruit up to half of all the suitably qualified women school leavers in order to maintain staffing and wastage levels in the National Health Service (NHS). In this context, the creation of a small, highly skilled nursing core, supported by a pool of cheaper workers, made for a more flexible workforce which could be deployed to meet changing demographic and social trends (Carpenter 1993; Naish 1993).

Second, Project 2000 afforded the opportunity to make efficiency savings. Managerialism in the NHS was rapidly gaining ground following the *Griffiths Report* (Department of Health and Social Security 1983) and was to be further consolidated by the 1990 NHS and Community Care Act. The emphasis on cost containment was strong and, in the context of market competition, issues of human resource management were brought center stage (Paton 1993). As the largest occupational group in a labor-intensive industry, nursing has always been a prime target for health service planners concerned with reducing expenditure, and government acceptance of Project 2000 was accompanied by an important rider: that nurses agree to a new training for health support workers which be determined by the National Council for Vocational Qualifications[4] Beardshaw and Robinson 1990). The health care assistant (HCA), as this new support worker came to be called, would undertake a wider range of work than the traditional auxiliary.

The "New Nursing" ideology, which infused the Project 2000 recommendations, reflected the aspirations of certain segments of the occupation to establish a domain of professional practice that was free from medical control. As a means to this end, efforts were being made to reintegrate intimate tending and caring activities into the professional nursing role, work that, in the past, had been devalued and delegated to support staff. The introduction of the HCA was clearly in tension with this professional vision and the conviction of the proponents of Project 2000 that all aspects of nursing should be carried out by qualified staff. As Celia Davies (1995) has observed, there was no explicit bargain struck at national level that the cost of educational reform was restructuring, and the question of who should do what in the caring division of labor was not explicitly addressed. Rather, the onus was shifted to the Regional Health Authorities to produce individual plans for replacement staff and for the numbers of admissions to the new Project 2000 programs. Responsibility for agreeing to the division of labor between qualified nurses and support workers was left to local determination.

A further key development at this time was the Junior Doctors' Hours Initiative which aimed to improve the working conditions and career opportunities of junior medical staff.[5] Local task forces were set up and given the power to remove educational approval from service providers if standards were not met. *The New Deal* (National Health Service Management Executive 1991) set firm limits on junior doctors' contracted hours (72 hours per week or less in most hospital posts) and working hours (56 hours per week). It called for an increase in the number of career grade posts and suggested new ways of organizing junior doctors' work. Of significance for the purposes of this article was the suggestion that key clinical tasks be shared by nurses and midwives.

Nationally, the nursing response to The New Deal was mixed. Many supported role expansion in principle but there was unease about the bracketing of role developments with the Junior Doctors' Hours Initiative. A number suggested that once again doctors were dumping their dirty work on an already overburdened group and that nurses risked becoming minidoctors, subject to medical direction. As we have seen, much of the impetus behind the Project 2000 reforms was the desire to differentiate the nursing contribution from that of medicine, and this entailed a rejection of the old hierarchy of prestige which elevated technical (medical) tasks over bedside (nursing) care. Others reasoned that The Junior Doctors' Hours Initiative offered an opportunity for nursing and argued that a high-profile political initiative commanded more resources and support than professionally driven change (Allen and Hughes 1993).

In was in this context that the UKCC published *The Scope of Professional Practice* (UKCC 1992). In the past, in order to undertake tasks not covered in basic training, nurses had needed extended role certificates which were signed by doctors to indicate they were proficient to practice. Eschewing the hierarchy implicit in the previous system, the new guidelines were based on a professional model in which the onus for defining the boundaries of nursing was shifted to individual practitioners. Nurses were cautioned that they should be competent to work in an extended role and that any boundary changes should not result in unnecessary fragmentation of patient care or lead to the inappropriate delegation of work.

The interactive effect of these developments was to create jurisdictional ambiguity at the medical-nursing and the nurse-support worker boundaries, raising many questions about the future shape of nursing work. My aim in undertaking the research was to capitalize on the natural experiment afforded by these policy developments and study the ways in which these changes in occupational frontiers were being managed by staff in the workplace. The study was framed by an interactionist perspective: occupational jurisdiction was conceptualized as a practical accomplishment.

The Study

The research was carried out between September 1994 and June 1995 at Woodlands, a large, district general hospital in the middle of England.[6] At the time it had an annual budget of £60 million, almost 900 beds and about 2,800 staff. It provided general, acute, obstetric, and elderly services to a population of 254,000. Together with two other local hospitals, it had acquired Trust status in 1993.[7]

I carried out field observations on a medical and a surgical ward (three months each) and elsewhere in the organization through attendance at meetings and in-service study days. As far as it was possible, field notes were recorded contemporaneously in a spiral-bound notebook and a behaviorist, low-inference style was adopted. That is, I recorded verbatim interactions rather than relying on my own interpretations of events. Certain activities were also tape-recorded: meetings, nursing handover, and study days. Data were also generated through fifty-seven tape-recorded, semifocused interviews with ward nurses ($n = 29$), doctors ($n = 8$), auxiliaries ($n = 5$), health care assistants ($n = 3$), and clinical managers ($n = 11$)[8] and spontaneous extended conversations. The latter were not tape-recorded but had a different flavor from the briefer discussions held with staff while they worked. I also employed documentary evidence.

Data were analyzed using a holistic approach. I compared material from different sources in order to make judgments as to how each piece should be interpreted. I then related individual segments of data to the emergent picture in order to evaluate their meaning and, on the basis of my analysis of these extracts, I reassessed the meaning of the whole. *Folio Views Infobase Production Kit version 3.1* was used to facilitate data handling.

Research Role

Although I am myself a nurse, I did not work as such during the field-work, but I did participate in hospital life when it felt appropriate to do so. I wore a white coat in the ward areas like other visitors to the clinical setting. I was overt about my nursing background, but I emphasized and de-emphasized this aspect of my personal biography according to the demands of the fieldwork. My badge was inscribed with the title "research student."

An issue frequently raised in the methodological literature (Burgess 1984) is of the relative advantages and disadvantages of researching settings with which one is familiar. Having a background in nursing had a number of advantages. First, I was well versed in nursing and medical speak and so, for the most part, did not have to grapple with understanding a strange language. Second, knowing that I had a background in nursing meant that the study participants perceived me as someone who knew what it was really like, a factor which I felt made respondents more inclined to give candid accounts of their actions. Third, in negotiating access to the wards, I was able to persuade gatekeepers that as a result of my nursing experience I had sufficient native wit to know when to keep a low profile so as not to disrupt the work.

The methodological literature suggests that familiarity with a setting may disadvantage researchers in that they may not be able to recognize cultural patterns other than those things that are conventionally there to be seen. The way in which I endeavored to deal with this was by making detailed field notes of my observations which, as I have indicated, had a behaviorist character. As Burgess (1984) has pointed out, however, the debate concerning the degree of familiarity or strangeness the sociologist may encounter in a cultural setting has been polarized in some of the literature. The assumption seems to be made that situations are either totally familiar or totally strange. This is clearly not the case. As a nurse researching nursing, I, like Robinson (1992), was not studying a strange tribe. Yet, I had not practiced as a nurse for some six years and I had never worked at the study site, so there were many things that were strange to me. But, as a nurse studying contemporary nursing issues, I could only play the naive researcher to a limited extent. Many of the interviews I carried out and the conversations that I had resembled a dialogue between two people grappling with the problems facing practitioners in the 1990s. This was particularly the case with many of the senior nurses who, because of the positions they occupied within the organization, had a special interest in the subject of my research. A more extensive description of the research methodology and the field-work process can be found in Allen (1996).

Changing the Division of Labor at Woodlands Hospital

During the research period, the formal division of labor between nursing, medical, and support staff in the study site was being reconfigured in response to national policy initiatives. A number of nurse practitioner posts had been founded which involved nurses undertaking work that had previously been the remit of doctors. All these new positions had been developed in the context of the "Junior Doctors' Hours Initiative." They covered a range of clinical areas such as urology, rheumatology, IV cannulation, pain control, colposcopy, and general surgery. The New Deal had also acted as the impetus for the more general realignment of the medical-nursing boundary: ward-based nursing staff throughout the organization were being encouraged to develop the scope of their practice. The principal areas in which nurses were developing their skills were the administration of intravenous antibiotics, venepuncture, ECGs, male urethral catheterization, and intravenous cannulation.

The boundary between nursing and support staff was also being redrawn with the introduction of the HCA. Formally distinct from the auxiliary, the HCA role embraced certain technical procedures – such as measuring and recording temperature, pulse, and blood pressure; collecting blood from the blood bank; taking patients to theater; removal of IV cannulae; and the removal of urinary catheters – which had previously been the remit of qualified nurses.

It was senior nurses and medical staff employed in clinical management positions who were responsible for taking these changes forward. This was a relatively small number of individuals who coalesced in different ways around a number of issues. The medical managers comprised the Director of Medicine (who was a member of the Trust executive board) and following eleven clinical directors, that is, consultants who managed specialty budgets.[9] The nurse managers included the Director of Nursing (also a member of the Trust executive board), four nurse managers of clinical directorates, and five specialist nurse managers.

In the UK, nursing has a long history of management hierarchy and nurse managers are often identified as a distinct segment within the occupation. Traditionally, this group has been associated with a "service" version of nursing work in contradistinction to the professional view (Strong and Robinson 1990).

I was somewhat surprised, therefore, to discover that the nurse managers at Woodlands employed a professional discourse and espoused many of the ideals of the New Nursing. Although their vision of nursing was tempered by a fair degree of pragmatism, it was clear that professional issues were very influential in their work. As such, the nurse managers acted as important mediators of the tensions between professional and service versions of nursing work in the study site. The one exception to this overall generalization was the Quality Manager who, unlike his colleagues, appeared to have embraced much of the rhetoric of managerialism. However, he had minimal involvement in taking role change forward.

Boundary-Work

In the following sections, I will analyze the strategies nurse managers employed in negotiating role realignment as examples of boundary-work. Gieryn (1983, 1999) developed this concept to refer to an ideological style employed by scientists in their attempts to create a public image for the discipline. They attributed selected characteristics to the institution of science for the purposes of constructing a social boundary that distinguished it from nonscientific or technical activities. Of course, scientists have access to considerable material and professional opportunities which are not available to nonscientists and thus the interactional work which is done in the social production of occupational boundaries has to be understood as a micro-political process. Gieryn focuses on "public science," that is, the kinds of claims which are made for science in public and political arenas. But as Abbott (1988) has pointed out, and Gieryn (1999) himself acknowledges, boundary-work processes are also found in the workplace, where the accomplishment of occupational jurisdiction is a routine feature of everyday practice. In this article, I extend the boundary-work concept to embrace the practices as well as the rhetorical devices nurse managers used in accomplishing demarcation. Moreover, I suggest that it can also be applied to the occupational identity work in which medical and nurse managers engaged in their accounts of role realignment.

It was through these different boundary-work processes that the formal division of labor was negotiated at Woodlands. Like all negotiation processes, however, they were constrained in important ways by key features of the negotiation context. Although the nurse managers felt deeply uncomfortable with many of the developments they were being asked to take forward within the organization, they felt powerless to resist them.

> Junior doctors' hours are going to reduce anyway whether we like it or not. It's something that Parliament is quite keen to do and it's going to happen. [. . .] If your patient needs an aminophylline drip there and then, I think it's inevitable and it's a must that we do do it. (Interview with Nurse Manager)

As we will see, one of the ways in which they appeared to have accommodated themselves to these constraints was by taking control of the initiatives as they arose and using them for professional purposes.

Accomplishing Nursing's Boundary with Medicine

The nurse managers in the research setting were equivocal about the changes in the nursing-medical boundary which were occurring. Although they supported nursing role development, they felt that it should be shaped by the holistic needs of patients. There was concern that jurisdictional change had become irrevocably linked with the "Junior Doctors' Hours Initiative" and was therefore being driven by the needs of doctors. Nevertheless, junior doctors' hours had a high political profile and nurse managers reasoned that it was preferable for nurses to expand their scope of practice than to allow another category of worker into the division of labor which would further fragment patient care.[10]

For the most part, the medical managers were happy to devolve certain technical tasks to nursing staff – intravenous antibiotic administration, venepuncture, ECGs, cannulation, and male urinary catheterization – although a number also felt these were key medical skills which they did not wish doctors to lose. Where an activity came closer to the focal tasks of medicine – such as taking a medical history – they became more ambivalent. Some expressed the view that nursing staff had the skills to undertake this work in a limited sense, providing they worked within clearly defined protocols. Others argued that this entailed nurses making diagnoses which was a responsibility that most doctors (and also nurses) believed should remain with the doctor.

Taking Control

Despite their reservations about its linkage with the Junior Doctors' Hours Initiative, it was nurse managers who took charge of the implementation of role development in the study site. This, in itself, may be seen as an example of boundary-work – albeit of a defensive kind – for, as the following extract indicates, it seems that the nurses were galvanized into action by the fear that their medical colleagues would take over the process.

> There was almost like a splinter group of the medical staff and they were going to be writing the protocols for us which was one of the big pressures for the nursing staff to get their act together and to produce these packages and things because otherwise it would have been imposed on us from the medics. It's been a hell of a struggle getting all the paperwork sorted out but we didn't want someone else setting it up for us. We wanted to do everything ourselves. (Interview with Nurse Manager)

In the light of their powerlessness to challenge government policy, the nurse managers decided it was preferable for them to seize the initiative. They may have had reservations about the overall direction of these developments, but this way they could at least exert some influence over the shape they were to assume in the local setting.

In managing the process of boundary realignment, nurse managers had developed a number of self-directed learning packages which nursing staff had to complete and then sign to indicate that they were competent to practice. At the time of the research, this rather bureaucratic approach appeared at odds with the UKCC guidance on nurses' scope of practice which had abolished the need for extended-role certification. Yet, faced with the prospect of protocols being written by medical staff, the nurses' action can be understood as a further piece of boundary-work. Control of education and training is vital in retaining professional jurisdiction (Abbott 1988; Jamous and Peloille 1970) and historically this has been a major obstacle to nursing's professional project (Dingwall, Rafferty, and Webster 1988; Rafferty 1996). By insisting on taking charge of the education and training of nurses for role development in the study site, the nurse managers were asserting the professional autonomy of nursing and resisting coming under the control of the medical profession.

Establishing Expertise

In developing the learning packages to support role expansion, the nurse managers underlined the need for ward staff to have an adequate knowledge base. At one level, this reflected risk management and litigation concerns; at another, it can be seen as further example of demarcatory practice. The following extract is taken from a meeting of senior nurses charged with responsibility for implementing nursing role developments at Woodlands. Two of the senior nurses in the group have expressed concern that the process was in danger of becoming bureaucratized.

> Nurse Manager: I take these points that Simon and Felicity made about it – we're being in danger of it becoming a bit cumbersome – but I mean what I would want to say is that the fact that the doctors and phlebotomists aren't trained how to do it doesn't make it right, does it?
>
> Nurse Practitioner (Felicity): No.
>
> Nurse Manager: I mean surely we ought to be putting ourselves in a better position than that.
>
> Ward Manager (Simon): I agree with you. (Tape recording of meeting)

By ensuring practitioners had the theoretical knowledge to support changes in their role, nurse mangers at Woodlands were attempting to differentiate the nursing contribution from the "see one, do one, teach one" training of medical

staff, and from other workers – such as phlebotomists and operating department assistants – who were also being trained to undertake similar activities.
Moreover, as textual representations of nursing knowledge, the learning packages may also be understood as important boundary markers in the social production of nursing jurisdiction in the study site.

The nurses' efforts to establish expertise were ridiculed by senior medical
staff, however, who, in undertaking boundary-work of their own, claimed that the
detailed knowledge included in the training packages was largely superfluous
and unnecessary for the needs of nurses. The following extract is taken from an
internal communication to the Director of Medicine by a consultant surgeon.

> re. *Scope of Professional Practice – Flushing of Central Lines [. . .]* I find this
> document exceedingly complex and probably overcomprehensive for the
> needs of nursing staff who may be required to flush a central line. In fact,
> it is so complex that I myself am unable to answer some of the questions
> required of the nursing staff, and I suspect that the majority of the medical
> staff within the hospital would also be unable to satisfactorily complete
> the questions. I feel that if the protocol is to be adopted within the hospital
> and I myself am unable to comply with it, then I must regard myself as
> being unsuitable for the insertion, let alone the flushing of central lines.
> On this basis, 1 would suggest that I am no longer a suitable person for
> the insertion of these lines, including of course Hickman and other central
> lines. I would, therefore, suggest that we no longer use central lines within
> this hospital.

This theme was also echoed in the interviews with medical managers.

> [It's] crazy – for what is a practical procedure with some theory behind it,
> actually putting it into a context where the theory is totally outstripping
> the practical nature that it's intended for. And nurses are practical people
> at the end of the day. (Interview with Medical Manager)

> They've produced a manual! [. . .] all they needed was to spend an after-
> noon in theater. If someone needs two hourly turns, they order her a
> special bed because there's a tissue viability nurse. (Interview with Med-
> ical Manager)

As a number of analysts (Abbott 1988; Hughes 1984; Jamous and Peloille
1970) have pointed out, the nature of an activity is not fixed, and, in the context
of jurisdictional disputes, the definition and meaning of task areas can become
the subject of intense conflict. According to Jamous and Peloille (1970), central
to this is the indetermination/technicality ratio. This refers to the part played
in the production process by skills which can be mastered and communicated in
the form of rules in proportion to those skills which, in a given historical context, are attributed to the individual talents of producers. The indeterminate
portions of a task area provide a more enduring basis for the maintenance of
exclusive control of an occupational domain due to their inaccessibility to the

uninitiated. Jamous and Peloille (1970) suggest that one of the ways in which a profession can defend the frontiers of its jurisdiction, when task areas are being taken over by other competing groups, is by reducing the role of their competitors to that of "technicians" or operatives. The boundary-work of the medical managers can be seen as micro-political processes of precisely this kind, that is, as an attempt to recast nurses in the subordinate role of technician in the face of their claims to a more elevated status.

Identity Work

The contested nature of these activities at the medical-nursing boundary was also evident in the ways in which the task area was rhetorically constructed in field actors' accounts of boundary realignment. Although I did not interview all the clinical managers, my transcripts are characterized by distinctive discursive repertoires. Medical staff typically downgraded the tasks that were being devolved to nursing, emphasizing their repetitive, practical nature and their relative safety.

> It is not difficult to put in a cannula and the more that you do, the better at it you get. (Interview with Medical Manager)

> [A] lot of what the juniors were doing were these repetitive tasks which were no good for their educational training [. . .] nurses are good at doing repetitive tasks ((laughs)). So you know, to be able to get nurses to do the tasks that were indicated like IV drugs, catheters, [. . .] and taking blood, giving intravenous injections was fine – the so-called drudgery. (Interview with Medical Manager)

Nurse managers' accounts, on the other hand, were permeated with the rhetoric of holism. This was a useful linguistic device through which they were able to bring the professional-client relationship into play so as to construct a higher margin of indeterminacy around the task area and fabricate a distinctive approach to patient care.

> Sarah [Nurse Practitioner] said that [. . . .] [The doctors] just want to shove an IV in. They don't think about the patient as a whole. (Field notes)

> [W]e're not developing our skills just to take off the menial jobs from the doctors [. . .] we're doing it because we want to and because it's more holistic individualized patient care. (Interview with Senior Nurse)

> I have a lot of excitement about The Scope because I think [. . .] nurses are in an ideal position to give more holistic care, not tasks. You know you ring the doctor up and it doesn't matter who the doctor is, but he'll come along and do the IVs for you. He might never have seen that patient. But if a nurse has got a relationship and understanding with the patient and she spends a bit of time giving an IV, then there's a lot of communication and relationship building going on there. (Interview with Nurse Manager)

At one level, the field actors' accounts may be understood as evidence of the broader micropolitics at work in the study site over the meaning and value of activities situated at the medical-nursing interface. At another level, however, these data arise in the interview context and so can also be understood in terms of the locally situated identity work they are rhetorically assembled to perform. The concept of identity work is widely used in the literature to refer to the impression management activities (Goffman 1959), in which individuals engage to accomplish a particular type of personal identity. Snow and Anderson (1987) suggest that the social construction of identity can entail management of physical settings and props, attention to personal appearance (see, for example, Phelan and Hunt 1998), selective association with individuals and/or groups, as well as the narrative construction of particular identities (see, for example, Antaki and Widdicombe 1998; Cohan 1997; Rosenfeld 1999; Snow and Anderson 1987). Hunt and Benford (1994) argue that identity talk is a "discourse that reflects actors' perceptions of a social order and is based on interpretations of current situations, themselves and others" (p. 492).

By constituting the nature of these devolved activities in such different ways, I suggest that the medical and nursing managers were attempting to construct accounts of shifts in the division of labor which were consistent with their respective occupational identities and their perceptions of the position of nursing and medicine within it. Doctors rhetorically constituted the task area so as to subordinate the nursing contribution to that of a technician, whereas nurses explicitly resisted the charge that they were unwilling recipients of doctors' dirty work and emphasized their distinctive professional contribution to care and the indeterminacy involved in the production process. The interactional work being done here relates to the identification of the nursing and medical managers with their respective clinical occupations and their associated professional rhetoric, and, as such, this occupational identity work may be considered a variant of boundary-work.

Accomplishing Nursing's Boundary with Support Workers

As we have seen, the division of labor between nursing and support staff was also being redrawn in the study site, as the hospital started to employ HCAs. Nurse managers accepted the need for better trained support staff in order to compensate for the loss of student nurses' service contribution following the introduction of Project 2000. They felt that a highly trained support worker would provide for a flexible division of labor and help to avoid the fragmentation of care that Project 2000 was designed to overcome. Nevertheless, working within a fixed budget, nurse managers had elected to staff wards with smaller teams but with a higher ratio of nurses to support staff. Moreover, they were also adamant that the parameters of the HCA role should be under the control of nurses, both in formal policy and in daily clinical practice.

Taking Control

It was the nurse managers who, in consultation with the ward sisters, defined the official parameters of the HCA role. A list of activities HCAs were permitted to undertake had been devised, which, like the learning packages, functioned as a textual marker of the limits of support workers' occupational license. Yet the extent to which HCAs practiced within these formally defined boundaries was to be determined by staff at the point of service delivery according to the requirements of the ward and the exigencies of the work.

> Nurse Manager: [Y]ou are working in very different areas and your areas have very different needs of you and those needs will vary from time to' time and I can't go along and say to you, "You will be doing this, this, this, and this." All I can do is say to you, "As an organization [. . .] we have things that have been agreed for you to actually start to undertake." (Tape recording of training day)

This is a very powerful boundary-work strategy for defending nursing jurisdiction because it effectively denies HCAs a clearly defined area of practice. Officially, at least, the role of the HCAs is what the registered nurse decides that it is on a given occasion.

Another strategy nurse managers employed in defense of nursing jurisdiction was to exert control over the education and training of HCAs. When Project 2000 was implemented, it was agreed that HCA training was to be taken forward under the auspices of the National Council for Vocational Qualifications (NVQ). At the time of the research, however, there had been little national guidance on the introduction of HCAs and it became apparent that there was local variation in the ways in which the role was being implemented. There was no compulsion for the HCAs to gain NVQ qualifications in the study site – but they had to undertake a 25-day training program provided in-house. This gave the nurse managers control over HCAs' knowledge base and also created an opportunity for them to undertake boundary-work of other kinds. This was important because, despite their careful policing of boundaries, the senior nurses knew that pressures of work on the wards presented a powerful countervailing force. They recognized that ward nurses were concerned with responding to the vicissitudes of daily practice and had little interest in the wider professional implications of devolution to support staff.

Cautionary Tales

The nurse manager responsible for HCA training had a number of well-rehearsed "atrocity stories" (Bosk 1979; Dingwall 1977) which she employed on training days for support workers and qualified staff which highlighted the strain towards dilution on the wards.

Nurse Manager: I still get phone calls now saying – I had one not too many weeks ago – "What else can the health care assistant do" and I said, "Well what are they doing?" Thinking, "I don't really want to know." So she proceeded to tell me – this is a ward manager – proceeded to tell me this, that, and the other and she said "In fact they do everything." So I thought, "Ah Ha! So what is the registered nurse then doing?" (Tape recording of HCA training program)

My field observations revealed these stories to have some substance. Work pressures could result in HCAs undertaking work for which they were not trained or in-staff working with inadequate supervision.

Authoring the Landscape

The nurse managers also used the training days as opportunities to counteract the strain toward dilution and to shore up occupational frontiers. These were "orchestrated encounters" (Dingwall 1980) which enabled them to author the organization (Shotter 1993) by formulating the landscape of enabling constraints (Giddens 1979, cited by Shotter 1993, 149) and moral positions relevant to HCAs. One of the ways in which they did this was to emphasize the possible legal implications of HCAs crossing the legitimate limits of their jurisdiction.

Nurse Manager: Now it's very easy for me to stand here and say "You don't do this, you do that, you do the other," very easy. But what I'm saying is "This organization will not support you if you go ahead and do these sorts of things." (Tape recording of Training day)

In addition, in-service training days for qualified nursing staff underlined their professional accountability for HCA practice. At the time of the research, concern with litigation and risk management was strong at all levels of the organization. This provided senior staff with a powerful discourse on which to draw in their efforts to encourage frontline workers to police the parameters of their practice in the face of contrary pressures from the ward.

On the HCA training program considerable effort also went into differentiating the role of qualified nurses from that of support staff. An entire day of the course was devoted to the role of the registered nurse. Although the HCAs questioned its relevance, from the perspective of nurse managers it represented an opportunity to make the nursing contribution visible, representing an important piece of boundary-work. Here is a typical example of the kind of rhetorical devices employed by the nurse manager responsible for HCA training.

Senior Nurse: Right – you are there to *assist* the registered nurse. You're not there to do the registered nurse's job. You're there to *assist* [. . . .] You will not be involved in assessing patients [. . . .] You are there to *assist* in the implementation of care. Assessing patients can be anything from admitting a patient to doing a bed-bath and looking at them. As a registered nurse, I can assess the situation there and then. It doesn't matter if it's the beginning of the patient's stay, the middle, or the end. I am assessing all the time because that's what I have been trained to do. If you're in a position to assess, then you're in the wrong position. Just let us take the TPR [temperature, pulse, and respirations] situation [. . .] from a registered nurse's point of view there is more to doing a pulse than just counting. I've got to know the rate, the rhythm, the depth of that pulse. By me putting my hands on that patient, I am assessing that patient. I'm assessing all those different things there. If that's what is required, then the registered nurse should be going in there and doing that, but if all that is required is a number then I don't see a problem with you getting in there. Assessment is a very fine line and it makes it very difficult to explain to you what you can and can't do. (Tape recording of Training day)

The extract begins with an explicit attempt to differentiate the support worker contribution from that of qualified staff. Notice the way in which the nurse emphasizes that the role of HCAs is to assist the registered nurse and the explicit statement that they will not be doing "the registered nurse's job" which, in this instance, is formulated in terms of "assessment." There are also clear parallels with the boundary-work we observed in relation to the nursing-medical interface. For example, the senior nurse's appeal to the indeterminacy of nursing skills – "assessment is a very fine line and it makes it very difficult to explain to you what you can and can't do" – which she contrasts with the narrow technical role of support staff – "if all that is needed is a number." In the same way the medical staff attempted to diminish the nursing contribution to that of technician, the senior nurse imputes a subordinate role to HCAs: "If you're in a position to assess, then you're in the wrong position."

Discussion and Conclusions

In this article, I have examined the boundary-work nurse managers employed in accommodating jurisdictional change at the medical-nursing and nursing-support worker interfaces. I have argued that these processes may be understood as micropolitical strategies through which work identities and occupational margins are negotiated. I have described the practices through which nurse managers attempted to accomplish professional autonomy by taking charge of the realignment of the medical-nursing interface and the development of training packages for nurses. We also saw how the support worker role was defined in ways which prevented him or her from developing an area of autonomous practice. In addition, I have highlighted the rhetorical devices field actors employed in talking their work boundaries and the demarcatory and identity work purposes to which they were oriented. Nurses employed a discourse of holism which differentiated their approach to care from that of medicine, whereas doctors' accounts were linguistically assembled in order to cast nurses in the subordinate role of technician. Nurse managers employed an analogous type of rhetoric in relation to the nurse-support worker interface. HCAs were constituted as mere technicians lacking theoretical knowledge in contrast to the indeterminacy of nursing practice.

The empirical focus of this article is relatively unusual within the tradition of interactionist studies of hospital work because it centers on the social production of work boundaries in organizational arenas other than the "shop floor." As Dingwall and Strong (1997) have observed, if one focuses solely on the activities of grassroots personnel, there is a danger of missing the co-ordinating and disciplining devices which bind their actions together. I have concentrated on what is micro-sociologically interesting in the fine grain of nurse managers' boundary-work and for what they reveal of the interpretative horizons (Gubrium and Holstein 1995) and discursive domains within which they practice. As I have indicated, however, the study also examined the negotiation of work roles at the ward level and it seems appropriate in bringing this article to a close to briefly comment on the relationship between the social production of work boundaries in these two domains.

Like the nurse managers, ward nurses also expressed concern about the general thrust of national policy, yet they accomplished their work with little explicit face-to-face negotiation of jurisdiction or reference to formal organizational rules. Moreover, contrary to the situation in the management arena, there was little evidence of overt boundary disputes at ward level in respect of the changes which were taking place.

One way of understanding these findings is in terms of the extent to which formal role realignment had been preempted at ward level in the informal work practices developed by staff in response to the daily requirements of practice. For example, the social organization of ward work at Woodlands frequently created space for experienced nurses to exert influence over junior doctors in relation to treatment decisions and led to them informally undertaking certain medical tasks (Allen 1997).

> I do blood forms and things like that even though I know I shouldn't. Because it's an easier life and I know things are going to get done. (Interview with a Junior Sister)

Boundary blurring was also a routine feature of the nurse-support worker interface. The organization had a long history of staff shortages and this had resulted in experienced auxiliaries informally extending the scope of their practice to include many of the activities assigned to the new HCA role. Moreover, nursing care was organized according to routines which resulted in support workers frequently working without supervision.

> HCA: [Y]ou get a lot of pressure – because you're the ones that are actually with the patients, so they [nurses] come to you all the time and asking you if the patient's all right. (Tape recording of an HCA training)

Clearly, this routine breaching of jurisdictional boundaries was not without limits, but it is difficult to assess the extent to which staff oriented to the formal organizational plan as an external constraint on action. Ward personnel certainly shared many of the discursive resources employed by nurse managers. Nurses made reference to support staff having an inadequate knowledge to undertake certain activities, and HCAs, nurses, and doctors all employed a vocabulary of "risk" in talking about role change. Furthermore, on occasion, staff also employed explicit "vocabularies of structure" (Meyer and Rowan 1977, 349) in explaining their work practices. Nevertheless, they also had access to alternative discourses which were not shared by nurse managers and which were more frequently used in accounting for their actions. For example, they were more likely to refer to personal skills and experience and invoke the rhetoric of "a fair wage" in legitimating the edges of their practice than they were the formal organizational rules.

> I would decide individually not as a job, not as a "Well, she's a D grade staff or she's a health care assistant"; I would take it as who they are and what experience they've got behind them. (Interview with a Junior Sister)

> She told me that Sister had decided that because the auxiliaries and HCAs removed catheters and IVs, then they might as well amend the care plans. . . . She said . . . "I don't see why I should take on that sort of responsibility when I'm not paid for it." (Field notes)

One way of conceptualizing organizations is as a configuration of interrelated interpretative domains composed of the "local knowledge" (Garfinkel 1967; Geertz 1983; Gubrium 1989, all cited by Miller 1997) that setting members employ in making sense of their experiences (Miller 1997). These normative frameworks (Gubrium 1988) furnish discursive resources through which social reality is routinely interpreted and accomplished. In this study, although members of the same organization and profession, nurse managers and ward-level staff were clearly located within separate interpretative domains or social worlds (Strauss 1982). They had disparate interests, priorities, and concerns; access to different vocabularies of motive; and operated within different constraints. This led them to accomplish jurisdiction in distinctive ways: nurse managers were concerned with the social production of formal organization and related professional issues, whereas ward staff were preoccupied with the practical accomplishment of caring for the sick.

It may be difficult to explicate the precise nature of the relationship between the social constitution of jurisdiction in these different domains in the study in question, but what these data do indicate is that the interactional accomplishment of work boundaries is profoundly situated. Heimer (1998) has suggested that frontline workers are far more likely to comply with regulatory structures when they are closely articulated with indigenously developed organizational routines. The degree of fit between the formal and social organization of work is therefore crucial. Further sociological research is clearly needed in order to identify the different interpretative realms in which work roles are routinely produced and the way in which these different normative frameworks are articulated in the doing of demarcation. Only then can we hope to develop a better understanding of their interrelationships in hospital workplace settings and beyond.

Author's Note

The study on which this article draws was supported by a Department of Health Nursing and Therapists Research Training Award. The views expressed here are my own and do not represent those of the Department of Health. Thanks are due to Professor Robert Dingwall (School of Sociology and Social Policy) and Professor Veronica James (School of Nursing and Midwifery Studies) at the University of Nottingham, who supervised the original research. I am also grateful to Professor Robert Dingwall, Professor Julia Evetts, Rob Benford and three anonymous reviewers for their helpful comments on earlier drafts of the manuscript. I would also like to express my gratitude to the research participants who found time in their busy lives to talk to me; without their support none of this would have been possible. An earlier version of this paper was presented at the BSA Medical Sociological Group Annual conference, University of York, September 1998.

Notes

1. The United Kingdom Central Council for Nursing, Midwifery and Health Visiting (UKCC) is a statutory body responsible for the establishment of standards for training and professional conduct and the protection of the public from unsafe practice. It is charged with the responsibility for maintaining a single register of all practitioners and determining the conditions of entry. It is supported by four national boards of the four countries of the UK: England, Wales, Scotland, and Northern Ireland, who all have responsibility for implementing the policies and rules of the UKCC.
2. Prior to the Project 2000 reforms nurses could undertake a two-year-hospital-based training to become an enrolled nurse or three years to become a registered nurse, although there was a growing number of college-based degree programs. The SEN/RGN distinction in the UK has parallels with the LPN/RN distinction in the U.S.
3. In the past, the need to deliver nursing care with a variable skill mix – qualified staff and learners at different stages of training – had resulted in the development of a system of hierarchical task allocation. This skills hierarchy was implicitly based on a medical model. Junior nurses were allocated all hands-on care activities and senior staff undertook medically derived technical tasks and ward management. New Nursing aimed to replace this with a patient-centered model of care in which all patient-care needs are provided by one nurse, and the value of intimate tending was underlined.
4. This is a generic, non-nursing, accrediting body responsible for a wide range of work-based vocational and technical education.
5. In the UK, junior doctors are those doctors in training – preregistration house officers, senior house officers, registrar and senior registrar. This is roughly equivalent to interns in the U.S.
6. A District General Hospital is a nonteaching hospital which provides a range of services to a local population.

7. Trust hospitals were established in the UK as a result of the 1990 National Health Service and Community Care Act. Hospitals and community units which were able to satisfy specified management criteria were allowed to apply for self-governing status. They remained publicly owned but were, in theory, no longer subject to direct bureaucratic control by the National Health Service (NHS). Services were provided under contract to the NHS purchasers in an arms-length relationship (Le Grand 1990).
8. These figures do not add up because one person was interviewed more than once and two auxiliaries were interviewed together.
9. The involvement of doctors in general management is a relatively new feature of health care systems in the UK. Medical dominance (Freidson 1970) has long presented problems for health service governance on both sides of the Atlantic and the introduction of general management into the NHS in the 1980s was in large measure an attempt to control doctors (Strong and Robinson 1990). When attempts to bring doctors under the sphere of influence of general managers brought only limited success, the reverse tactic of involving doctors in management was introduced (Packwood et al. 1991). The extent to which these developments have been successful in incorporating doctors into the new management ethos remains empirically moot.
10. Similar arguments were made in the United States in the 1970s. Nurses' initial resistance to the development of the nurse practitioner role was overcome in the face of the threat posed to them by the development of the non-nursing physician's assistant role.
11. I am grateful to Lesley Griffiths for drawing my attention to Shotter's work.

References

Abbott, A. 1988. *The system of professions: An essay on the division of expert labor*. Chicago: University of Chicago Press.

Allen, D. 1996. The shape of general hospital nursing: The division of labour at work. Unpublished PhD diss., University of Nottingham.

———. 1997. The doctor-nurse boundary: A negotiated order? *Sociology of Health and Illness* 19 (4):498–520.

Allen, D. and D. Hughes. 1993. Going for growth. *The Health Service Journal* 103 (5372): 33–4.

Anspach, R. R. 1987. Prognostic conflict in life-and-death decisions: The organization as an ecology of knowledge. *Journal of Health and Social Behavior* 28:215–31.

———. 1993. *Deciding who lives: Fateful choices in the intensive-care nursery*. Los Angeles: University of California Press.

Antaki, C., and S. Widdicombe., eds. 1998. *Identities in talk*. London: Sage Ltd.

Beardshaw, V., and R. Robinson. 1990. *New for old? Prospects for nursing in the 1990s*. London: Kings Fund Institute.

Benson, J. K. 1977a. Organizations: A dialectic view. *Administrative Science Quarterly* 18:5–18.

———. 1977b. Innovation and crisis in organizational analysis. *The Sociological Quarterly* 18:5–18.

———. 1978. Reply to Maines. *The Sociological Quarterly* 19:497–501.

Bosk, C. L. 1979. *Forgive and remember: Managing medical mistakes*. Chicago: University of Chicago Press.

Brown, P. 1989. Psychiatric dirty work revisited: Conflicts in servicing nonpsychiatric agencies. *Journal of Contemporary Ethnography* 18 (2):182–201.

Burgess, R. G. 1984. *Into the field: An introduction to field research*. London and New York: Routledge.

Carpenter, M. 1993. The subordination of nurses in health care: Towards a social divisions approach. In *Gender work and medicine: Women and the medical division of labour*, edited by E. Riska and K. Wegar. London: Sage Ltd.

Chambliss, D. 1997. *Beyond caring: Hospitals, nurses and the social organization of ethics*. Chicago: University of Chicago Press.

Cohan, M. 1997. Political identities and political landscapes: Men's narrative work in relation to women's issues. *The Sociological Quarterly* 38 (2):303–19.

Davies, C. 1995. *Gender and the professional predicament in nursing*. Milton Keynes, England: Open University Press.

Day, R. A., and J. V. Day. 1977. A review of the current state of negotiated order theory: An appreciation and critique. *The Sociological Quarterly* 18:126–42.

Day, R. A., and J. V. Day. 1978. Reply to Maines. *The Sociological Quarterly* 19:499–501.

Department of Health, 1989. *Working for patients: The health service caring for the 1990s*. London: HMSO.

Department of Health and Social Security. 1983. *Inquiry into NHS management* (The Griffiths Report). London: HMSO.

———.1987. *Hospital medical staff (Achieving a balance) – Plan for action*. Health Circular 87, 25. London: HMSO.

Dingwall, R. 1977. Atrocity stories and professional relationships. *Sociology of Work and Occupations* 4:317–96.

———.1980. Orchestrated encounters: A comparative analysis of speech-exchange systems. *Sociology of Health and Illness* 2:151–73.

Dingwall, R., A. M. Rafferty, and C. Webster. 1988. *An introduction to the social history of nursing*. London: Routledge.

Dingwall, R., and P. M. Strong. 1997. The interactional study of organizations: A critique and reformulation. In *Context and method in qualitative research*, edited by G. Miller and R. Dingwall. London: Sage Ltd.

Emerson, R., and M. Pollner. 1976. Dirty work designations: Their features and consequences in a psychiatric setting. *Social Problems* 23:243–54.

Evers, H. 1982. Professional practice and patient care: Multidisciplinary teamwork in geriatric wards. *Ageing and Society* 2:57–76.

Freidson, E. 1970. *Medical dominance*. Chicago: Aldine.

———.1976. The division of labor as social interaction. *Social Problems* 23:304–13.

Garfinkel, H. 1967. *Studies in ethnomethodology*. Engelwood Cliffs, NJ: Prentice Hall.

Geertz, C. 1983. *Local knowledge*. New York: Basic Books.

General Medical Council. 1993. *Tomorrow's doctors*. London: GMC.

Giddens, A. 1979. *Central problems in social theory: Action, structure and contradiction in social analysis*. London: Macmillan.

Gieryn, T. 1983. "Boundary-work" and the demarcation of science from non-science: Strains and interests in professional ideologies of scientists. *American Sociological Review* 48:781–95.

———.1999. *Cultural boundaries of science: Credibility on the line*. Chicago: University of Chicago Press.

Glaser, B., and A. S. Strauss. 1964. Awareness contexts and social interaction. *American Sociological Review* 29:669–79.

Goffman, E. 1959. *The presentation of self in everyday life*. Harmondsworth, Middlesex: Penguin.

Gubrium, J. 1988. *Analyzing field realities*. Beverly Hills, CA: Sage.

Gubrium, J. 1989. Local cultures and service policy. In *The politics of field research*, edited by J. F. Gubrium and D. Silverman. London: Sage Ltd.

Gubrium, J., and J. A. Holstein 1995. Biographical work and new ethnography. In *Interpreting experience: The narrative study of lives*, edited by R. E. Josselson and A. Llieblich. Thousand Oaks, CA: Sage.

Guillemin, J. H., and L. L. Holmstrom. 1986. *Mixed blessings: Intensive care for newborns.* New York: Oxford University Press.

Heimer, C. A. 1998. The routinization of responsiveness: Regulatory compliance and the construction of organizational routines. *American Bar Foundation Working Paper*: 9801.

Hughes, D. 1980. The ambulance journey as an information generating process. *Sociology of Health and Illness* 2 (2):115–32.

———.1988. When nurse knows best: Some aspects of nurse/doctor interaction in a casualty department. *Sociology of Health and Illness* 10 (1):1–22.

Hughes, E. C. 1984. *The sociological eye.* New Brunswick, NJ: Transaction Books.

Hunt, S. A., and R. D. Benford. 1994. Identity talk in the peace and justice movement. *Journal of Contemporary Ethnography* 22 (4):488–517.

Jamous, H., and B. Peloille. 1970. Changes in the French university-hospital system. In *Professions and professionalization*, edited by J. A. Jackson. Cambridge: Cambridge University Press.

Le Grand, J. 1990. *Quasi-markets and social policy.* Bristol: School for Advanced Urban Studies.

Maines, D. R. 1977. Social organization and social structure in symbolic interactionist thought. *Annual Review of Sociology* 3:235–59.

Maines, D. R., and J. C. Charlton. 1985. The negotiated order approach to the analysis of social organization. In *Foundations of interpretative sociology: Original essays in symbolic interaction*. Studies in symbolic interaction, supplement 1, edited by H. A. Faberman and R. S. Perinbanayagam. London: JAI.

Mesler, M. A. 1989. Negotiated order and the clinical pharmacist: The ongoing process of structure. *Symbolic Interaction* 12 (1):139–57.

———. 1991. Boundary encroachment and task delegation: Clinical pharmacists on the medical team. *Sociology of Health and Illness* 13 (3):310–31.

Meyer, J. W., and B. Rowan. 1977. Institutionalized organizations: Formal structure as myth and ceremony. *American Journal of Sociology* 83:340–63.

Miller, G. 1997. Towards ethnographies of institutional discourse: Proposals and suggestions. In *Context and method in qualitative research*, edited by G. Miller and R. Dingwall. London: Sage Ltd.

Miller, G., and J. A. Holstein. 1993. Disputing in organizations: Dispute domains and interactional process. *Mid-American Review of Sociology* XVII 2:1–18.

Millman, M. 1976. *The unkindest cut: Life in the backrooms of medicine.* New York: William Morrow.

Naish, J. 1993. Power, politics and peril. In *Project 2000: Reflection and celebration*, edited by B. Dolan. London: Scutari Press.

National Health Service Management Executive. 1991. *Junior doctors: The new deal.* London: NHSME.

Packwood, T., J. Keen, and M. Buxton. 1991. *Hospitals in transition: The resource management experiment*. Milton Keynes, England: Open University Press.

Paton, C. 1993. Devolution and centralism in the National Health Service. *Social Policy and Administration* 27 (2):83–108.

Phelan, M. P., and S. A. Hunt. 1998. Prison gang members' tattoos as identity work: The visual communication of moral careers. *Symbolic Interaction* 21 (3):277–98.

Porter, S. 1991. A participant observation study of power relations between nurses and doctors in a general hospital. *Journal of Advanced Nursing* 16:728–35.

Rafferty, A. M. 1992. Nursing policy and the nationalization of nursing: The representation of "crisis" and the "crisis" of representation. In *Policy issues in nursing*, edited by J. Robinson, A. Gray, and R. Elkan. Milton Keynes, England: Open University Press.

———.1996. *The politics of nursing knowledge.* London: Routledge.

Robinson, J. 1992. Introduction: beginning the study of nursing policy. In *Policy issues in nursing*, edited by J. Robinson, A. Gray, and R. Elkan, Milton Keynes, England: Open University Press.

Rosenfeld, D. 1999. Identity work among lesbian and gay elderly. *Journal of Aging Studies* 13 (2):121–44.

Rosenthal, C., R. S. Marshall, A. S. Macpherson, and S. E. French. 1980. *Nurses, patients and families*. London: Groom Helm.

Roth, J., and D. J. Douglas. 1983. *No appointment necessary: The hospital emergency department in the medical services world*. New York: Irvington.

Shotter, J. 1993. *Conversational realities: Constructing life through language*. London: Sage Ltd.

Snow, D. A., and L. Anderson. 1987. Identity work among the homeless: The verbal construction and avowal of personal identities. *American Journal of Sociology* 92 (6): 1336–71.

Strauss, A. L. 1978. *Negotiations: Varieties, contexts, processes and social order*. London: Jossey-Bass.

———.1982. Social worlds and their segmentation processes. *Studies in Symbolic Interaction* 5:123–39.

Strauss, A. L., S. Fagerhaugh, and B. Suczet. 1985. *Social organization of medical work*. Chicago: University of Chicago Press.

Strauss, A. L., L. Schatzman, R. Bucher, D. Ehrlich, and M. Sabshin. 1964. *Psychiatric ideologies and institutions*. London: Free Press.

Strauss, A. L., L. Schatzman, D. Ehrlich, R. Bucher, and M. Sabshin. 1963. The hospital and its negotiated order. In *The hospital in modern society*, edited by E. Freidson. New York: Free Press.

Strong, P., and J. Robinson. 1990. *The NHS under new management*. Milton Keynes, England: Open University Press.

Sudnow, D. 1967. *Passing on*. Englewood Cliffs, NJ: Prentice-Hall.

Taylor, C. 1970. *In horizontal orbit: Hospitals and the cult of efficiency*. New York: Holt, Rhinehart and Winston.

United Kingdom Central Council for Nursing, Midwifery and Health Visiting. 1987. *Project 2000: The final proposals*. London: Author.

———.1992. *The scope of professional practice*. London: Author.

Zerubavel, E. 1979. *Patterns of time in hospital life*. Chicago: University of Chicago Press.

32

The Ethnographic Approach and Nursing Research

Antoinette T. Ragucci

I n utilizing the ethnographic approach for the investigation of cultural phenomena related to health, the method of participant-observation, used by anthropologists to study peoples of non-Western cultures, was adapted for the investigation of cultural continuity and change in the concepts of health, curing practices, and ritual expressions of women living in an ethnic enclave of a large American city.

The focal point of the research described here centered on the discovery of "conceptual models" of health and illness of peoples who represent variants of Western and Eastern European civilization. Attention was directed toward the identification of so-called "folk" health systems, usually associated with an agrarian mode of life, as viable and functional entities within an urban milieu. The scope of interest, then, was similar to that of anthropologists who engage in research in the more recently developed areas of the science of man – medical and urban anthropology.

The old and new approaches are not mutually exclusive. Both methods may be utilized in the same field experience. Frake (1961), for example, discovered that effective communication with the Subanun people depended upon the anthropologist's mastery of the terminology of folk medicine and botany before he could proceed to a systematic study of other cultural and structural elements.

The concept underlying ethnoscience is not a new idea. Malinowski expressed a similar view 50 years ago:

Source: *Nursing Research*, 21(6) (1972): 485–490.

The final goal of which the Ethnographer should never lose sight ... is briefly to grasp the native's point of view, his relation to life, to realize *his* vision of *his* world (Malinowski, 1954, p. 25).

The size and complexity of American communities have been cited as obstacles for attaining the ethnographic ideal of studying cultures as wholes. However, the study of one aspect, for example, health, within the context of the community will allow the investigator to gain an understanding of its spatial or ecological patterns and social and cultural processes. For example, in my study (Ragucci, 1971) of the health beliefs and practices of women in an Italian-American enclave, the structure of social relationships at the level of kin, ritual kin and neighborhood were analyzed according to the functional nature of the social links in events concerned with illness and death. In like manner, the dominant value orientations were studied according to their fit with cultural behavior during periods of crisis.

The Participant-Observation Method

A strategy was devised to insure the researcher's maximum exposure to a number of situations in which the beliefs and behaviors about health and healing were more likely to be expressed. The method of participant-observation is synonymous with the ethnographic approach. The observation process itself is part of what Nagel (1961) referred to as "controlled investigation" (p. 452).

Scientific observation is deliberate search, carried out with care and forethought, as contrasted with 'the casual and largely passive perceptions of everyday life. It is this deliberateness and control of the observation process which is distinctive of science, not merely the use of special instruments (Kaplan, 1964, p. 126).

The major instrument for the collection of data is the investigator himself. Thus, the successful employment of the method of participant-observation is predicated upon one's ability to establish rapport and relationships of mutual trust and respect with his informants. The way in which the investigator defines his role may facilitate or hinder his entry into the community. For example, in collecting data for my study of the cognitive orientations and basic premises about health held by women in an Italian-American enclave, the decision about the role in which I wished to be perceived was made prior to my initial reconnaissance in the community to rent an apartment. The role had to be congruent not only with the type of research questions that I intended to ask, but also with the residents' expectations of those who occupy the role. After much deliberation, I decided that the most plausible explanation for my presence in the community was that of a graduate student who was interested in studying health and the "old traditions" and customs associated with health and curing. This definition was congruent with the role I assumed for the 15-month period of residence in the enclave.

The type and location of living quarters, too, determined the quantity and quality of primary or face-to-face relationships. I rented modest living quarters in an apartment complex which had a larger number of units than the typical tenement. After moving into the community, I discovered my decision had been a fortunate one. Rental of a cold water flat, one of the choices, would have lowered my status with my neighbors. On the other hand, occupancy of a re-modeled luxury-type apartment rented to middle-class professionals considered "outsiders" by the older residents would have increased social distance.

The time table and circumstances relative to entry in the social world of the women varied according to generation. Four months elapsed before I was accepted as a neighbor and friend. Some factors which facilitated acceptance by the women in the oldest age class, the established base line group, were my identity as a second-generation Italian who could communicate in the native tongue and the ascription of the role of "literati" by those women who lacked literary and language skills in English. The strategy of using the quotations of Italian proverbs, the repositories of folk wisdom, was particularly effective in establishing rapport with women who were initially resistant to the researcher's attempts to elicit information about their traditional and contemporary customs and beliefs. This resistance might be viewed from the perspective of women who probably were sensitive to the criticism of their children for holding "superstitious" ideas.

Status differentials delayed entry into the social world of second-generation women. The problems associated with social distance decreased as I immersed myself in neighborhood and community activities. The establishment of a sym-metrical dyadic relationship with a neighbor was probably the most important single factor for my eventual acceptance within the established neighborhood social structure. In the community, the principle which defined the social rela-tionships of the first- and older second-generation women, for example, those above 50 years of age, was that derived from the model of the dyadic contract. According to Foster (1961), this model is consistent with the form of interper-sonal relationships which prevail in some European Mediterranean peasant societies. Reciprocity is the basic integrative principle of the implicit dyadic contract which serves to link a person to certaining hypotheses were formu-lated as guides for future inquiry. Significant events and interactions were recorded according to two categories, "act meaning" and "action meaning." As used here, "act meaning" refers to the people's explanation or definition of an event or behavior, that is, the semantic explanation. "Action meaning" refers to the meaning of the event or behavior from the perspective of the investigator, that is, the theoretical explanation of the event (see Kaplan, 1964, pp. 358–363).

The personal diary functioned as a "dialogue with self." It provided a means by which observations were insulated by focusing attention upon those factors which might have interferred with the achievement of the necessary detachment or objectivity. Most notations dealt with problems associated with value conflicts between those being observed and the observer, overidentification with the group, doubts about the ethical validity of collecting data by means of an essentially indirect and unobtrusive method, and conflicts relative to the exploitation of relationships as means to an end not always fully understood by my informants. One of the most problematic issues was the role conflict engendered by the constraints imposed upon a health professional when incorrect or irrelevant health beliefs or practices were noted. Deliberate and planned intervention occurred when the occasion demanded it, that is, when a belief or practice was known to be potentially or actually harmful.

These records of field research provide the raw materials from which data are selected for the ethnography. A qualitative inductive method of data collection presents a formidable challenge for the organization of the final account. The task of separating interpretations from descriptions is difficult, and the report of findings does not always yield elegant explanations.

Uses for Ethnography

However, the advantages in the use of this method outweigh its costs. The ethnographic approach is most effective for the study of groups whose members do not have the literary and language skills characteristic of the dominant white middle-class culture. The method of participant-observation permits entry into cultures which would otherwise be inaccessible by reason of their marginality or style of life. For example, the child psychiatrist, Robert Coles (1970), adapted the methods of the social anthropologist for the study of the early life of migrant workers. The method of participant-observation allows the investigator to look beyond reports of behavior and to observe the behavior itself so that he can assess the correspondence or the discrepancy that exists between the real and the ideal cultural statements. Finally, prolonged residence in a community and the continuing relationships provide more opportunity to check the reliability of informants.

The ethnographic study of urban communities will probably best be accomplished by means of the coordinated efforts of a research team. In the division of labor within the fields of medical and urban anthropology, the basic task of the nurse-anthropologist appears to be that of the ethnographer of the "health cultures" of the various subcultural groups which make up the population of large urban centers.

The investigation of the functional relationships and the interconnections of health, social structure, and culture need not be restricted to the community. Ethnographies of the natural settings in which behaviors and attitudes related to health and illness are more likely to be expressed – namely, the hospital, the clinical division, the health center, or the nursing home – need to be compiled. The ethnography of these samples of social and cultural systems should be written from the point of view of the people who are recipients of health services.

An alternate approach, the ethnoscientific, will enable the nurse-ethnographer to describe adequately the phenomena associated with health and illness according to the conceptual systems of the people she is studying. Having identified a culture's or a patient's model for perceiving, relating, or otherwise interpreting health phenomena, she can inductively construct a theory of how her informants or patients have organized the same phenomena (see Goodenough, 1964).

The ethnoscientific method is most effectively used within the context of the natural setting. In the study of the women residents of an ethnic enclave, I constructed theories of how people perceived health and illness by listening to their conversations and eliciting information within the context of situations specifically oriented to illness experiences.

An interesting area of ethnoscientific exploration is ethnophysiology, a domain which refers to the classification of human physiology by the folk or laymen. Because I hold an appointment as associate in nursing, I can explore this area while engaging in the administration of nursing care on the medical-surgical clinical divisions. The ultimate objective is to devise a method which can be replicated for the study of intracultural and intercultural similarities and differences in the classification of the same phenomena. The use of a three-generation design in this area may pose formidable problems in eliciting information from non-English-speaking people because the introduction of a translator will change the natural research setting. A more immediate problem concerns the framing of the research questions. Therefore, I am currently concentrating on the task of phrasing the eliciting questions without the imposition of my own preconceived categories of human physiology.

The ethnographic is an appropriate methodological approach to the study of the cognitive and affective orientations of diverse urban subcultural groups and the mode of their responses to the processes of acculturation considered within the perspective of health and medical systems. It has a place in nursing science. For, the final goal – of which the nurse-ethnographer should never lose sight – is to grasp the patient's point of view, his relation to life, to realize his vision of the phenomena of health and illness.

References

Ackerknechi, E. H. Problems of primitive medicine *Bull Hist Med* 11: 503–521, May 1942.
———. Natural disease and rational treatment in primitive medicine. *Bull Hist Med* 19:467–497, May 1946.
Arensberg, C. M. and Kimball, S. T. *Culture and Community. New York*, Harcourt, Brace and World, 1965.

Coles, Robert, *Uprooted Children.* New York, Harper and Row Publishers, 1970.

Forster, G. M. What is folk culture? *Am Anthropologist* 55:159–173, Apr.–June 1953.

———. The dyadic contract: a model for the social structure of a Mexican peasant village. *Am Anthropologist* 63: 1173–1192, Dec. 1961.

Frake, C. O. Diagnosis of disease among Subanun of Mindanao. *Am Anthropologist* 63:113–132, Feb. 1961.

Freidson, Eliot. *Patient's Views of Medical Practice.* New York, Russell Sage Foundation, 1961.

French, David. The relationship of anthropology to studies in perception and cognition. In *Psychology; a Study of a Science,* edited by Sigmund Koch. New York, McGraw Hill Book Co, 1963, Vol. 6, pp. 388–428.

Gans, Herbert *The Urban Villagers.* New York, Free Press, 1962.

Goodenough, W. H. Cultural anthropology and linguistics. In *Language in Culture and Society,* edited by Dell Hymes. New York, Harper and Row, 1964, pp. 36–39.

Hymes, Dell, ed. *Language in Culture and Society.* New York, Harper and Row, 1964.

Kaplan, Abraham. *The Conduct of Inquiry.* San Francisco, Chandler Publishing Co., 1964.

Lévi-Strauss, Claude. *The Savage Mind.* London, Wiedenfeld and Nicholson, 1966.

Malinowski, Bronislow. *Argonauts of the Southern Pacific.* New York, E. P. Dutton and Co., 1954. (Originally published in 1922)

Murdock, G. P. *Ethnographic Atlas.* Pittsburgh, University of Pittsburgh Press, 1967.

———, and others. *Outline of Cultural Materials.* New Haven, Human Relations Area File, 1967.

Nagel, Ernest. *The Structure of Science.* New York, Harcourt, Brace and World, 1961.

Pike, Kenneth. Toward a theory of the structure of human behavior. In *Language in Culture and Society,* edited by Dell Hymes. New York, Harper and Row, 1964 pp. 54–62.

Pitré, Giuseppe. *Biblioteca delle Tradizione Popolare Siciliane.* 25 Volumes, Palermo, Italy, L. Pedone-Lauriel di Carlo Clausen, 1871–1913.

———. *Medicina Popolare Siciliana.* Torino-Palermo, Italy, L. Pedone-Lauriel di Carlo Clausen, 1896.

Radcliffe-Brown, A. R. On the concept of function in social science. *Am Anthropologist* 37:394–402, July–Sept. 1935.

Ragucci, A. T. *Generational Continuity and Change in the Concepts of Health, Curing Practices and Ritual Expressions of the Women of an Italian-American Enclave.* Boston, Mass., Boston University, 1971. (Unpublished Ph.D. dissertation)

Redfield, Robert. The folk society *Am J Sociol* 52:293–308, Jan 1947.

Sturtevant, W. C. Studies in ethnoscience. In *Theory in Anthropology,* edited by Robert A. Manners and David Kaplan. Chicago, Aldine Publishing Co., 1968, pp. 475–500.

33

Ethnographic Evidence: The Value of Applied Ethnography in Healthcare

Jan Savage

Introduction

One of the main planks of recent NHS policy, the promotion of evidence-based healthcare, has prompted debate about the most credible forms of evidence and the most appropriate methodologies for its acquisition. Until recently, it was usually only studies that used an experimental methodology (such as randomised controlled trials) that were afforded scientific credibility. There is now growing recognition of the value of other, more qualitative kinds of evidence (Mays and Pope, 2000) and, as discussed more fully below, increasing interest in ethnographic evidence indicated, for example, by a move towards increased funding for ethnographic studies in the field of healthcare.

However, despite this, there remains considerable confusion about what ethnography is or is not, and limited understanding of how ethnography can be applied to healthcare issues (Brink and Edgecombe, 2003). This paper, which provides a context for the other papers on ethnography in this issue, will first briefly outline what is meant by ethnography and how it relates to qualitative research more broadly. It then provides examples of the application of ethnography in both commercial and public sectors, before moving on to look at the nature of evidence that ethnography can provide and its relevance to healthcare issues.

Source: *Journal of Research in Nursing*, 11(5) (2006): 383–393.

The Place of Ethnography within Qualitative Research

Qualitative research is difficult to define with any precision. Very broadly, it is concerned with the study of social life in naturally occurring settings. This naturalistic approach tends to be contrasted with positivist social research, which assumes that it is possible to use the principles and methods associated with natural science to measure social phenomena. Traditionally, such quantitative approaches have been more widely accepted than qualitative research in the healthcare context.

Qualitative research is informed by one of a range of methodologies or broad theoretical and philosophical frameworks. The choice of methodology then influences the kind of methods chosen for a particular qualitative study: in other words, the method and methodology are inseparable (Brewer, 2000). Some researchers argue that qualitative research involves the use of multiple methods in an attempt to secure an in-depth understanding – a form of triangulation that provides an alternative to validation (Denzin and Lincoln, 1994). While a multi-method approach is characteristic of ethnography, much qualitative research, particularly in the health services, relies on a single method such as the use of focus groups. What is characteristic of all qualitative research, though, is that researchers study phenomena in their everyday context, and attempt to make sense of these phenomena in terms of the meanings that research participants bring to them.

Ethnography sits like a chameleon within the tradition of qualitative research. It is a form of naturalistic enquiry that may, if appropriate to the research problem and chosen methodology, incorporate quantitative as well as qualitative methods. For some, the term 'ethnography' is synonymous with fieldwork (what Brewer (2000) calls 'the little tradition'), while others use it to refer to the whole spectrum of qualitative research ('the big tradition'). To confuse matters further, the term 'ethnography' is sometimes mistakenly used interchangeably with 'participant observation' (Savage, 2000).

What is Ethnography?

The absence of a single, fixed understanding of ethnography has probably contributed to its under-utilisation in healthcare research. At its simplest level, 'ethnography' can refer to a way of collecting data (a set of research methods); the principles that guide the production of data (a methodology); and/or a product (the written account of a particular ethnographic project).

Yet, at another level, ethnography can be understood as a composite of theoretical principles, method and written account: these different elements of ethnographic research are generally closely interwoven, as is made evident by the features that characterise ethnography. These features – not all of which are necessarily present, or given the same emphasis, in all ethnography – include recasting everyday understandings and practices that are taken for granted, or turning the familiar into the strange (Dixon-Woods, 2003). Ethnography is also typified by the priority placed on gaining an emic perspective: the ethnographer tries to gain the insider's view of a particular group or community (or what Ong (1993) has referred to as 'getting under the skin of participants'). More recently, ethnographers have also been concerned with gaining the perspectives of numerous and differently positioned individuals, giving attention to questions of power, inequality and how some voices are heard above others. Historically, ethnographic research has tended to focus on 'culture' and to explore what people say, what they do, and the relationship between these. In doing so, the ethnographer draws on a number of methods, traditionally involving immersion in the life of research 'subjects' over a prolonged period of time. Typically, the researcher acts as the primary tool for data collection, although there is some dispute as to whether he or she needs to employ some form of observation for the study to be deemed ethnographic (Bloor, 2001). What, for many ethnographers, is centrally important is that findings are presented in a way that conveys a sense of 'being there', or indicates the nature of the relationship/s between the researcher and the researched, and how this may affect the research process and findings. Fieldwork may focus on a single, bounded community or explore the connections and relationships between different sites (Marcus, 1998). Usually, data collection does not follow a detailed, pre-determined study design, but is responsive to what is found in the field, while analysis is primarily concerned with understanding meaning or providing detailed description: there is generally little emphasis on quantification.

Yet, while all ethnographic research will incorporate some of these features, it is arguably the way in which ethnography makes links between the micro and macro, between everyday action or interaction and wider cultural formations through its emphasis on context, that most clearly distinguishes ethnography from other approaches (and makes it particularly valuable for researching healthcare issues). The ethnographer's approach can therefore be described as

> a curious kind of cross-eyed vision, one eye roving ceaselessly around the general context, any part of which may suddenly reveal itself to be relevant, the other eye focusing tightly, even obsessively, on the research topic.
> (Hirsch and Gellner, 2001: 7)

Just as there is no single understanding of ethnography, the use of an ethnographic approach is not limited to one disciplinary field. Sociologists, for example, have a long tradition of ethnographic work. In the United States, the Chicago School was hugely influential during the 1920s and 1930s in developing the use of ethnography to study small communities (such as street gangs) at the margins of industrial society, and later in exploring complex organisations, work practices and collective behaviour such as labour strikes.

However, ethnography is widely regarded to have originally sprung from social anthropology, at a time when the discipline was concerned with creating a comparative archive of the cultures of pre-industrial societies or groups, particularly those made subject to European and American colonialist rule (Marcus, 2003). Within anthropology, ethnography was initially characterised by long-term participatory fieldwork in small-scale and often remote communities, followed by an intensive period of writing, during which fieldnotes were transformed into a monograph. This provided a supposedly authoritative and unbiased account of the beliefs and practices of the group under study, preferably before these were contaminated by Western influences. Significantly, in a post-colonial age, ethnographers have become more aware of their ambiguous political and ethical position, and of the need to give more attention to the relationships between knowledge, society and power. This awareness, together with changing views about the nature of knowledge, has led to both new areas of focus (such as healthcare) and new forms of ethnographic practice.

Different forms of Ethnographic Practice

A number of different types of ethnography have emerged in recent years, largely differentiated by the epistemology (theory of knowledge) and ontology (theory of being) that inevitably inform an ethnographer's approach. A useful but not exhaustive typology of these is provided by Skeggs (2001), who draws out the distinctions between naturalist, realist, modernist, social constructionist and postmodernist ethnography. Much of the ethnography carried out by anthropologists, Skeggs suggests, has been naturalist ethnography, which is underpinned by an ontological assumption that people can only be known through observing them in their 'natural' or everyday world. Realist ethnography is in many ways similar, but is perhaps more clearly premised on the belief that there is a single reality that can be discovered and described, and in which community, coherence and structure are key features. Rather differently, Hammersley (1992) proposes a more subtle form of realism, premised on an acceptance that research does not aim to reproduce reality, but merely to represent it. Moreover any representation will inevitably arise from a particular perspective in which some things are assumed to be pertinent and others extraneous.

Other forms of ethnography, while still shaped by assumptions regarding the nature of reality, also focus on issues of power, knowledge and identity. For example, Skeggs (2001) suggests that modernist ethnography is less concerned with community, and more with the construction of identity and what, or who, controls identify formation. While naturalistic ethnography has tended to report on those it studies, critical ethnography generally aims to speak on behalf of research participants, with a view to lending more authority to their voice (Thomas, 1993: 46) and, in some contexts, leading to the development of new ethnographic methods such as Participatory Rural Appraisal (Spencer, 2001). Along similar lines, feminist ethnography is concerned with questions about power and interests, although it may focus particularly on the way these shape women's experience. A more consistent focus of feminist ethnography, however, has been on the nature of the research process, how the ethnographer can best ensure that this is informed by a feminist ethics of care, and that knowledge is elicited in ways that can be used by research participants to change the exploitative conditions of their society (Skeggs, 1994).

These different approaches to ethnography can be understood to reflect a succession of phases, marked by changing assumptions about the relationship between researchers' aims and the knowledge they may produce, and changing mores governing the relationship between the researcher and the researched (Denzin, 1997). Yet, as Taylor (2002) has argued, these phases continue to exist, and often co-exist, in current research practice and might therefore be more accurately depicted as competing ideas that can shape social research.

The Application of Ethnography

Ethnography has a long been used to study the everyday, such as organisational life or industrial relations. Wright (1994), for example, identifies three periods – the 1920s, the 1950s and 1960s, and the present time – when anthropologists have made significant contributions to organisational studies. However, these sorts of ethnographic studies were still largely rooted in academic departments and, although they may have provided insights for the managers of various institutions or corporations, at heart they were generally concerned with the development of ideas about social organisation and culture, or with developing research methodology. Traditionally, those who plied their trade as ethnographers beyond the academy have been regarded by their colleagues as beyond the pale, and ethnography applied to the problems or requirements of industry and the public sector has often been viewed as 'impure' (Roberts, 2004).

Such a derogatory view of applied ethnography is, however, under review. To some extent, this change of heart within disciplines such as anthropology comes at a time of upheaval and uncertainty for university departments, indicated for example by declining student enrolment and course closures (Mars, 2004). At the same time, there is growing interest in the potential that ethnography offers amongst those outside the social sciences. Ethnography, it seems, has become something of a 'buzz word' and many businesses, institutions and organisations are now commissioning ethnographic research or employing anthropologists on their staff (Roberts, 2004). However, in the world of applied ethnography, academic debate on issues such as representation, multiple voices and so on tends to be set aside (Marcus, 2003). In other words, there is a new approval for ethnography, but generally in its more conventional or pragmatic forms.

The trend towards increased acceptance of ethnography is also driven in part by a growing resistance on the part of many key informants to continued co-operation with more traditional research procedures. Chapman (2001), for instance, suggests that there is particular disenchantment with the research questionnaires employed in business studies, partly because of the huge numbers of these that managers are asked to complete, as well as doubt about the quality of the data that these generate. There is a feeling on the part of participants that questionnaires ask the wrong questions, and as a result, response rates are low. In contrast, according to Chapman, an ethnographic approach can have the advantage of allowing managers a rare, and often highly valued, opportunity to talk about the complexity of what they do and to formulate and pursue problems in their own terms through discussions with someone who is genuinely interested. The value placed on this kind of opportunity can be evident, in Chapman's experience, in the way that interviews are not quickly terminated by participants, but often last longer than intended and sometimes only end because of exhaustion on the part of both parties.

Ethnography is useful in many contexts. For example, it is widely recognised as a form of pilot testing for a broader survey, or for clarifying hypotheses. It is particularly useful where information is new and unfamiliar, or when the information required is too subtle or complex to be elicited by questionnaires or similar techniques (Brewer, 2000). Ethnographic methods have been used to understand how people negotiate the sometimes competing demands of efficiency and quality (Smith, 2001). In addition, ethnographic research has been effective in uncovering the tacit skills, decision rules and subtleties in jobs labelled as routine, unskilled or deskilled, or even trivial (Smith, 2001). One area in which the value of ethnography is often overlooked is in helping programme developers (that is, those who introduce interventions with the aim of bringing about change) and programme evaluators (those who assess the effectiveness of an intervention programme) to improve the quality of their programmes. Nastasi and Berg (1999), for instance, claim that ethnography can contribute to all stages of a programme, as well as facilitating the involvement of stakeholders. They argue that ethnography is crucial in describing and monitoring the process of change, and can help to describe the evolution of an intervention and its effect both on individuals and their social context. Moreover, ethnography is characterised by an iterative process of continuous data collection, analysis and reflection that makes it possible to strengthen or otherwise adapt interventions in a continuous manner and ensure a close relationship between intervention and assessment.

However, the application of anthropology to non-academic fields such as the worlds of business, or indeed healthcare – if traditional in terms of its epistemology – has involved a certain amount of adaptation and responsiveness on the part of ethnographers. Chapman (2001), for example, did not carry out classic fieldwork, but relied instead on long, unstructured and much-repeated interviews that he claimed remained within the ethnographic tradition, partly because of maintaining a focus on context, and because there was sufficient involvement to develop sustained and relatively 'close' relationships with participants.

With applied ethnography, the time available for fieldwork tends to be briefer than usual in ethnographic research; the nature of the relationship between the researcher and study participants may be differently structured (for example, informed by commercial interests rather than the pursuit of knowledge for its own sake); and there is often more, possibly multidisciplinary, collaboration on projects (Ortleib, 2004). In response to new types of research opportunities and new audiences, ethnographers have expanded their traditional tool kit of methods. These include techniques for rapid appraisal, and the development of 'quick ethnography' that integrates conventional methods of data collection and analysis with more novel approaches, such as successive pile sorts or multivariate statistical procedures (Handwerker, 2001). A further way of adapting ethnography to the tight deadlines of applied research is through team ethnography, rather than the employment of the traditional, solitary ethnographer or 'Lone Ranger' (Erickson and Stull, 1998). For example, some team ethnographers use the methods and iterative process of ethnography, albeit in a retracted way, together with the triangulation of findings to carry out rapid assessments for policy-makers and programme planners (Beebe, 2001). In addition, ethnography may be 'focused' in that it deals with a relatively narrow field of inquiry: in contrast to traditional ethnography, fieldwork may be premised on clearly formulated research questions (Kleinman, 1992). Yet while there may be differences between traditional and applied ethnography, these differences have been described as differences of degree, rather than of kind, with key features of an ethnographic approach, such as the focus on context, still central (Hart, 2004).

The Application of Ethnography to Healthcare

Classic ethnographic studies of illness, health and healthcare include Goffman's (1961) exposition of patients' experiences of mental health institutions, Roth's (1963) study of how patients renegotiated treatment regimens in a TB sanatorium, and Strong's (1979) work identifying the tacit rules governing clinical interactions. A more recent example is provided by Lawton's (2000) study of patients' experiences of palliative care. Lawton carried out fieldwork in both a day care service and a hospice providing respite care, pain or symptom control, and 'terminal care' for patients with advanced disease (mostly cancer). One of the main findings concerned the way that patients' conception of self changed once they lost their physical ability to act for themselves and, more fundamentally, once the physical boundaries of their bodies were irreversibly eroded. The findings thus make a significant contribution to understandings of the modern, Western self as well as providing important insights into the experience of terminal illness.

Although the findings from 'mainstream' sociological or anthropological studies can be made use of by healthcare practitioners, the nature and purpose of these studies – rather like the early ethnographic studies of organisations – have been shaped to a large extent by a social science agenda, particularly the development of social theory, and reported in the sociological or anthropological literature.[1] However, the usefulness of ethnography, either as the sole research approach or as an adjunct to others, is increasingly recognised within the field of healthcare research, with ethnography more and more applied to essentially practical concerns that have been identified, for the most part, by policy-makers, managers or practitioners, and reported primarily in professional rather than academic journals.[2] For example, ethnography has been recognised to be useful in the study of safety and quality in healthcare, being well suited to identifying conditions of risk, particularly where these are rooted in organisational dynamics, human performance or interactions between staff and technology, and in complex areas where there are long chains of causation (Dixon-Woods, 2003). As Dixon-Woods (2003: 326) puts it, ethnography 'can capture the winks, sighs, head shaking, and gossip that may be exceptionally powerful in explaining why mistakes happen, but which more formal methods will miss' (Dixon-Woods, 2003: 326).

The Value of Ethnographic Evidence

Despite its potential, however, those who fund healthcare research, for the most part, have continued to shy away from ethnography. This is partly because, along with other qualitative approaches, it attempts to explain rather than measure, offers insight rather than generalisable findings, and generates rather than tests hypotheses (Jones, 1995). There remains scepticism about the usefulness of ethnography in the healthcare context, endorsed to some extent by controversy over whether or how qualitative research in general can be rigorously assessed, and a belief that ethnography, as a form of qualitative inquiry, inevitably provides a lower order of evidence than more quantitative types of research.

For example, whether or how qualitative research can be evaluated is highly contested, even amongst researchers in this field, with some arguing that qualitative research is premised on anti-realism (that is, that there is no reality that exists independent of our awareness of it), and therefore cannot be evaluated by any standardised set of criteria. Conversely, others suggest that, if qualitative research is to have any practical application, criteria need to be developed in order to allow evaluation, but because qualitative and quantitative research are located in essentially different research paradigms, the criteria they use will necessarily be different (Mays and Pope, 2000). Murphy et al. (1998), however, suggest that, whilst a rigid set of checklists is inappropriate, certain practices are helpful in ensuring the validity of qualitative findings[3] and help readers to assess the trustworthiness of qualitative evidence. These practices include providing a clear account of how data has been collected, analysed and interpreted, with sufficient display of the data to allow the reader to assess whether the researcher's interpretation is supported, and an indication that researchers have not discounted data that contradicts their interpretation. In addition, there should be signs of in-depth reflection on the ways in which the research data are influenced by the research process.

Despite arguments that there are ways of evaluating qualitative research, the findings produced by ethnography, along with the findings of qualitative inquiry more generally, tend to be assigned an inferior position in the hierarchy of evidence that increasingly shapes decision-making in the health services. In industrialised economies, evidence-based practice has become one of the central means of assuring that clinicians base their clinical decisions on the 'best' available evidence, to the point that it has become a key factor in the allocation of healthcare resources (Forbes and Griffiths, 2002). However, what is agreed as 'evidence' is contentious: as Larner (2004) has noted, who controls the definition of evidence is a political matter. Evidence-based practice, which has emerged from the tradition of clinical epidemiology, has been accused of focusing only on variables that can be easily measured, and of recognising only certain kinds of evidence, predominantly evidence generated by experimental studies such as randomised controlled trials (RCTs). While RCTs represent a powerful method of testing which treatments have the greatest effect, they have certain limitations. For example

> the constraints on the patients entered into trials are often very tight, which means that the result of the trial may not be applicable to the population from which they are drawn, or at least to the patients seen in the clinic or hospital ward.
>
> (Goodman, 2000: 38)

As Goodman (2000) points out, although evidence-based medicine is now widely regarded as the safest form of practice, there is a lack of evidence that it is reliable or testable. Nonetheless, the emphasis placed on the findings of experimental research means that alternative forms of evidence arising from qualitative inquiry – evidence, for example, that may still contribute to the reduction of morbidity and mortality, or demonstrate efficacy (Morse, 2005) – has been largely overlooked. Moreover, although 'evidence' is often interpreted as information concerning the best course of treatment, decision-making in the healthcare context is also informed by other forms of knowledge (for instance, knowledge about the nature of health beliefs, the impact of organisational and cultural issues, or patient experiences that impact on treatments or services) that is more likely to be derived from qualitative rather than quantitative research (Pope and Mays, 1995).

On a more positive note, there are signs of a new openness to the various forms of evidence beyond that provided by experimental research with, for example, growing acceptance of the contribution that qualitative inquiry can make to systematic reviews (Dixon-Woods and Fitzpatrick, 2001). Indeed, recent guidance concerning systematic reviews of research on effectiveness (NHS Centre for Reviews and Dissemination, 2001) includes a consideration of qualitative research and recognises the range of different types of evidence that can be included in research synthesis. In addition, the remit of evidence-based practice topics has recently been extended to include phenomena such as 'experience' and 'perceptions' (Forbes and Griffiths, 2002), topics amenable to ethnographic inquiry.

However, research synthesis is a contentious issue for many qualitative researchers as qualitative inquiry appears incommensurate with the traditional rules of evidence and with the hierarchy of research designs advocated by evidence-based practice. For example, the principles informing qualitative inquiry are concerned with induction rather than deduction, subjective perceptions rather than objective quantification, and description and interpretation rather than inferential testing (Giacomini, 2001). Moreover, the synthesis of qualitative studies assumes that it is possible to generalise beyond individual qualitative studies, an assumption that many in the qualitative research community do not accept (Campbell et al., 2003). Thus many take the stance that, rather than attempting to apply the conventional processes for synthesis to qualitative evidence, or trying to reconcile the different standards of evidence associated with quantitative and qualitative traditions, the kinds of findings generated by qualitative and quantitative approaches to synthesis are generally considered complementary rather than commensurate in nature, and cannot therefore be incorporated into the same reviews (Morse, 2005).

It is still early days in exploring whether, or how, it is possible to develop a system for synthesising qualitative research findings that remains true to the tenets underlying qualitative inquiry. As Morse (2005) has pointed out, there has been considerable effort to 'shoehorn' qualitative inquiry into the framework of evidence-based practice, despite the awkwardness of the fit. The danger remains of trying to stretch qualitative inquiry to meet the criteria developed for other types of research design that are considered more scientific or more objective, at the expense of the alternative kinds of evidence that qualitative inquiry can generate. The contribution of qualitative inquiry to healthcare lies in its potential to explore complex issues, such as those shaping the context of care, or the nature of care provided (Morse 2006). Within the paradigm of qualitative inquiry, ethnography, with its multi-method approach and attention to context, is particularly well suited to tackling such complexity.

In addition, the scope of ethnography means that it can make an important contribution to the debate about evidence itself, and, for instance, the extent to which protocols based on evidence arising from systematic reviews may impact on practice. For example, Smith et al, (2003) used an ethnographic approach to study the nature of anaesthetists' expert practice, and the role of different kinds of knowledge in accomplishing this. They found that varying and sometimes competing forms of knowledge were learned and employed in anaesthetic practice, namely knowledge of the patient as a person; knowledge derived from case notes; knowledge from direct observation and indirectly from electronic monitors; formal theoretical knowledge; and knowledge from experience. Findings suggested that instructional knowledge (that is, knowledge from sources such as textbooks or protocols) did not help practitioners to address the uncertainties they faced in practice, and did not lead to expertise. Deciding what was happening and how to respond to any particular situation was a matter of interpretation based partly on experience and what felt 'normal'. Indeed, in relation to a specific patient, experience could suggest that the most appropriate course of action ran counter to what protocols might propose, even though protocols are now the 'tool of choice' for clinical decision-making.

Conclusion

Curiously, the scope for ethnographic inquiry within healthcare research is currently shaped both by increasing receptiveness on the part of funders and others towards its potential *and* dismissal of its findings on the basis that it offers low-order evidence. While this contradictory stance is particularly noticeable towards ethnography, it is also experienced by qualitative researchers more generally. Those who resist this approach to evidence argue that qualitative research has inherently different aims, subjects and methods to quantitative research, that it can reach the areas that quantitative research cannot reach, and moreover, that continuing refusal to accept the kind of evidence that qualitative research provides will undermine improvements in healthcare. Ethnography is especially suited to advancing the cause of qualitative inquiry within healthcare research. Its particular strengths, such as its multi-method approach (including its capacity to incorporate a varying range of methods to address research aims) and its attention to context, while giving voice to individual experience, provide a counter for the totalising tendencies of evidence-based practice. Finally, ethnography offers a holistic way of exploring the concept of evidence itself, or the interaction of different kinds of evidence, within the various contexts in which evidence-based practice is promoted.

Notes

1. For an overview of ethnographic research in medical sociology, for example, see Charmaz and Olesen (1997).
2. Indications of this include tendering by the National Patient Safety Agency (www. npsa.nhs.uk) for an ethnographic study of the practice of recycling single-use medical devices, and the commissioning of an ethnographic study of violence in the accident and

emergency setting by the Service Delivery and Organisation Research and Development panel (www.sdo.lshtm.ac.uk).
3. Although 'validity' may have a slightly different meaning for quantitative researchers.

References

Barbour, R. (2001) Checklists for improving rigour in qualitative research: a case of the tail wagging the dog? *British Medical Journal* **322**: 1115–1117.

Beebe, J. (2001) *Rapid Assessment Process: an Introduction.* Walnut Creek, CA: Alta Mira Press.

Bloor, M. (2001) The ethnography of health and medicine. In: Atkinson, P. Coffey, A., Delamont, S., Lofland, J., Lofland, L, (eds) *Handbook of Ethnography.* London: Sage, pp. 177–187.

Brewer, J. (2000) *Ethnography.* Buckingham: Open University Press.

Brink, P., Edgecombe, N. (2003) What is becoming of ethnography? *Qualitative Health Research* **13**:7, 1028–1030.

Campbell, R., Pound, P., Pope, C., Britten, N., Pill, R., Morgan, M., Donovan, J. (2003) Evaluating meta-ethnography: a synthesis of qualitative research on lay experiences of diabetes and diabetes care. *Social Science and Medicine* **56**: 671–684.

Chapman, M. (2001) Social anthropology and business studies: some considerations of method. In: Gellner, D., Hirsch, E, (eds) *Inside Organisations: Anthropologists at work.* Oxford: Berg, pp. 19–33.

Charmaz, K., Olesen, V. (1997) Ethnographic research in medical sociology. *Sociological Methods and Research* **25**: 542–494.

Denzin, N. (1997) *Interpretive Ethnography: Ethnographic Practices for the 21st Century.* Thousand Oaks, CA: Sage Publications.

Denzin, N., Lincoln, Y. (1994) Introduction: entering the field of qualitative research. In: Denzin, N. and Licoln, T. (eds) *Handbook of Qualitative Research.* Thousand Oaks, CA: Sage Publications, pp. 1–17.

Dixon-Woods, M. (2003) What can ethnography do for quality and safety in healthcare? *Quality and Safety in Health Care* **12**: 326–327.

Dixon-Woods M., Fitzpatrick, R. (2001) Editorial: qualitative research in systematic reviews. *British Medical Journal* **323**: 765–766.

Egger, M., Davey Smith, G. (1997) Meta-analysis: potentials and promise. *British Medical Journal* **315**: 1371–1374.

Erickson, K., Stull, D. (1998) *Doing Team Ethnography.* Qualitative Research Methods Series 42. Thousand Oaks. CA: Sage Publications.

Forbes, A., Griffiths, P. (2002) Methodological strategies for the identification and synthesis of 'evidence' to support decision-making in relation to complex healthcare systems and practices. *Nursing Inquiry* **9**:3, 141–155.

Giacomini, M. (2001) The rocky road: qualitative research as evidence. *Evidence-based Medicine* **6**: 4–6.

Goffman, E. (1961) *Asylums: Essays on the Social Situation of Mental Patients and Other Inmates.* New York: Doubleday

Goodman, N. (2000) NICE and the new command structure: with what competence and with what authority will evidence be selected and interpreted for local clinical practice? In: Miles, A., Hampton, J., Hurwitz, B. (eds) *NICE, CHI and the NHS Reforms: Establishing Excellence or Imposing Control?* London: Aesculpius Medical Press: 33–50.

Hammersley, M. (1992) *What's Wrong with Ethnography?* London: Routledge.

Handwerker, P. (2001) *Quick Ethnography.* Walnut Creek, CA: Altamira Press.

Hart, E. (2004) Applications of anthropology in the National Health Service. *Anthroplogy in Action* **11**:1, 21–23.

Hirsch, E., Gellner, D. (2001) Introduction: ethnography of organisations and organisations of ethnography. In: Gellner, D., Hirsch, E. (eds) *Inside Organisations, Anthropologists at Work.* Oxford: Berg, pp. 1–15.

Kleinman, A. (1992) Local worlds of suffering: an interpersonal focus for ethnographies of illness. *Qualitative Health Research* **2**:2, 127–134.

Lawton, J. (2000) *The Dying Process: Patients' Experiences of Palliative Care.* London: Routledge.

Larner, G. (2004) Family therapy and the politics of evidence. *Journal of Family Therapy* **26**: 17–39.

Marcus, G. (1998) *Ethnography Through Thick and Thin.* Princeton, NJ: Princeton University Press.

Marcus, G. (2003) On the problematic contemporary reception of ethnography and the stimulus for innovations in its forms and norms in teaching and research. *Anthropological Journal on European Cultures: Shifting Grounds – Experiments in Doing Ethnography* **11**: 191–206.

Mars, G. (2004) Refocusing with applied anthropology, Guest editorial. *Anthropology Today* **20**:1, 1–2.

Mays, N., Pope, C. (2000) Qualitative research in healthcare: assessing quality in qualitative research. *British Medical Journal* **320**: 50–52.

Morse, J. (2005) Beyond the clinical trial: expanding criteria for evidence. *Qualitative Health Research* **15**:1, 3–4.

Murphy, E., Dingwall, R., Greatbatch, D., Parker, S., Watson, P. (1998) Qualitative research methods. *Health Technology Assessment* **2**: 1–273.

Nastasi, B., Berg, M. (1999) Using ethnography to strengthen and evaluate intervention programmes. In: Schensul, J., LeCompute, M., Hess. G.A., Nastasi, B., Berg, M., Williamson, L., Brecher, J., Glasser, R. (eds) *Using Ethnographic Data: Interventions, Public Programming and Public Policy.* Ethnographer's Toolkit 7. Walnut Creek, CA: AltamMira Press, pp. 1–56.

NHS Centre for Reviews and Dissemination (2001) *Undertaking Systematic Reviews of Research on Effectiveness: CRD's Guidance for Those Carrying Out or Commissioning Reviews.* Report 4 (2nd edn). York: CRD.

Ong, B. (1993) Ethnography in health services research. *The Practice of Health Services Research.* London: Chapman Hall, pp. 42–64.

Ortleib, M. (2004) Applications of anthropology I: professional anthropology in the C21 – Seminar report. *Anthropology in Action* **11**:1, 24–26.

Pope, C., Mays, N. (1995) Qualitative research: researching the part other methods cannot reach: an introduction to qualitative methods in health and health services research. *British Medical Journal* **311**: 42–45.

Robert, S. (2004) The pure and the impure? Applying anthropology and doing ethnography in a commercial setting. *Anthropology in Action* **11**:1, 9–10.

Roth, J. (1963) *Timetables.* New York: Bobbs-Merrill.

Savage, J. (2000) Participative observation: standing in the shoes of others? *Qualitative Health Research* **10**:3, 324–339.

Skeggs, B. (1994) Situating the production of feminist ethnography. In: Maynard, M., Purvis, J. (eds) *Researching Women's Lives from a Feminist Perspective.* PLACE?: Taylor and Francis, pp. 79–92.

Skeggs, B. (2001) Feminist ethnography. In: Atkinson, P., Coffey, A., Delamong, S., Lofland, J., Lofland, L. (eds) *Handbook of Ethnography.* London: Sage Publications, pp. 426–442.

Smith, A., Goodwin, D., Mort, M., Pope, C. (2003) Experts in practice: an ethnographic study exploring acquisition and use of knowledge in anaesthesia. *British Journal Anaesthesia* **91**:3, 319–328.

Smith, V. (2001) Ethnographies of work and the work of ethnographers. In: Atkinson, P., Coffey, A., Delamong, S., Lofland, J., Lofland, L. (eds) *Handbook of Ethnography.* London: Sage Publications, pp. 220–233.

Spencer, J. (2001) Ethnography after postmodernism. In: Atkinson, P., Coffey, A., Delamong, S., Lofland, J., Lofland, L. (eds) *Handbook of Ethnography.* London: Sage, pp. 443–452.

Strong, P. (1979) *The Ceremonial Order of the Clinic: Parents, Doctors and Medical Bureaucracies.* London: Routledge.

Taylor, S. (2002) Researching the social: an introduction to ethnographic research. In: (eds?) *Ethnographic Research: a reader.* London: Sage Publications in association with the Open University, pp. 1–12.

Thomas, J. (1993) *Doing Critical Ethnography.* Qualitative Research Methods Series 26. Newbury Park: Sage Publications.

Wright, S. (1994) *The Anthropology of Organisations.* London: Routledge.

34

Ethnomethodological Insights into Insider–Outsider Relationships in Nursing Ethnographies of Healthcare Settings

Davina Allen

E thnography is growing in popularity as a method of choice for nursing research. It is particularly effective for researching health and social care provision in the context in which it occurs. Although ethnographic studies are typically methodologically pluralistic, the central method of data generation is participant observation using the researcher as the principal research tool. The practice of ethnography therefore requires careful attention to issues of identity and social status and the role of the researcher in the generation of data.

This article re-examines insider–outsider relationships in nursing ethnographies of healthcare settings as a case study in the wider sociological debate around reflexivity in field research. There has been some discussion of this issue in the nursing literature, but our understanding of the impact of nurse researchers' identities on the research process remain partial. Whilst we have a developing understanding of some of the ethical dilemmas encountered by nurse ethnographers (Gerrish 1997, 2003), the advantages and disadvantages of familiarity and distance (Pugh, Mitchell and Brooks 2000; Bonner and Tolhurst 2002), and the relationship between the biography of the researcher and the research process (Pellat 2003); the practices through which the field-work role is accomplished remain opaque. If we are to realize fully the value of ethnography in understanding healthcare and counter claims that our studies are biased in professionally self-serving ways (see, for example, Aguilar 1981;

Source: *Nursing Inquiry*, 11(1) (2004): 14–24.

Silverman 1998), then a more systematic approach is needed. This report shows how insights derived from ethnomethodology can promote a more rigorous and theoretically informed orientation to the conduct and reportage of ethnographic fieldwork.

Reflexivity and the Insider–Outsider Dialectic

Orthodox histories of ethnography identify its roots in social anthropology and the tradition of studying unfamiliar social groups. As ethnographic methods have come to be utilized by researchers to understand their own society, there has been a growth in studies that use the researcher's insider status as the basis for the research (cf. Burgess 1984). Within nursing, ethnographic methods are being increasingly utilized to explore various dimensions of healthcare practice (James 1989, 1992; Savage 1995; Latimer 2000).

Developments of this type have stimulated examination of the relative advantages and disadvantages of 'insider' and 'outsider' research in the general sociological literature on ethnography. Advocates of the 'insider' view argue that it is only those who are closely immersed in the field of study who can ensure an authentic account. Others make the counter claim, that the 'outsider' position is a preferable stance as it is free from the potential for bias that arises from too close an affiliation with the research subjects or 'going native'. As Burgess (1984) observes, however, the debates about familiarity and strangeness have become polarized in the literature. Situations are neither totally familiar nor totally strange, and the researcher's insider–outsider status changes at different points in a research project and is different with different groups and different individuals. Moreover, both poles of the argument are predicated on assumptions about the existence of an objective reality that can be scientifically observed. As Hammersley and Atkinson (1983) observe, it is an unavoidable existential fact that we are part of the world that we study. This overall insight has found expression in the notion of researcher reflexivity (Clifford and Marcus 1986; Van Maanen 1988; Wolf 1996; Reed-Danahay 1997), which recommends that a more fruitful way forward is to work towards a better understanding of the role of the researcher and the impact of the research process on the research findings.

Despite its widespread currency within the literature, however, 'reflexivity' is often an imprecisely used term that has a: 'diverse range of connotations, and sometimes (. . .) virtually no meaning at all' (Atkinson and Coffey 2002). For current purposes we can concentrate on those dimensions of reflexivity that are directly relevant to the fieldwork role. This comprises several elements:

- a concern with how the field of study is filtered through the very particular interpretative lens of the researcher and, as such, reflects their individual history and biography as well as their theoretical perspective;

- an acknowledgement that in actively participating in the field, the researcher will have an effect on the phenomena being researched (Hammersley and Atkinson 1983); and
- a recognition that the field will have an effect on the researcher (Coffey 1999).

The practice of researcher reflexivity requires that these processes are made transparent in order to augment the rigour of qualitative research and enable both the researcher and the reader to assess the validity of the study findings. Thus far, however, these reflexive insights have made only a modest contribution to current understanding of the insider–outsider dialectic in nursing ethnographies of healthcare settings. The nursing literature concentrates on a different set of themes.

Impact of the Research Process on the Researcher

Some authors have focused attention on the impact of the research on the researcher. Pellat (2003) explored how undertaking a study into patient participation in rehabilitation enabled her to acknowledge her own taken-for-granted assumptions and how they had influenced her research and clinical practice. She writes:

> Perhaps as a researcher this is the firs time that I have had the opportunity to really confront what patients are feeling and to experience those feelings myself, which begs the question, 'what have I been doing for the last 35 years? (Pellat 2003, 33).

Such accounts are undoubtedly insightful; however. they have a tendency to emphasize psychological introspection over sociological reflexivity, and, as a consequence, the relationship between such accounts and the execution of the research remains hidden from view (Emerson. Fretz and Shaw 1995; Coffey 1999).[1]

Dilemmas of the Dual Practitioner–Researcher Identity

Nurse ethnographers have also explored the dilemmas they face by virtue of their dual practitioner–researcher identity. At one level, there are clear linkages here with the researcher accounts considered above, but the focus of this literature is also practical, in as much as it highlights the implications that such dilemmas have for the individual researcher and their field relationships. For example, Gerrish (1997, 2003) explores the ethical dilemmas that she encountered daily in her ethnographic study of individualized nursing care in a multiethnic society. Reflecting on the 'thorny issue of intervention', Gerrish writes:

> Throughout fieldwork I was acutely aware of the dissonance between my responsibilities as a nurse towards patients should I observe nursing practice that I considered detrimental to their wellbeing, and the effect I would have on the research should I challenge a particular nurse's practice (Gerrish 1995, 90).

Others have also drawn attention to these concerns (see, for example, Johnson 1992; Rudge 1995; Fitzgerald 1997) and have highlighted how nurses' individual professional identities confer upon them moral responsibilities that may be in tension with the norms of the social groups they are trying to access and understand. The situational ethics typical of ethnographic fieldwork strain against the deontological ethics that are more characteristic of professional nursing practice.

Familiarity and Distance

It is, however, the tension between familiarity and distance which has thus far received the greatest attention within nursing scholarship. In general, this body of work tends to draw heavily on the debates in the realist literature about the relative advantages and disadvantages of insider and outsider perspectives, to consider how these tensions were managed in a particular project. For example, Pugh, Mitchell and Brooks (2000) examined how, in a study of shared governance, the 'insider' perspective of the nurse researcher was balanced by the 'outsider' perspective of the principal investigator in order 'to make the strange familiar' and 'the familiar strange'. In a similar vein, Bonner and Tolhurst (2002) examined the advantages and disadvantages of insider–outsider perspectives and the strategies they employed to manage these in their respective studies. Bonner analysed her research role as an 'insider' nephrology nurse exploring the world of nephrology nursing. She argued that her 'insider' status gave her a privileged understanding of 'the fundamentals of what was going on', a prior knowledge of where to gather data, and sensitivity to changes in the normal clinical practices of the research participants. Conversely, she acknowledged that familiarity with a setting carries with it the risk that the significance of certain routine behaviours could be overlooked and assumptions made about the meaning of events without clarification being sought. Bonner's account is juxtaposed with that of Tolhurst, who writes from the perspective of an 'outside' researcher. Reflecting on her research into the attributes of clinical teachers in the acute setting, she argued that because she was a non-regular member of the ward team, the research participants were more inclined to entrust her with potentially sensitive information. In addition, Tolhurst argued that the 'outsider' position enabled her to be more attuned to 'subtle differences in certain events'. Tolhurst also claimed that her 'outsider' status excused her from the obligation to practice as a nurse, which was more conducive to the objective observation of events. Nevertheless, as an 'outsider', she found it difficult to assess the impact of her presence on the clinical setting and establish trusting field relationships.

Beyond 'Insiders' and 'Outsiders'

All the studies reviewed here treat the terms 'insider' and 'outsider' in an a priori manner. The account of Savage (2003), of her attempt to 'stand in the shoes of others' whilst researching nursing and intimacy, challenges such assumptions. Taking a 'participative' approach to observation, she charts her efforts to get inside nursing through participating in nurses' bodily practices in order to access embodied practitioner knowledge. Her analysis draws attention to the epistemological problems with this kind of approach and underlines the difficulties of effacing the personal histories and biography of the researcher:

> (T)he researcher's body is not a *tabula rasa* on which the experiences of others can be inscribed, unmodified by those of the researcher. (. . .) (However) (i)n some ways, deliberately mimicking the practices of nurses on the ward served to highlight some of the differences between us, rather than allowing me access to nurses' subjective worlds. yet, becoming aware of what constituted otherness in this context helped me to make aspects of these nurses' practice more explicit (Savage 2003, 70–71).

Although she does not address these directly, the account of the fieldwork practices of Savage (2003) raises a number of key questions:

(1) What does it mean to be an 'insider' or an 'outsider' in a given setting?
(2) How is the researcher's status negotiated and accomplished throughout the research process?
(3) What are the implications of (1) and (2) for the study objectives and the study findings?

These are important issues because, irrespective of whether our aim is for 'detached observation' or 'embodied understanding', our role in the research setting is inherently connected with what we 'find out'. However, despite an obvious preparedness to adopt a more reflexive orientation to the research process, discussions of the researcher's insider–outsider status within the field tend, for the most part, to be founded on taken-for-granted common-sense assumptions derived from the researcher's intuition and feelings. The interactions and social practices on which such claims are based remain opaque. There is, I think, a need to be much more systematic in our accounts of the fieldwork process. Having reinstated the researcher as the creator of ethnographic texts, this reflexive positioning needs to be underwritten with an empirically substantiated and theoretically informed treatment of their social interaction within the field.

Theorizing the Research Role

Despite recognition of the social nature of fieldwork practice and its strong resemblance to the routine ways in which people make sense of their every-day life (Hammersley and Atkinson 1983), it is only relatively recently that efforts have been made to develop a theoretical basis for the fieldwork role. For example, Ashworth (1995) looks to phenomenology in order to develop such an understanding, arguing that participant observation should be predicated on the phenomenology of 'participation'. According to Ashworth, 'participation' entails:

> ... attunement to the others' stock of knowledge at hand, emotional and motivational attunement to the group's concerns, taking for granted that one can contribute properly to the group, and becoming relatively un-threatened concerning one's identity in the group.

He goes on to explore the practical aspects of participant observation in re-lation to these four areas.

Notwithstanding the value of the contribution of Ashworth (1995), there is a danger that the uncritical adoption of a phenomenological approach to ethnographic practice will lead to an exclusive focus on the meaning of participation and excessive psychological introspection on the part of the researcher. In order to address these concerns, I suggest a framework in which equal weight is given to social practices. As we have seen, the value of such an approach is illustrated in the work of Savage (2000, 2003), in which she draws attention to the dissonance she experienced whilst participating in the bodily practices of the nurses she studied and, in so doing, highlighted her sense of difference from those whose experiences she was at pains to access.

Savage's work is an important contribution to the literature as it draws attention to: (i) embodiment; and (ii) the practices of a particular group. Researcher reflexivity is an important way of accessing such processes and making them visible. However, it is also the case that the research role is ac-complished through rather more mundane social practices which, because they are so taken-for-granted. are less open to retrieval. This is where an ethnomethodological orientation may prove more fruitful than Savage's reliance on the work of Bourdieu (1977) and his concept of 'habitus'. In the second half of this article, my aim is to build on the work of Ashworth and Savage and suggest how an ethnomethodological orientation may enhance our understanding of the fieldwork role. First, the underlying theory is outlined, then examples from my own research are considered in order to illustrate the potential of such an approach.

Theorizing the Fieldwork Role: Insights from Ethnomethodology

The term ethnomethodology, which was invented by Garfinkel literally means 'people's methods' and the focus of the perspective is on the practices through which members construct their social world. Garfinkel built on the phenomenology of Schutz (1967) and set out to develop: 'a generalized social system built solely from the analysis of experience structures' (Heritage 1984). At the heart of the ethnomethodological perspective is the 'lived order'.

> The term 'lived order', then, calls our attention to both the contingent and socially structured ways that societal members construct/enact/do/inhabit their everyday world. Ethnomethodologists have generally noted that the lived orders of the everyday world are both relied upon and ignored by societal members. Every American English-speaking adult, for example, knows in incredible detail, and as a matter of practical production and recogntion, the structures involved in taking turns in conversation, or in supplying the necessary 'continuers' to allow conversation to proceed. In this sense, the everyday orderliness known. But, it is not known in a way that is conscious and reportable, (Goode 1994, 127–8).

The aim of ethnomethodology is to investigate the methods that people use in creating this lived orderliness. Emerson and Pollner (2001) have suggested that there are aspect of ethnomethodology which might be applied to the practice of ethnography. They cite an example (Pollner and Emerson 1988, 242–51) in which they examined how an ethnographer, despite feeling as if he or she is 'just an observer', must achieve and sustain the role of 'observer' in the face of diverse pressures to participate more fully in unfolding events:

> Ethnographers may, for example, anticipate and attempt to preclude overtures for consequential involvement, evade such overtures through vague and ambiguous responses and even periodically 're-mind' themselves of their research goals and priorities in the face of inclusive tendencies.

The insights of ethnomethodology can also heighten our sensitivity to how insider–outsider status is managed in the field. In contrast to a phenomenological perspective which prompts the researcher to consider what it means to be a member of a particular group or how the fieldwork role feels, such an approach would also alert nurse ethnographers to the need to consider the processes through which the fieldwork role is accomplished and group membership is achieved. Such an approach suggests that 'identity' (i.e. 'insider' or 'outsider') is: 'an interactional accomplishment that is socially constructed, interpreted and communicated via words, deeds and images' (Hunt and Benford 1994, 491).

A large body of ethnomethodological literature could be used as a theoretical basis for developing understanding of the fieldwork role, covering topics such as: the accomplishment of group membership; how inclusion and exclusion is achieved; and how identity is managed (see, for example, Emerson and Pollner 1976; Cohan 1997; Dingwall 1977; Gieryn 1983; Antaki and Widdicombe 1998). As a number of authors have pointed out, the theories we develop to explain the behaviours of others should also, where relevant, be applied to our own activities as researchers in order to aid the development of our research practice (Hammersley and Atkinson 1983; Ashworth 1995).

Case Study: The Changing Shape of Nursing Practice

The study I am going to draw on was my first experience of ethnography. The research was concerned with the practical accomplishment of nursing juris-diction and was carried out in a large District General hospital in the north of England. I had never worked at the hospital previously and my only prior contact was as a service user attending the Accident and Emergency depart-ment with one of my children. At the time of the research I was a full-time PhD student at a university which had no formal relationship with the hospital and I had been absent from clinical practice for almost 5 years. I elected to be open about my nursing background, and my fieldwork role was informed, *inter alia*, by my own identity, the aims of the research and my underlying theoretical perspective.

The study was informed by ecological theories of the division of labour (Durkheim 1933; Hughes 1984; Abbott 1988), which are predicated on the assumption that the world of work is a social system. Accordingly, it is not possible to understand the role of one individual or occupation without reference to those with whom they interact. Informed by interactionist soci-ologies and ethnomethodology, in particular, the aim of the research was to document and explain how the boundaries of nursing work were constituted at the point of service delivery through social interaction. My epistemological stance was to observe and document actions and practices in the context of the workplace, rather than to access research participants' experiences by at-tempting to stand in their shoes. At the same time, in order to understand why nursing jurisdiction was carried out in the ways that it was, I wanted to develop an appreciation of a range of occupational perspectives: nurses, doctors and healthcare assistants (HCAs) and, as far as possible, to not privilege one view over another. The development of high-quality trusting field relationships was therefore essential. Given these considerations, I entered the field setting with a heightened sensitivity to the significance of social divisions and how these impacted on my insider–outsider status. Moreover, the analyses I have undertaken since the cessation of the fieldwork have further developed this awareness (Allen 2000, 2001a). The following discussion focuses on the nego-tiation of my fieldwork role and my insider–outsider status vis-a-vis the nursing staff on the first of the two wards studied.

Initial Presentation of Self and General Orientation to the Fieldwork Role

Appearance is a powerful marker of group identity, and this is especially true in healthcare settings in which uniform and mode of dress are important signifiers of group membership, status and rank. Attending to the physical presentation of self – dress, appearance and non-verbal means – is one way in which 'impressions' can be managed (Goffman 1959) and the social construction of a particular identity can be accomplished (Snow and Anderson 1987: Phelan and Hunt 1998). In his famous study of the managed achievement of sex status in an intersexed person, Garfinkel (1967) describes how scrutiny to her outward appearance was one of the practical methodologies Agnes deployed in 'passing' as a 'normal natural female' and, in so doing, reveals something of the taken-for-granted ways in which membership of this social group is achieved. Phelan and Hunt (1998) have also explored prison gang members' tattoos as a medium for the visual communication of moral careers.

Given my concern not to align myself with any particular occupational group, careful consideration needed to be given to my outward appearance. Taking advice from the Director of Nursing, I elected to wear a white coat inform in the style worn by hospital voluntary workers and had the title 'research student' inscribed on my badge. The Director of Nursing believed that my self-presentation would make the reasons for my presence on the ward clearer to patients, enable me to participate in mundane ward activities and differentiate me from 'visitors'. I was rather ambivalent about the white coat, given its powerful symbolic association with the medical profession, but had no wish to unsettle the smooth progress of my access negotiations, so capitulated. However, in the early days in the field, a number of ward staff confirmed my anxieties and teased me about my appearance, indicating that I was likely to be mistaken for a doctor. In actuality, the fabric and cut of the coat was subtly different to that worn by medical staff (it was also pristinely clean!) and I lacked the other outward symbols of group membership adorned by this occupational group (stethoscope, pharmaceutical formulary, neurological-torch and tourniquet). Generally speaking, my appearance allowed me to blend into the ward scene, whilst, for the most part, resisting any obvious alignment with a particular occupational group. My impression of management did, however, fail me on two occasions and, as the nurses predicted, I was mistaken for a medical student. In one instance, this resulted in my being pulled into the inner circle attending a cardiac arrest so as 'to get a better view of things' and, in another, saw me grilled by an overbearing consultant on the generic name of an antibiotic. In both of these examples, I had been shadowing house officers and, during the course of my observations, had found myself in contexts in which my research identity was unknown to a number of people present.[2] Given the circumstances, I elected to 'pass' in my perceived identity, rather than disrupt the scene by explaining my researcher identity. In neither case was the data subsequently used for research purposes.

As Hunt and Benford (1994) argue, social boundaries and identity are also accomplished through deeds and actions. A key issue in discussions of the insider–outsider dialectic relates to the researcher's mode of participation in the field. It is commonplace to see Gold's (1958) continuum of research participation rehearsed in methods books to capture the range of roles that may be adopted. Frequently, however, this reference is followed by the caveat that in real life the ethnographer's role is more complex than Gold's continuum allows and that, in a given study, a researcher may adopt different roles along this range. Moreover, as Atkinson and Hammersley (1994) point out, Gold's framework is of limited value in understanding the fieldwork role. He does not consider how this relates to the researcher's orientation as an insider–outsider and he fails to specify the activities in which the researcher will engage in a given setting and how such participation will position them in relation to different social groups.

Selective association with particular individuals or groups is one way in which identity is accomplished and, from an ethnomethodological perspective, participation in work activity is a clear marker of membership of an occupational group and one's status within an occupational group (Emerson and Pollner 1976; Hughes 1984). For example, I have noticed that when nurse ethnographers talk and write about not participating in a field setting or having an 'outsider' status, what they actually mean is that they are not going to participate as a practitioner. There are, of course, many other modes of participation available to the nurse ethnographer, but this observation is interesting for what it reveals about the centrality of clinical practice to nurses' identity.

In this particular study, I did not want my role to include significant participation in the ward work as this would have aligned me more clearly with certain occupational groups and restricted my access to others. Nevertheless, as an 'insider' of sorts to healthcare settings. I was acutely aware of the pressures on clinical staff and, given my occupational socialisation, of how difficult it would be for me to remain unoccupied if the ward was busy. I therefore decided to In flexible, anticipating that I would help out with the more mundane ward work when it seemed appropriate to do so, but would otherwise adopt more of an observer stance. In actuality, in the early days in the field I was so uncomfortable with the research role that I spontaneously volunteered to do a range of things, with little consideration of my ability to actually carry them through.

On reflection I think that unconsciously I was trying to find a role in the field that I felt at ease with because the research role felt so alien to me. A number of studies have highlighted the importance within nursing culture of 'getting through the work' (Melia 1987) and the research field was no different (Allen 2000b, 1: 64). Feeling very much an 'outsider', participation in the ward work was a way of fitting in and overcoming my initial sense of social isolation, even though, from an ethnomethodological perspective, it contradicted my original objectives not to participate in the field in ways which aligned me with any one particular group. This highlights the fact that the role we adopt in a field setting will, at times, be driven by our own psychological and emotional needs. To think that we can totally avoid this is naive, but we do need to have a critical awareness of its consequences and be honest about the reasons for our actions. In my case, as I became more comfortable with my research status, I was better able to adopt a role that was compatible with the aims of the research.

Initial Reception

My identity as a nurse clearly influenced my relationships in the field, and critically shaped my interactions with the different groups I was studying and my own emotional responses to them. I had last worked in healthcare as a staff nurse and I began the study expecting that I would be accepted by ward nurses in those terms.[3] Having rotated around a succession of clinical areas as part of nurse training, and during a subsequent period of agency nursing, I was accustomed to fitting in with new teams. In a number of respects the nurses clearly treated me as an insider. This was evident, for example, in the language they used to explain things to me. Access to esoteric and specialist language is an important marker of group boundaries. For example, Meehan (1981) has argued that one of the ways in which the health professions maintain a boundary with lay people is through the use of medical jargon. Medical jargon provides an efficient way of communicating shared knowledge and provides a common sense of identity for health professionals. In my interactions with them the nurses' use of language signified that they assumed that I had access to this specialist vocabulary and body of knowledge; they did not choose to elaborate or translate the meaning of their utterances. It was also evident that they saw me as someone who understood the architecture of hospital wards and the significance of ward routines, as these too were referred to unproblematically, thereby indicating assumptions about our presumed shared stock of knowledge.

Yet, whilst the nurses treated me as someone with insider knowledge, it was also clear that they did not see me as one of them, and this came as a tremendous shock. I was ascribed the role of 'expert academic' and there was concern that I would be making judgements about the quality of their practice and reporting this back to management:

> Just as I was leaving after I had been discussing the project with the nurses there was some reference made by Petra to 007. I picked up on this comment and jokingly asked if I was being accused of spying. [Fieldnotes]

> Alison was having difficulty in finding some of the drugs on the trolley. She said: 'you'll he going back to Nottingham University and telling them all about those thick nurses at Woodlands'. I assured her that I was not

> in the hospital to make judgements – that wasn't what my research was about. [Fieldnotes]

This next extract is more subtle and layered.

> I was introduced by Sister: 'This is Lavinia (sic) the research nurse, well she used to be a nurse, research person'. The night sister said she had seen a circular about my work. I said that I imagined that she knew what it was I was interested in. She gave me a puzzled and embarrassed look and to my horror it became clear that she thought I was testing her. She said she wasn't sure she could remember exactly now. I quickly said that I did not expect her to remember what it was about. [Fieldnotes]

Here, my status as 'outsider' is constituted in a number of ways. First, the need for an introduction defines me as somebody who is a stranger to the night sister. Second, the incorrect recall of my name signals a lack of familiarity. Third, the continued relevance of my nursing identity is problematized, thereby according me a marginal status. Fourth, the night sister's non-verbal response, when she cannot remember the details of the research outline, indicates an orientation to my assumed academic role and my status as a 'guest' in this hospital who might reasonably expect studied politeness from hospital staff. The night sister's response was also one of a number of powerful reminders of the fact that, however, important it may have been to me, my research did not figure very highly in her over overall scale of priorities!

My 'outsider' status was also exemplified by what was not said by the ward nurses. Close relationships are typical based on reciprocal trust and intimacy. Openness and the disclosure of private thoughts are mechanisms through which such familiarity is accomplished and there was little evidence of this between myself and the nursing staff in the early days of my fieldwork. Instead, in their conversations with me, the nurses displayed an over-reliance on careful public accounts of their work and took care to exclude me from 'backstage' (Goffman 1959) conversations. Similarly, it was custom and practice for ward staff to congregate at the nurses' station at quiet times on the ward, despite the had that this practice is discouraged by certain sectors of the profession, including nurse educators. From the perspective of the ethnographic fieldworker, such occasions are rich opportunities to learn about the culture and norms of the field setting. However, in the early days of the fieldwork, I noticed that if I were to approach such social gatherings, the individuals concerned would suddenly disperse to the different corners of the ward.

Negotiating the Insider–Outsider Dialectic

Field relations are central to any ethnographic study and the quality of the data depends crucially on the quality of the relationships established in relation to the research objectives. As I have described, my aim was to both observe the processes through which occupational boundaries were established in daily practice and combine this with an understanding of the relevant occupational perspectives. It was therefore necessary to take measures to overcome the perceived social distance between myself and the nurses, and this entailed the self-conscious management of self-presentation.

I worked hard to demonstrate my roots in ordinary practice. I attended the wards at unsociable times of both day and night, and at weekends, and undertook work involving the handling of body products. As Hughes (1984) has noted there are different degrees of honour and prestige associated with different kinds of work and 'body products work' occupies an ambiguous place in nursing culture. On the one hand, new nursing ideologies revere hands-on-nursing care as central to the nursing role. On the other, the body's boundaries are symbolically polluting and therefore morally unclean (Douglas 1966). in the study site, this tension created a particular sensitivity to the division of labour in relation to 'body products work'. Whereas other mundane work could be legitimately delegated by a senior nurse to a more junior colleague, physically dirty work tended to be managed according to the principle of 'whoever finds it, deals with it' (Allen 2001b). The delegation of work of this kind by a certain senior members of staff was berated by the other ward staff as evidence of the exercise of their power and status. Accordingly, I self-consciously involved myself in work of this kind in order to level the perceived status differential between myself and the rest of the ward staff:

> I was contemplating giving out lunches when Dawn was looking for help in clearing a patient up who had diarrhoea. I donned an apron and volunteered my services. The nurses were surprised, but grateful. Dawn joked, saying that I'd 'done it now' and that they'd be getting the involved in 'all sorts of things'. [Fieldnotes]

A key thread in ethnomethodological thought is the constitutive power of talk. As Heritage (1984) has observed, at its most fundamental level, social reality is talked into being. From this perspective, rather than the words, statements and stories used by social actors being understood as direct reflections of their identities, they are conceptualized as tools through which identities are constructed (Cohan 1997). A number of authors have examined how stories and story-telling function to define the boundaries of social groups (Dingwall 1977; Allen 2001a). They are a way of narrating 'insiders' and 'outsiders', and a mechanism for communicating shared experiences and moral concerns. In his study of the occupational socialisation of health visitors, Dingwall (1977) argues that the acquisition of a repertoire of stories and the ability to identify appropriate occasions for telling them are important requirements in order to become a competent member of a particular occupational group. In developing my relationships with the ward nurses I was able to draw on my own repertoire of occupational narratives. For example, I told self-effacing stories as part of an overall strategy of managed self-disclosure in order to develop trust and as a way of discouraging nurses' careful public accounts of their practice by indicating that I was someone who 'knew how things really were'.

> Alison was talking about how threatened nurses were to have other nurses observing them. She referred to their dislike of having nurses on the ward as patients. I told her that I'd nursed the Regional Director of Nursing Services when I was a student nurse and that we'd all been very nervous [Everybody gasps]. I said that we had scored some 'Brownie points' by remembering to offer her milk to take her anti-inflammatory drugs with, which she declined [Laughter].

These strategies for accomplishing rapport were partly successful in promoting good field relationships. This was exemplified by my gradual inclusion in 'backstage' talk and conversations at the nurses' station, the research participants' greater willingness to 'tell it as it is', and increased levels of intimacy and self-disclosure. There was also a noticeable improvement in my field relations after I started undertaking interviews with the ward staff. Although methods books typically devote considerable attention to the importance of developing rapport in qualitative interview research, little has been written about the impact of interviews on field relationships in ethnographic research. There may have been a number of reasons for the effect of the interviews on field relations. First, I suspect, that the nurses were rather intimidated by the whole idea of research which, in part contributed to the social distance I experienced and, as the informal nature of the interviews became more widely known, they treated me with less caution. Second, the interviews, which typically lasted from 1–2 hours, were arguably more conducive to the establishment of good field relations than the more fleeting encounters that had been possible in the context of the daily work, given the predominantly observational stance I elected to adopt. Third, during their interviews the nurses talked about the existence of interpersonal tensions on the ward and thus I became privy to an important unspoken undercurrent which influenced much of ward activity and became somebody who was 'in the know'.

In orthodox debates about the pros and cons of insider–outsider positions, it is argued that research participants are more willing to divulge sensitive information to an outsider researcher (Griffiths 1998) and similar claims have also been made in the nursing literature (see, for example, Bonner and Tolhurst 2002). Yet, in the context of this study, despite experiencing a degree of discomfort with different participants' disclosures, I felt as if my relationships with the nursing staff had become closer and did not interpret this as a reaffirmation of my 'outsider' status. Moreover, to have been positioned or to have positioned myself as closer to one perspective over another would have been counter-productive given the research objectives. There are resonances here with the work of Savage (2003), in which she draws attention to how her immersion in the physical practices of the ward amplified her sense of difference from the nurses she was studying. This underlines the importance of ensuring that in our fieldwork accounts, we clearly distinguish our personal emotional responses to relationships in the field from the social interactions which prompted them. Having done this, however, we need also to explicate the relationship between the two. Whilst it is now more common for ethnographers to keep a reflective account of the research process, the usual practice is to separate the narrative of the field from the narrative of the self (Coffey 1999). Such a separation is misleading, however, and is in danger of distorting the meaning of field data (Emerson, Fretz and Shaw 1995). In order to ensure that researcher accounts are reflexive (rather than simply reflective), then the two narratives need to be integrated. I have endeavoured to do this in this admittedly brief and selective account.

Discussion and Conclusion

In this report I have attempted to make a contribution to the development of a more theoretically informed understanding of the research role. Building on the work of Ashworth (1995) and Savage (2003), I have argued that insights from ethnomethodology can help us to develop a sensitivity to the taken-for-granted practices through which the fieldwork role is accomplished. An ethnomethodological approach rejects a priori assertions about the researcher's insider–outsider status in the field and views this as something to be discovered, negotiated and renegotiated as part of the research process. Although we are not free to make our identities in any which way we choose, an ethnomethodological orientation also encourages experimentation with the fieldwork role to test out different observer effects on the field setting. This is exemplified by the insights generated by the breaching experiments of Garfinkel (1967) in which he asked his students to go home and behave as if they were lodgers. Disrupting the social order brought into view the taken-for-granted assumptions underpinning family life. In the same way, proactively managing the insider–outsider dynamic in studies of healthcare settings and analysing its effects might further enhance our understanding of the routine grounds of everyday activities in healthcare settings.

I have endeavoured to illustrate the potential value of an ethnomethodo-logical perspective in making visible the practices through which the fieldwork role is accomplished by drawing on my doctoral research experience. In this article, owing to limitations of space, I have focused attention on my relationships with the nursing staff, but the same approach might also have been applied to the analysis of my field relations with the other key occupational groups in the study (doctors and HCAs). In analysing my field relations I have purposively avoided using the terms 'insider' and 'outsider' in an essentialist sense. Rather, I have taken a dual approach, which combines my own expectations, feelings and emotional responses to the field with an analysis of the social practices that gave rise to them. It is the latter which for the most part, is currently absent from the research literature and, as a result, an individual's insider–outsider status remains something that exists in the heads of researchers rather than founded on empirical evidence and open to critical scrutiny. Ethnomethodology offers a theoretical basis for increasing our sensitivity to these everyday social practices and provides a framework through which they can be systematically described, thereby allowing the researcher and the critical reader to assess the relationship between the fieldwork role and the aims and objectives of the research:

> When we self-consciously apply the reflexive lens to ourselves it can help us to see and appreciate how our renderings of others' worlds are not, and can never be, descriptions from outsider those worlds. Rather, they are informed by and constructed in and through relationships with those under study. Hence, in training the reflexive lens on ourselves we understand our own enterprise in much the same terms remains that we understand those we study (Emerson, Fretz and Shaw 1995, 216).

There is, however, a need for some final words of caution. First, as a number of its critics have pointed out, ethnomethodology has some inherently deconstructing elements. Taken to extremes, there is a danger of descending into a state of hyper-reflexivity, in which the production of an ethnomethodologically informed analysis of the fieldwork role becomes the subject of yet-to-be articulated practices (Woolgar 1988). This is certainly not what I am advocating in this report. My aspiration is to increase the rigour with which we describe the research process, rather than encourage further navel gazing. As Spencer (2001) notes, it is important to be clear that, on the whole, the people we are talking to are more important than the person asking the questions. Second, adopting an ethnomethodological orientation to the fieldwork role does not necessarily commit nurse researchers to applying this kind of perspective to the research project in question. Rather, I am arguing that its application should increase our awareness of the mundane process through which the fieldwork role is conducted and encourage nurse researchers to provide empirical evidence for what has hitherto remained at the level of intuition. The notion of reflexivity is now finding widespread acceptance in qualitative research. Unless we make its actual practice more explicit, however, there is a real danger that it will remain little more than a device for according studies the appearance of academic rigour, and its potential to enhance understanding of the research process and strengthen the quality of our studies will be lost.

Notes

1. This criticism is not confined to nursing. As ethnography research has developed its methodological self-consciousness, there has been a tendency to pursue reflection rather than reflexivity (Pollner 1991).

2. See Moore and Savage (2002).
3. Although I did not appreciate it at the time, my fieldnotes indicate that I had very different expectations of the reletionships that were likely to be possible with HCAs and doctors. My initial sense of being on outsider was never as acute in relation to these social groups, but I had not entered the field with the same expectations of being treated as an insider, nor did I have the same understanding of and sensitivity to what being an insider to these groups comprised.

References

Abbott A. 1988. *The system of professions: An essay on the division of expert labour.* Chicago: University of Chicago Press.

Aguilar JL. 1981. Insider research: An ethnography of a debate. In *Anthropologists at home in North America*, ed. DA Messersschmidt, 15–26. Cambridge: Cambridge University Press.

Allen D. 2000. Doing occupational demarcation: The 'boundary work' of nurse managers in a District General Hospital. *Journal of Contemporary Ethnography* 29: 326–56.

Allen D. 2001a. Narrating nursing jurisdiction: Atrocity stories and boundary work. *Symbolic Interaction* 24: 75–103.

Allen D. 2000b. *The changing shape of nursing practice: The role of nurses in the hospital division of labour.* London: Routledge.

Antaki C and S Widdicombe. 1998. *Identities in talk.* London: Sage.

Ashworth PD. 1995. The meaning of 'participation' in participant observation. *Qualitative Health Research* 5: 366–87.

Atkinson P and A Coffey. 2002. Revisiting the relationship between participant observation and interviewing. In *Handbook of interview research*, eds JF Gubrium and JA Holstein, 801–14. Thousand Oaks: Sage.

Atkinson P and M Hammersley. 1994. Ethnography and participant observation. *In Handbook of qualitative research*, eds N Denzin and Y Lincoln, 248–62. Thousand Oaks: Sage.

Bonner A and G Tolhurst. 2002. Insider–outsider perspectives of participant observation. *Nurse Researcher* 9: 7–19.

Bourdieu P. 1977. *Outline of a theory of practice.* Cambridge: Cambridge University Press.

Burgess RG. 1984. *In the, field: An introduction to field research.* London and New York: Routledge.

Clifford J and GE Marcus. 1986. *Writing culture: The politics and poetics of ethnography.* Berkley, CA: University of California Press.

Coffey A. 1999. *The ethnographic self: Fieldwork and the representation of identity.* London: Sage.

Cohan M. 1997. Political identities and political landscapes: Men's narrative work in relation to women's gender issues. *Sociological Quarterly* 38: 303–19.

Dingwall R. 1977. Atrocity stories and professional relationships. *Sociology of Work and Occupations* 4: 317–96.

Douglas M. 1966. *Purity find danger: An analysis of concepts of pollution and taboo.* London: Routledge and Kegan Paul.

Durkheim E. 1933. *The division of labour in society.* London: Collier-Macmillan.

Emerson RM, RI Fretz and LL Shaw. 1995. *Writing ethnographic fieldnotes.* Chicago and London: University of Chicago Press.

Emerson R and M Pollner. 1976. Dirty work designations: Their features and consequences in a psychiatric setting *Social Problems* 23: 243–54.

Fitzgerald M. 1997. Clinical report: Nursing and researching. *International Journal of Nursing Practice.* 3: 53–56.

Garfinkel H. 1967. *Studies in ethnomethodology.* Cambridge: Polity Press.

Gerrish K. 1995. Being a 'marginal native': Dilemmas of the participant observer. *Nurse Researcher* 5: 25–34.

Gerrish K. 2003. Sell and others: The rigour and ethics of insider ethnography. In *Advanced qualitative research for nursing*, ed. J Latimer, 77–94. Oxford: Blackwell Publishing.

Gieryn T. 1983. 'Boundary-work' and the demarcation of science from non-science: Strains and interests in the professional ideologies of scientists. *American Sociological Review* 48: 781–95.

Goffman E. 1959. *The presentation of self in everyday life.* New York: Doubleday.

Gold RL. 1958. Roles in sociological fieldwork. *Social Forces* 36: 217–23.

Goode D. 1994. *A world without words: The social construction of children born deaf and blind.* Philadelphia: Temple University Press.

Griffith AL. 1998. Insider–outsider: Epistemiological priviledge and mothering work. *Human Studies* 21: 361–376.

Hammersley M and P Atkinson. 1983. *Ethnography: Principles in practice.* London and New York: Routledge.

Heritage J. 1984. *Garfinkel and ethnomethodology.* Oxford: Polity Press.

Hughes EC. 1984. *The sociological eye.* New Brunswick, NJ: Transaction Books.

Hunt SA and RD Benford 1994. Identity talk in the peace and justice movement. *Journal of Contemporary Ethnography* 22: 488–517.

James N. 1989. Emotional labour: Skill and work in the social regulation of feelings. *Sociological Review* 37: 15–41.

James N. 1992. Care = organisation + physical labour + emotional labour. *Sociology of Health and Illness* 14: 488–509.

Johnson M. 1992. A silent conspiracy? Some ethical issues of participant observation in nursing research. *International Journal of Nursing Studies* 29: 223.

Latimer J. 2000. *The conduct of care: Understanding nursing practice.* London: Blackwell Science.

Mechan AJ. 1981. Some conversational features of the use of medical terms by doctors and patients. In *Medical work realities and routines*, eds P Atkinson and C Heath, 107–27. Westmead: Gower.

Melia K. 1987. *Learning and working: The occupational socialisation of nurses*, London: Tavistock.

Moore L and J. Savage. 2002. Participant observation and ethical approval. *Nurse Researcher* 9: 58–69.

Pellat G. 2003. Ethnography and reflexivity: Emotions and feelings in fieldwork. *Nurse Researcher* 10: 28–37.

Phelan MP and Hunt SA. 1998. Prison gang members' tattoos as identity work: The visual communication of moral careers. *Symbolic Interaction* 21: 277–98.

Pollner M. 1991. Left of ethnomethodology: The rise and decline of radical reflexivity. *American Sociological Review* 56: 370–80.

Pollner M and RM Emerson. 1988, The dynamics of inclusion and distance in fieldwork relations. In *Contemporary field research: A collection of readings*, ed. RM Emerson, 235–52. Prospect Heights, IL: Waveland.

Pollner M and RM Emerson. 2001. Ethnomethodology and ethnography. In *Handbook of ethnography*, eds P Atkinson, A Coffey, S Delamont, J Loftland, L Loftland, 118–133. London: Sage.

Pugh J, M Mitchell and F Brooks. 2000. Insider/outsider partnerships in an ethnographic study of shared governance. *Nursing Standard* 14: 43–44.

Reed-Danahay DE. 1997. *Auto/ethnography: Rewriting the self and the social.* Oxford: Berg.

Rudge T. 1995. Response: Insider ethnography: Researching nursing from within. *Nursing Inquiry* 2: 58.

Savage J. 1995. *Nursing intimacy: An ethnographic approach to nurse–patient interaction.* London: Scutari Press.

Savage J. 2000. Participative observation: standing in the shoes of others? *Qualitative Health Research* 10: 324–39.

Savage J. 2003. Participative observation: Using the subject body to understand nursing practice. In *Advanced qualitative research for nursing*, ed. J Latimer, 53–76, Oxford: Blackwell Publishing.

Schutz A. 1967. *The phenomenology of the social world* [translated by G Walsh and F Lehnert]. Evanston, IL: Northwestern University Press [Originally published in 1932].

Silverman D. 1998. The quality of qualitative health research: The open-ended interview and its alternatives. *Social Sciences in Health* 4: 104–18.

Snow DA and L Anderson. 1987. Identity work among the homeless: The verbal construction and avowal of personal identities. *American Journal of Sociology* 92: 1336–71.

Spencer J. 2001. Ethnography after post-modernism. In *Handbook of ethnography*, eds. P Atkinson, A Coffey, S Delamont, J Loftland, L Loftland, 443–52. London: Sage.

Van Maanen J. 1988. *Tales of the field: On writing ethnography.* Chicago: University of Chicago Press.

Wolf DL. 1996. Situating feminist dilemmas in fieldwork. In *Feminist dilemmas in fieldwork*, ed. DL. Wolf, 1–55. Colorado: Westview Press.

Woolgar S. 1988. *Knowledge and reflexivity: New frontiers in the sociology of knowledge.* London: Sage.

35

Applications of Performance Ethnography in Nursing

Carrol A.M. Smith and Agatha M. Gallo

Performance ethnography has the potential to be employed widely in nursing research, education, and practice. This method of ethnography has grown out of cross-disciplinary work in sociology, anthropology, communication studies, performance arts, and cultural studies. In this article, we elaborate on the origins and theory behind performance ethnography, describe some of its forms, and discuss how it can be used effectively in nursing. We include as an example the text of an ethnographic performance written by one of the authors (CS) based on research interviews conducted with parents of children with genetic conditions. The purpose of this example is to demonstrate the aims of performance ethnography and its effective use in presenting research findings.

Performance Ethnography and the Seventh Moment

Denzin and Lincoln (2000) have described historical "moments" during which qualitative researchers have searched for and expressed knowledge. A moment is a demarcation of a time when new sensibilities appear or when researchers and scholars begin to imagine and produce new forms of their work. The moments described by Denzin and Lincoln are the traditional, from the beginning to the middle of the 20th century; the modernist, from midcentury through the 1960s, to the postmodern and postexperimental, at the

Source: *Qualitative Health Research*, 17(4) (2007): 521–528.

end of the 20th century. The current, or seventh, moment in the 21st century is "the methodologically contested present" (Denzin & Lincoln, 2005, p. 1116), a time of tension between conservative and quantitative researchers and their qualitative counterparts, and a time when qualitative researchers are exploring varied methodologies, paradigms, and perspectives for their inquiries. No matter how diverse these contested methods might seem, the driving force of the current qualitative focus is toward more feminist, ethical, communitarian, democratic, engaged, performative, and social justice–oriented research (Denzin & Lincoln, 2005).

In this current moment, performance ethnography is gaining attention. Often, it is presented as a performance text that one or more people write and read for an audience. The material on which the text is based can be empirical research results, autobiographical stories, ethnographic field notes, reflexive journal entries, or specific memories of a life event. The purpose of the text is to engage the audience fully, so that performer and listener meet in the liminal (or threshold) space that lies between them. Listeners understand the text slightly differently based on their gender, ethnicity, social class, or historical or cultural background. Ultimately, the text brings the listeners to new understanding or knowledge, or moves them to action based on their own interpretation of the text. The text often tells a story of the lived experience of others, a story that involves the listeners fully in the moment created by the text (Denzin, 2003; Denzin & Lincoln, 2000; Madison, 2005).

Historical Perspective on Performance Ethnography

Performance ethnography is a broad descriptor for a number of performative methods used by qualitative researchers. Performance has long been a part of the human behavioral repertoire. In certain periods of history (Renaissance and Baroque), the theatricality of regular social life was recognized and used in performance (Carlson, 2004). Many sociologists and anthropologists have argued that in our postmodern world, we are all performing and constructing our social lives as we live them (Denzin & Lincoln, 2005). In the mid 20th century, anthropologists Turner (1969) and Geertz (1973), and sociologist Goffman (1974) each developed theories related to performance. Turner worked with the liminality (that which is barely perceptible, at the edge of a threshold of consciousness) (Mish, 2003) of performance as an opportunity for new cultural forms, models, or paradigms to arise, whereas Geertz theorized about the relationship between performance and cultural critique. Goffman contributed "framing" to performance theory; a frame sets apart certain social events, such as a performance. Within the frame of performance, there is a performer who places a set of activities before an audience, whose sole obligation is to observe the performer.

Contemporary Performance Theorists

Taking these early theories of performance and combining them with ethnographic research is the purview of contemporary social scientists Conquergood (2002), Denzin (1997, 2003), and Madison (2005). These researchers have provided skillful overviews of theory as well as relevant discussions of practice. All three view performance ethnography from the perspective of critical social theory, a theory that highlights issues of power, justice, and the ways in which the economy, gender, race, ideologies, education, and culture interact in the production of social systems (Denzin & Lincoln, 2005).

Conquergood had ethnographic interests that ranged from the Latin Kings street gang to Chicago's diverse immigrant neighborhoods. Over his lifetime of work, he gradually moved from traditional ethnography into ethnographic performance by way of plays, performed texts, and films. He emphasized the importance of meanings expressed through intonation, silence, and body tension, and saw performance as stories that struggle "to open the space between analysis and action . . . and to pull the pin on the binary opposition between theory and practice" (2000, p. 145). He sought to define and bridge the hierarchical divide between artists and practitioners, and scholars and researchers, believing that performance could draw together many types of knowledge.

Another of Conquergood's emphases was the ethical stance of performance. He hypothesized four morally problematic stances toward the persons being researched that could lead to dishonorable performance: Selfishness, wherein the researcher is merely looking for good performance material; the Enthusiast's Infatuation or overidentification with the research participant, resulting in superficial performances; the Curator's Exhibitionism, or dehumanization of the participants by overemphasis of the exotic or primitive; or Skepticism, when the researcher detaches from the participant in a way that creates a cynical or cowardly stance. Researchers and performers need to pay careful attention to themselves and their motives for using the research material, lest they find themselves using it in these potentially unethical ways (Conquergood, 1985).

A student of Conquergood, Madison teaches myth and popular culture, performance ethnography, performance of literature for social change, and the political economy of performance. Many of her ideas are similar to those of Conquergood, but in her recent book. *Critical Ethnography: Method, Ethics, and Performance* (2005), Madison has emphasized the roles of the subjects, the audience, and the performers. She stated that each group gains something from the performance. The subjects benefit when voice experience, and history are brought together in the presentation; once the subjects are voiced, their presence is acknowledged among us as constructed beings that are real and are not alone. The performer communicates the world of the subjects, such that meanings and intentions are amplified; the audience is affected by what it sees and hears, and is motivated to "act and think in ways that now beneficially affect (directly and indirectly) either the subjects themselves or what they advocate" (p. 174). The audience travels into the world of the participant, where a profound meeting of the two takes place; the audience (outsiders) fuses with the participants (insiders).

Denzin (1997, 2001, 2003) has written extensively about performance texts and performance ethnography. He has thoroughly infused his notions of performance with politics and confronted the issues of racism and democracy in postmodern America (Denzin, 2003). He has not only described how to construct rhetoric into performance texts but also demonstrated this by re-constructing and adding to his performance text about the small town in Montana, where he and his wife own a cabin and vacation every year. In "Per-forming Montana" (1999), Denzin tells stories of their activities as they "perform Montana" (fishing, quilting, volunteering at the local library, attending town celebrations.) He also attended to the geographic racism present with regard to Native Americans (Denzin, 2003).

In his book *Performance Ethnography*, Denzin (2003) evaluated critical ethnography in the seventh moment. He defined *performance* as an inter-pretive event involving actors, scripts, stories, and interactions, and *perform-ance texts* as poems, plays, staged or improvised readings, or texts of natural conversations. Autoethnography is lifted up as additional material for perform-ance. Performance texts can be seen as complimentary forms of research pub-lication, "an alternative way of interpreting and presenting the results of an ethnographer's work" (p. 13).

Denzin (2003) has defined terms that are important to his description of per-formance texts: liminality, ritual, and the epiphany. Denzin, like Turner (1969), has used *liminality* to describe the space between performer and audience. Rituals and personal epiphanies are moments in peoples' lives when they are particularly vulnerable; these are often the ethnographic sites that draw an audience in. The performance text allows for the everyday relationship in which "we are all co-performers in our own and others' lives" (p. 56.)

Much of our information comes to us by way of stories elicited through inter-views: News stories, television news magazines, and market research studies are examples. There are many kinds of interviews taking place all the time, and ethnographic interviews are among them. Denzin (2003) sees the reflex-ive interview as appropriate for performed stories. The reflexive interview is not one-sided; it draws all parties into a dialogue in which each attempts to understand the other by carefully attending to the verbal and nonverbal com-munication. Material from reflexive interviews creates dialogue that leads to performances in which multiple voices can be heard, dichotomies are resisted, differences are brought to the foreground, and the audience is responsible for interpreting the performance. The interpretation might be different for each audience member, depending on such factors as cultural background, social class, and gender; each interpretation creates new knowledge for listeners or might move them to action on behalf of the persons represented in the text.

Although each of these three scholars gives it a different name, they share a common vision of the substance of performance ethnography: Conquergood (2002) named it dialogical performance; Madison (2005), excellent representation; and Denzin (2003) described interpretive sufficiency, representational adequacy, and authentic adequacy. All agree that the performer must clearly and adequately represent the participants being studied. The performance must be free from stereotyping by race, class, or gender. Interpretive sufficiency allows for varied worldviews, voices, value systems, and beliefs to come together, to meet in dialogue such that an intimate conversation can occur between the self and the "other" that goes beyond differences (Denzin & Lincoln, 2005). When these criteria are achieved, performance ethnography is at its best.

Performance ethnography is primarily used in the social sciences: sociology (Stevens & Delamont, 2006), anthropology (Turner, 1982), communication studies (Alexander, 2005; Ellis & Bochner, 2004; Jago, 2006), women's studies (Lather, 2000), education (McClaren, 1999), performance studies (Conquergood, 1988), cultural studies (Smith, 1993, 1994), and even the field of English (Weems, 2002). Performance ethnography has not been formally used in the fields of nursing, medicine, or other allied health professions. Researchers in these fields have conducted ethnographic research (Hall & White, 2005 [social work]; Harrison, 2005; Hoppes, 2005 [occupational therapy]; Manderson, 2005; Perry, Lynam, & Anderson, 2006; Stevens, 2006; Tsai, 2006 [nursing]; Weeks et al., 2006 [medicine]), but they have not connected their research with the performative. Had they taken their research a step further, performance of their findings would be available to an audience in another way.

A Sample Performance Text

An example of the "how" of performance ethnography is drawn from one of the authors' work (CS) for the past 5 years as a research assistant on a project supported by a grant from the Ethical, Legal, and Social Issues (ELSI) research program of the National Human Genome Research Institute (NHGRI). The aim of the research was to describe how parents of children with genetic conditions manage the child's illness and the information about the condition. Semistructured interviews were completed with 86 families (143 parents and caregivers), at which time the parents also completed structured measures evaluating individual and family functioning.

I conducted many of the interviews with parents about their children with sickle cell disease, phenylketonuria, cystic fibrosis, neurofibromatosis, thalassemia, hemophilia, Marfan syndrome, and von Willebrand's disease. The stories parents told kept circling in my memory. Having recently learned about performance text, I decided these parents' stories would make an excellent resource for an ethnographic performance. I used material from transcripts of the recorded interviews to write a text that represented the experiences of many of the families. The verbatim transcripts had been coded such that answers to specific interview questions could easily be retrieved. I chose several broad themes evident across transcripts and then located quotes that demonstrated those themes. Specifics of situations and all given and place names were changed to preserve confidentiality. Parents had previously given their consent for the material to be used in publications based on the study findings.

Please read the following text aloud to yourself, or have someone read it aloud to you. The human voice adds to the text in a way that is not present with silent reading.

Stories of Parents of Children with a Genetic Condition

For those of us who have borne children and those of us who have not … and for those of us who care for children and families.…

Please make a sojourn with me to a place much closer than any of us wish it to be. Imagine the anticipation of a baby on the way – a baby planned or un-planned, joyfully conceived or not – anticipated nonetheless as a beautiful, healthy child.

Imagine the shock when the anticipated healthy child is not.

Due to understood or not-yet-understood processes within our genes, some human babies are born with irregularly shaped red cells, with tenacious mucous in their lungs and guts, with metabolic disturbances, with neurological conditions, with fragile hearts and eyes – these children may be well loved, but it's not quite that simple. And who is to say they are not healthy? The more we learn about genetics, the more we know that many of us have genetically based conditions that will catch up with us sooner or later. Who's to say what "perfect" or "healthy" are?

But, journey with me now to hear the words of parents of these children and how they speak to us of fear and pain, of misunderstanding, of difficult deci-sions, and sometimes of death; and the joys of family love and support, children who defy the odds, children developing even with dysfunctional bodies and terrible pain, maintaining hope along the way.

> When the doctor told me my baby had sickle cell I just didn't know what to do. I really didn't even know what it was. I was too young and I already had one baby, and now I had a sick one. I almost gave him up for adoption.

> How did I find out my baby had the sickle cell? They sent me a letter in the mail and said I needed to come in because of something they had found. When I got there, the doctor said, "Your baby has sickle cell anemia." My baby was just three months old. I knew I had the trait, but his daddy had never admitted to me that he did. I was hurtin' with this news. When ladies have babies they look for all the fingers and toes and eyes and ears … make

sure everything's in place and no outside marks and then they never think to ask, "How is the inside? How is the blood? How is the heart?" Unless it comes up and you get a letter in the mail that says, "We have something we want to talk to you about," and it's not nothing to talk to you about on the phone.

When Joey was 8 days old I got at call from a doctor at the pediatrician's office who said there was an abnormality in the screening and the indication was that he had PKU. They said it was a treatable disorder but it was imperative that we make an appointment that very afternoon to take him to the clinic. I was devastated, but I'd had a premonition that something would go wrong. Everyone at the clinic was great and I remember feeling very surprised and overwhelmed that there were so many people who were specially trained to help me deal with a child that needed special help. I was not in a caring profession and I did not know people did this.

How did I feel? I was mad – hurt – upset. I was ignorant because I didn't know exactly what it was. I thought my baby was gonna die. And everybody came at me with something negative. Your baby's gonna die. She's gonna have terrible pain and her limbs will swell up, you're gonna have to have them removed. I was hurt, I was crying all the time and I was depressed. I just didn't know what to do.

Once parents hear the difficult news they usually share it with others. Most tell their own parents immediately. Then siblings and other family members learn. The information may mean that others in the family should be tested, but they don't always want to hear that. What *does* it mean to learn that a child in your family has a genetic condition?

When we told our families they both kind of did, the "It must come from the other side of the family" thing. We don't have that in our family. But it was from both of us. Both families have to take the blame.

When I got home I was crying and I told my baby's father and his father's mother. The doctor had said that both his father and I should come in for testing. But his father was pretty unresponsive. He just said, "There's nothing wrong with my side of the family, so I don't know what you're talkin' about." And after that his father just gradually disappeared.

And then others are told: friends, playmates of the child …

I can't say honestly that I remember how I told most people because it was such a painful time and an awkward thing to bring up. You know, people said, "Oh how's your baby?" And you wanna say, "He's perfect! He's fine!" And at the same time there's this other thing that you have to say, and um … it's difficult to sort of manage people's reactions, too. Because most people don't know about the condition until you tell them what it is.

When the families learn how they must care for these special children, how do they cope? How does the family envelop the child and manage the care?

I have accepted the basic information about the care for her condition. I don't like to get too much into the research studies, though. There's just a lot that I don't want to know. I just want to know that I'm doing what I'm supposed to be doing, and the children are doing what they're supposed to be doing, and together we'll have a happy life ...

At first I was very paranoid. I didn't want her to go outside and play. I didn't want her to get dirty. I used to make her sit right up under me, 24/7. I would wake up in the middle of the night and go pinch her to make sure she was breathing. But I have changed a lot. She does everything now from tap dance to field hockey, basketball, and track.

I would like to be more restricting, but then my husband says, "Let him be a child. Let him grow. Don't hinder him. If he can do like the rest of the children, let him get out there. Let him get hit. Let'em knock him down and see he gets back up. That's what children do. Don't take the growing up away from him because you know he has a life-threatening disease" ... So ... it took a little while, but I try to bend.

What do parents do about getting information and dealing with health care providers on a frequent basis ....?

In 1986, it was like, sickle cell was a secret Black peoples disease that nobody talked about. Where now, it's like. OK. It's out there. People discuss it. It's easy to obtain information when I need to.

I'd say, the doctors and nurses, they're gonna pretty much give you medical, and sometimes you need a little bit more than that. It's like, okay, with her and her illness. I worry about her development. You know, growing up well. They're not worried about that. They're concerned with the illness. It's like, not her, the person, but the illness. Whereas I'm more concerned with her. Her growing up, and her life, and just everything. We wanna deal with the illness, 'cuz we have to, but we still wanna deal with her. We don't wanna lose her in the illness. And I think with the doctors, sometimes, they kind of do.

And then there are the decisions about having other children ...

After our baby was diagnosed we decided to try for another baby with the idea that we would have prenatal testing and terminate the pregnancy if [the genetic condition] was present. I terminated two pregnancies that way. Then I had a surprise pregnancy. My husband just wanted me to terminate again without even testing, but I'd had enough. I said I was keeping this baby no matter what ... and we had a perfectly healthy baby.

Finally, what do parents of these children say about the future?

I finally began to get a little perspective on things. But before that I had already planned Sissy's birthdays, her dating, her wedding, her funeral, I mean, you know, do we serve low protein wedding cake? What do we do?

I'm like, her funeral, now that she's gone, she can't eat it, but should we still have low protein food in honor of her? I mean I had her proms figured out, and her death … you know, she was only two weeks old and I had gone the whole gamut!

I know at this time she will probably die before I will. I don't look forward to what could happen in the future, but I'm very realistic about this, and it will probably happen. I focus on today and now, but I also try to keep in mind that her health will decline as time goes on and that eventually I will lose her. If I did not think this way, when the end comes I would be too devastated to function.

I think it's more important for my kids and my son to know that even though he has this disease, that he could be whatever he wants to be. I want him to get a good education and I will let him know that. It's just like breaking a curse. And I want him to break that curse of his disease because I know that it's something that he could do, he could be whatever he wants to be. If he wants to be a doctor, he can be a doctor, he can do that. And I always let him know that if he has a goal that he wants to set he could do it. Just keep that goal in mind and I will always stand with him to help him make that goal.

And how does it feel to be the person who does these interviews with parents of children with genetic conditions?

When I leave the interviews I always feel grateful that none of my children or grandchildren was born with genetic conditions … but it's kind of like having survivor's guilt. How come my family got off so easy? How come we did not experience any of this pain? Why do some have to bear this burden and I do not? Do I have to pay in some other way?

I am always amazed at what people will tell me. They throw the window into their hearts wide open.

Sometimes I cry when they do. Imagine listening to these stories. Each one is a little different, and these parents cope amazingly well … and they still weep when you ask them to "tell me the story about the time when you first found out your child had this condition."

I would have found it difficult to continue conducting these interviews if I did not think we were learning things that would assist health care providers to support these families better. The stories will help a great deal if we listen to them.

Evaluation of the Performance Text

Examination of this text shows that it meets the performance text criteria defined by Conquergood (1985, 1988, 2002), Madison (2005), and Denzin (1997, 2001, 2003). Voices of parents are brought together to name their shared joys and difficulties. The listener can experience parents' decisions, changes in attitude, surprise, self-appraisal, directness, and love for their children with genetic conditions; all lead to breadth of interpretive sufficiency. We have attempted to keep the dialogue free from stereotypes. Health practitioners have stated that from their experience the parents' voices are clearly representative. Many who have heard this text have reported that they had not previously understood the complexities of having children with genetic conditions. The intimacy of the parents' conversations moves us and encourages us to know more. Listening to this text shows us parental epiphanies; a parent who was surprised that health practitioners could be so caring; a mother who understood that she did not want to lose the child in the illness; the grandmother who held that her child could grow up to be anything he wanted to be and break the curse of the disease. These are the hoped-for outcomes when a text is performed. We see this performance text as Denzin (2003) considered it: a complementary form of research publication and an "alternative way of interpreting and presenting the results of an ethnographer's work" (p. 13). We took empirical knowledge gained from the interviews and created an ethnographic representation of how the parents view their lives and of how we responded to those stories. The text represents the authentic voices of the parents and brings different voices to bear on the same issues.

Implications for Nursing

How would a nurse go about using a performance text? I (CS) performed this text in June 2005 as part of a symposium at the Seventh International Family Nursing Conference in Victoria, British Columbia, Canada. The other two panel members used data from the same study to highlight the ways in which genetic conditions were disclosed to parents (Angst, Knafl, & Gallo, 2005), to analyze how parent data clustered on two of the structured measures (Knafl, Knafl, Gallo, & Angst, 2005), and to discuss how parents shared information with their children about genetic conditions (Gallo, Angst, Knafl, Hadley, & Smith, 2005). The symposium was slated as a mixed-methods presentation, each presenter focusing on a different aspect of the study with different methods of data analysis, so that the audience had the opportunity to learn about several facets of the study. The performance text provided a dialogical approach from which attendees could hear the voices of the parents speaking about their experiences, meet the parents in Denzin's (2001, 2003) liminal space, and, finally, experience the lives of the parents themselves.

Nursing students have responded positively to performance texts. Hearing and engaging with a text is a way for students to appreciate the lived experience of family members or how a family member deals with a major health issue, such as the birth of a child with a genetic condition. We all respond to and can learn from a storied text; an autoethnographic description of a nursing approach to patient education or care is a useful way for students to learn from a clinical instructor. Students can also learn that performance ethnography is a valid and powerful way of presenting research findings.

Our UIC College of Nursing had its second "Arts and Humanities Day" in February 2006. We decided to involve members of the community near the College, undergraduate and graduate students as well as faculty, in a presentation of performance texts. We shared the many ways in which we care for ourselves, for those with whom we work and learn, and for those in our community. There were texts highlighting ethnographic research as well as nursing's response to the war in Iraq. We heard veterans from the Veterans' Administration hospital across the street and young women with disabilities from a nearby rehabilitation program with whom one of our undergraduates volunteers. Nursing students and faculty hunger for forums where they can express the value and knowledge of their work in new ways. This was a chance for the entire College and surrounding community to enjoy its own talents and meaningful stories.

Nurses in clinical settings can use performance texts as a way of helping patients comprehend a newly diagnosed condition or teaching them management of their health when they are discharged from a clinical setting. This is the kind of conversation commonly seen in nursing practice and research where all parties contribute. These texts can be taken from memories of other patients for whom the nurse has provided care as well as from the nurse's clinical knowledge. With performance text, an individual does not necessarily need to stand up and declaim the story, nor does it mean that the text must be performed for a large audience. Sitting with a family member and telling him or her the story could lead to that "dialogical moment" when the storyteller, the story, and the listener meet, leading to enhanced knowledge or understanding.

The telling of a story through performance ethnography is a qualitative method that can be used readily in nursing. It draws the audience and the performer together in a shared moment of understanding and, in many cases, points the way to action. The received information fosters dialogue that can create new insights into more appropriate nursing responses with our clients or patients. Performance ethnography provides another means for nurses to achieve the goal of a clear understanding of human needs and conditions for improved quality of care.

Authors' Note

We thank team members. Denise Angst, DNSc, Suzanne Feetham, PhD, RN, FAAN, Emily Hadley, MS, RN, and Kathy Knafl, PhD, FAAN, for their review of previous drafts of the article. Research is funded by the Ethical, Legal, and Social Issues (ELSI) research program of the National Human Genome Research Institute (NHGRI), ROI HG0236.

References

Alexander, B. (2005). Performance ethnography: The reenacting and inciting of culture. In N. K. Denzin & Y. S. Lincoln (Eds.). *The Sage handbook of qualitative research* (3rd ed., pp. 411–441). Thousand Oaks, CA: Sage.

Angst, D., Knafl, K., & Gallo, A. (2005, June). *Uncovering a melody: Using thematic analysis to characterize parents perspectives surrounding diagnosis of a child with genetic condition.* Paper presented at the Seventh International Family Nursing Conference, Victoria, Canada.

Carlson, M. (2004). *Performance: A critical introduction* (2nd ed.). New York: Routledge.

Conquergood, D. (1985). Performance as a moral act: Ethical dimensions of the ethnography of performance. *Literature in Performance, 5,* 1–13.

Conquergood, D. (1988). Health theatre in a Hmong refugee camp: Performance, communication and culture. *Drama Review: A Journal of Performance Studies, 32,* 174–208.

Conquergood, D. (2002). Performance studies: Interventions and radical research. *Drama Review: A Journal of Performance Studies, 46,* 145–156.

Denzin, N. K. (1997). *Interpretive ethnography: Ethnographic practice for the 21st century.* Thousand Oaks, CA: Sage.

Denzin, N. K. (1999). Performing Montana. In B. Glassner and R. Hertz (Eds.), *Qualitative sociology as daily life* (pp. 147–158). Thousand Oaks, CA: Sage Publications.

Denzin, N. K. (2001). *Interpretive interactionism* (2nd ed.). Thousand Oaks, CA: Sage.

Denzin, N. K. (2003). *Performance ethnography: Critical pedagogy and the politics of culture.* Thousand Oaks, CA: Sage.

Denzin, N. K., & Lincoln, Y. L. (Eds.). (2000). *Handbook of qualitative research* (2nd ed.). Thousand Oaks, CA: Sage.

Denzin, N. K., & Lincoln, Y. L. (Eds.). (2005). *The Sage handbook of qualitative research* (3rd ed.). Thousand Oaks, CA: Sage.

Ellis, C., & Bochner, A. P. (2004). *The ethnographic I: A methodological novel about autoethnography.* Walnut Creek, CA: AltaMira.

Gallo, A., Angst, D., Knafl, K., Hadley, E., & Smith, C. (2005). Parents sharing information with their children about genetic conditions, *Journal of Pediatric Health Care, 19,* 267–275.

Geertz, C. (1973). *The interpretation of cultures: Selected essays.* New York: Basic Books.

Goffman, E. (1974). *Frame analysis.* Garden City, NY: Doubleday.

Hall, C., & White, S. (2005). Looking inside professional practice: Discourse, narrative and ethnographic approaches to social work and counselling. *Qualitative Social Work, 4,* 379–390.

Harrison, D. (2005). Context of change in community mental health occupational therapy: Part one. *International Journal of Therapy and Rehabilitation, 12,* 396–400.

Hoppes, S. (2005). Meanings and purposes of caring for a family member: An autoethnography. *American Journal of Occupational Therapy, 59,* 262–272.

Jago, B. (2006). A primary act of imagination: An autoethnography of father-absence. *Qualitative Inquiry, 12,* 398–426.

Knafl, G., Knafl, K., Gallo, A., & Angst, D. (2006). *Patterns of functioning in families having a child with a genetic condition.* Unpublished manuscript.

Lather, P. (2000). Against empathy, voice, and authenticity. *Women, Gender, and Research, 4,* 16–25.

Madison, D. (2005). *Critical ethnography: Method, ethics and performance.* Thousand Oaks, CA: Sage.

Manderson, L. (2005). Boundary breaches: The body, sex and sexuality after stoma surgery. *Social Science & Medicine, 61,* 405–415.

McLaren, P. (1999). *Schooling as a ritual performance: Toward a political economy of educational symbols and gestures* (3rd ed.). Lanham, MD: Rowman & Littlefield.

Mish, F. (Ed.). (2003). *Merriam-Webster online.* Retrieved August 18, 2005, from http://www. m-w.com/dictionary/

Perry, J., Lynam, M. J., & Anderson, J. M. (2006). Resisting vulnerability: The experiences of families who have kin in hospital – A feminist ethnography. *International Journal of Nursing Studies, 43,* 173–184.

Smith, A. D. (1993). *Fires in the mirror: Crown Heights, Brooklyn, and other identities.* Garden City, NY: Anchor.

Smith, A. D. (1994). *Twilight: Los Angeles, 1992.* Garden City, NY: Anchor.

Stevens, C. A. (2006). Being healthy: Voices of adolescent women who are parenting. *Journal for Specialists in Pediatric Nursing, 11,* 28–40.

Stevens, N., & Delamont, S. (2006). Balancing the *Berimban, Qualitative Inquiry, 12,* 316–339.

Tsai, J. H. (2006). Use of computer technology to enhance immigrant families' adaptation. *Journal of Nursing Scholarship, 38,* 87–93.

Turner, V. (1969). *The ritual process: Structure and anti-structure,* Chicago: Aldine.

Turner, V. (1982). *From ritual to theatre.* New York: Performing Arts Journal.

Weeks, M. R., Mosack, K. E., Abbott, M., Sylla, L. N., Valdes B., & Prince, M. (2004). Microbicide acceptability among high-risk urban U.S. women: Experiences and perceptions of sexually transmitted HIV prevention. *Sexually Transmitted Diseases, 31,* 682–690.

Weems, M. (2002). *I speak from the wound that is my mouth,* New York: Peter Lang.

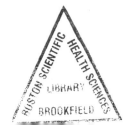

36

(Re)Writing Ethnography: The Unsettling Questions for Nursing Research Raised by Post-Structural Approaches to 'The Field'

Trudy Rudge

Introduction

A [researching nurse] is like a shipwrecked person who learns how to live in a certain sense *with* the land, not *on* it, not like Robinson Crusoe whose goal is to colonize his little island, but more like Marco Polo, whose sense of the marvellous never fails him, and who is always a traveller, a provisional guest, not a freeloader, conqueror, or raider (p 43–44).[1]

This is a story from the field that explores dynamics that are inherent in the research process and embedded in the 'texts' of ethnography. It outlines how, as a researcher, I came to recognize that I was not like Robinson Crusoe, rather I positioned myself, and was positioned by others, more like the guest and traveller suggested by Said.[1] As a nurse, researching nursing, it became only too apparent that 'the nurse' within me, a nursing subjectivity, was a crucial aspect of my participation in 'the field'. Such positioning frequently blurred and unsettled my, in hindsight, rather naive conceptualization of ethnographic research. How I wrote the observational record, how the nurses and patients used these notes, and how the notes recorded my positioning became a source of unsettling and challenging thoughts about the research process.

Source: *Nursing Inquiry,* 3(3) (1996): 146–152.

All of my studies, reading and preparation for this research did not prepare me for how these records told me as much about 'the researcher' as they did 'the researched'. Exploring my field notes for authorial positioning led to a fuller understanding of the ethics of research, the perspective and rhetoric embedded in the notion of participant observation, as well as a way in which to incorporate post-structural perspectives into the research process itself. What follows in this paper is some discussion of current understandings about participant observation and ethnographic research. I will then explore, through the examination of one field observation, the different positionings evidenced within the field notes. The observation that formed the basis of this paper was two and half hours in duration, due to part of the observation being some discussion with the patient and the nurse after the dressing procedure had been completed.

The Disappearing Field

As an undergraduate student of anthropology during the late 70s and early 80s, I witnessed what appeared to be the expansion of ethnography into the analysis of deviant, but colourful sub-cultures, or rural backwaters, of 'late monopoly capitalist' society. There was much soul searching on the ethics of applied anthropology (given its work with mining companies; more recently with various Land Councils), on the ethics of 'doing the natives', and on the ethics of covert research or the exploitation of the host culture as part of an academic career. Ethnography, as a research process and outcome, continued to cross disciplinary boundaries, forming alliances with psychology, medicine and law, as well as spawning enclaves of cultural analysis in geography, history, education, and even stronger links with its epistemological roots in philosophy.

Indeed, women anthropologists using feminist perspectives re-analysed exotic cultures from women's point of view, reconceptualized the concepts of the economic exchange of women, sexuality and social taboos, and kinship practices, and highlighted the importance of race and class as confounding and compounding factors on women's position. It was always obvious to me that the debates about knowledge construction and underpinning epistemological positions were central to anthropology's understanding of its 'field'. Was it appropriate to analyse primitive culture from the perspective of structural marxism? Were Western feminist perspectives, predicated as they were on different structural realities, the appropriate approach for 'island' cultures? How could ethnographers consistently deny the cultural imperialism of white ethnographies of African cultures, which disavowed the effect of tribal affiliations in Africa's political context or the central role of apartheid in the political economy of South Africa? Indeed, all of these questions challenged anthropology's assumptions.

(Re)Writing the Field

Writing in 1992, Hammersley questioned where ethnography was going and the problematic nature of it assuming a critical inflection.[2] Hammersley doubted whether such moves would overcome the problems of validity and relevance, which he considered accompanied the ethnographic method. He suggested, similar to Simon and Dippo[3] and Carr and Kemmis,[4] that participant or practitioner research may overcome ideological distortions and power imbalances currently embedded in this research process. In summing up ethnography's future. Hammers-ley suggested that both participant observation and ethnographies might need to be re-thought, or even renamed, to more accurately represent the form of research entailed. Furthermore, Hammersley suspected that the deconstruction of the dichotomy of quantitative/qualitative research methods would further destabilize its position within the domain of qualitative research.

Even such 'classical' ethnographers as Geertz[5] are currently challenging how interpretation of discourses of informants occurs and how the field notes are considered, as well as the ethnography itself. In opening up 'the field' for consideration as a text, Clifford welcomed this critique of empiricism and its attendant privileging of the 'ethnographic gaze' (see also Clough,[7] Van Maanen,[8] Clifford[9]).[6] Further, Clifford asserted, the time that it has taken for this critique to surface is indicative of how strong the belief is, within the social sciences, in ethnography's purported transparency and congruence with reality and experience. The role language played in the method was masked by a position that asserted that ethnography was simply 'writing reduced to method: keeping good field notes, making accurate maps, "writing up" results' (p. 2).[6] As Geertz,[10] Clifford[6] and Pratt[11] all suggested, ethnography is as much about writing as it is participation in the 'field'. Such writing contains the personal narrative of the participants, both direct and interpreted by the researcher, the narrative of the researcher's journey and the narrative of the research outcomes themselves.[11] As such, Clifford contended that ethnography, as text, invents culture rather than fully representing cultural reality described within its texts.[6] He further argued, along with Tyler,[12] that ethnographies are constructed according to particular textual rules set by the academy, and represent 'ethnographic fictions' (see Geertz[10]), which cannot claim to be 'truth' or to accurately correspond with the culture written about in the text Consequently, ethnographic writings can, at best, claim to be partial in that they are 'something made or fashioned',[6] but also in the sense put forward by Gore[13] and Ellsworth[14] that they are representations both partial and partisan.

As Clough asserted with regard to the current textual practices and narratives in sociology, not only does the narrative construction of ethnography construct an empirical reality, it 'enacts for sociological discourse the authority of the storyteller, in the figure of the *heroic ethnographer* ... Ethnography is the productive icon of empirical scientific authority' (p. 2, emphasis added).[7]

With the dissolution of its colonial 'field' as I outlined earlier,[6] ethnography, both as process and outcome, has been problematized for its ethnocentric focus; for its unquestioning belief in the unitary nature of the ethnographer 'subject'; and for the primacy afforded the knowledge produced by such a unitary 'subject' ethnographer.[7]

Clough considered that while acknowledging the dissolution of the field of ethnography, Clifford did not sufficiently extend his analysis to explain the interrelationship between narrative and empirical reality. She claimed that the desire for unity of the subject remains unacknowledged within ethnographic works. Clough highlighted how postmodern reflections on desire, which has embedded within it an awareness of how such desire is unconsciously motivated, suggests that both ethnographer and informant are motivated by unconscious desire in the 'picture' they present (see Bourdieu[15]). To conceive of these texts as unaffected by such desire, Clough argued, is to deny how we construct such narratives. Further, Pratt suggested that the dominant metaphors of ethnography, that is participant observation, data collection and cultural description, are imbued with unconscious desires of mastery over knowledge and appropriation of the cultures described within them.[11] More problematically for nurses researching nursing, these metaphorical positions assume continuation of 'the outsider' standpoint.

But can we, as Clough suggested, open ethnography and its textual records if we view them as but textual mediations of reality? Does this open paths to new forms of text, new forms of resistance to the hegemonic discourses that seek closure and empirical certainty? Would such contestation and constitution of the various subject positions open to the 'ethnographic hero' prevent premature closure of the textual record of such inquiry? The result she suggested would be 'textual fields' of resistant knowledges, openly partial and partisan. What follows is an attempt to open up one such record, to explore the positionings evident within it and to detect the influences upon that record. Voices within a particular text are evidence of positions afforded within them.[16] Similarly, they are evidence of the power relations underpinning language use in the formation of knowledge or truth claims as they relate these to espoused positions. In exploring my field notes for positionings within them, I will raise more questions than answers. Marcus suggested that application of postmodernism and poststructuralism result in 'messy texts'.[17] These texts resist totalizing effects of traditional ethnography, and in opening field notes to this critique I suggest that this record, even before analysis, conveys much about the messiness of research.

Researcher Presence: Positioned by the Researched and the Research

The notes are from an observation of a dressing procedure for a patient in a burns unit. The patient had been in the unit for two months, and six days prior to my observation he had undergone his third debridement and skin grafting. He had been showered, clean dressings had been applied to his still burnt skin, and he was back in bed to have his recent skin grafts receive their second radical trimming and clean up. In the case notes, it was noted that the patient's newer areas of grafting needed trimming, and some assessment was made of the areas that required further grafting. The nurse doing this had worked in the unit for six years. I had been present in the unit for three months and focusing on this patient since the first week of his admission to the ward. At this stage, I had several informal discussions with the nurse, and had been present at most of the dressings this patient had undergone since his first week in hospital. What follows is an excerpt from my records for this patient.

> Today Gary's dressing is to be done by Susan. The first parts of the dressing were done in the bathroom, that is Gary washed under the shower and parts of the dressing were then done in his room. The areas that had recently been operated on now these new grafts could be more extensively trimmed and cleaned up as they were more stable and therefore need to be attended to by a more senior nurse. The parts which needed to be attended were his flanks and the areas on his arms. Susan waited until Gary was back in bed to do them as they were quite extensive. She explained to me that what she is doing is an extended clean up of the areas of graft which were over some are is which were granulating, areas of graft which were in fact doubled up and radical trimming and cleaning up of serous ooze which had built up around some grafts. She explained to Gary that these areas needed to be cleaned up as they could become infected or would not heal properly. I asked her why she was doing it because a GNP had helped Gary with his shower. She said that it needed a practised eye, one that could see the difference between the various types of skin that were now evident on Gary's grafted areas. Some of the areas might need new skin grafts or would need some attention which unless you knew what you were looking at you would not see that it actually needed cleaning up. Also some of the grafts were quite fragile and easily damaged and this took some practice to work out whether they should stay or be cleaned up.

Nursing Researcher or Nurse–Researcher

This extract from my field notes shows some of the voices evident in the notes, and the positioning afforded within them. This was the first time that I had worked with this nurse, but certainly not the first time that we had talked. I have largely written the observation in narrative form: a story of a particular nurse doing a particular patient's dressing. Within the talk at the beginning of the dressing, the nurse positioned herself as someone who needs to provide information to both the patient and to me. She has provided different types of information though. For me, she has provided information that suggests that I understand the language of wound care, speaking to me about serous ooze, granulating tissue and trimming grafts. Her assumption is that I understand the scientific framing of the dressing and the actual timing of this extensive 'trimming'. Such talk positions me as informed with the basic understanding of the process, and with an understanding of wound healing and graft care requirements. At the same time, she is also aware of my 'information' needs as a researcher, explaining why she had come to do this dressing even though that day the patient was cared for by a first-year registered nurse.

It is this desire for information that of course drives most research that we undertake. To be aware of how we use this information is perhaps the key issue here. The notes contain a signal to me of an aspect of the care which I need to take note of; its primacy indicated by its situation at the beginning of the observation notes. The idea of experience and knowledge alluded to in the nurse's use of the term 'the practised eye' came to be one of the key aspects of care that differentiated nurses from each other. However, my noting of difference and positioning, as well as experience, does not surface unintentionally – it is loaded with desire. I am searching for such occurrences because of the post-structural theoretical perspectives and literature about nursing practice informing my research. But as is also evident, this was solicited by my inquiry as to why this nurse was doing this dressing. As Clough suggested it is difficult to explicate whose desire is surfacing here.[7] Why did I ask the question? Was I seeking to confirm something I had noted before? Why did the nurse answer in the way that she did?

There are other influences evident in this section of the record. Indeed, in the record it is apparent that I am observing the wound as well as the dressing process itself. I explain in the field notes about grafts and how the wound looks in that areas which were granulating, areas of graft which were in fact doubled up and needed radical trimming and cleaning up of serous ooze which had built up around some grafts'. But the question I ask of this record is, 'who is talking here'. Is it nurse, researcher or nurse–researcher? All through the field notes, I find instances of this blurring of boundaries in my positioning within the textual record. It seems that at times, I am positioning myself within the knowledge system of wound care 'science' and that my notes speak with this voice. At other times, the nurses position me as co-worker with 'special' information needs about the processes within the unit. In this observation record, the nurse assumes some form of knowledge, but when I ask her why she is actually doing the dressing she provides me with vital confirmation, not only about what the dressing entails but about an element of the nurses' work which would come to be pivotal in differentiating what was happening on the unit.

Moreover, in 'traditional' ethnography, there is a position for this nurse. She is a 'key' informant, someone who assists the ethnographer to mark out the significant parts of the research observations, as well as assist in discussion about these observations. These moments of insight are evident in the observational record by the way in which I privilege them at the beginning of the record, or highlight them by turning my record from a description of the observation into an interpretation of what I see and hear.

Researcher Absence: Silencing by the Research

It is also evident from this observational record and the discussion afterwards that I actively change my own positioning. At times, my presence in the notes disappears. When and how this happens is the key to understanding the position of researcher.

> While she was cleaning the areas with saline, forceps and fine scissors, the nurse took the opportunity to point out to the patient the sorts of things that he needed to do to get going again. Susan: For example, because your hands have been grafted, you need to use your hands. One of the ways you can do this is to put the cream on yourself (this was the Nutra-D cream that is used to keep the grafted skin supple and moisturized). When you do this you will have to get used to opening the jar, and used to the feel of putting on the cream and having to reach behind to stretch your arms and shoulders. This will help to get your body used to moving again. You'll get used to how your new skin feels and to learn how much pressure it can take as well as what feels right and what doesn't. It's all part of getting used to the way things would feel like now … This will double up as good exercise for your hands and help to get the fine movement back in your fingers. Having to stretch to get to awkward areas will help in getting the movement back into your arms and shoulders. Gary: Yes I have started to do that a bit more. But it still hurts and I don't really know what I can do. Susan: I know. But the longer you leave it, the longer it will take to get moving again. You might have to work against some of the pain. We can give you some lighter pain relief to help and each day will get easier because you will be able to move easier than the day before.

The Paradox of Researcher Silence

The notes relate the conversation in detail (only an excerpt is shown here), with the voices of the nurse and patient taking the main part of the notes. My presence is recorded only in my observation of what they were doing at the time they were having this conversation. Such absences can be identified throughout my observational field notes. This raises the question of how and why I disappear. My main aim in this research was to observe and analyse nurse–patient interactions during the processes of wound care, thus to intervene with my own observations or talk would be to prejudice this aspect of the research process. My silence is essential so that I can analyse, as an outsider, an interaction between nurse and patient. Evidenced within the observation is a nurse at work with a patient, seeking to have him understand his role in his recovery, but at the same time providing him with information about the recovery process and how the nursing staff can assist with this. I noted the talk in order to provide evidence of the textually mediated practice of nurses and patients; to explore the discursive framing of their talk as social practice to uncover the assumptions and taken-for-granted background to their work,[18] just as I am observing to see how this impacts on nursing practice.

But what of the post-structural researcher who would insist that the researcher, and their paradigmatic influence, is never absent. Well, it is evident I am not. Paradoxically, I am present in my absence, because this is a central focus of my research. I am present by the special position accorded to such interactions within my research notes; in the record of nurses discussing a particular patient's wound care, psychosocial needs, pain relief measures; in the detail of conversations between nurses and patients; in the detail of conversations I had with patients about the care provided for them. I am present in how I talk about the climate of the interaction, how I observe the reaction of the patient or nurses within the conversations, and in the questions I ask about the observation or in more formal interviews. The questions come from my research perspective and the focus that my observations came to take. I am apparent also in the focus on not so much what explicitly happened in each dressing but the noted differences, how each nurse approached the dressing, and what they and the patients said to each other and to me.

In informal discussion with this nurse, she picked up on the idea of experience and how this allowed her to provide the patient with examples of what could happen and how he could help himself. This nurse was able to identify, when we talked later, how she has changed her practices to take opportunities to talk with patients about their treatment, their progress and what they can do to help themselves – in effect, how she negotiates interaction with patients. Discussion based around the observational record also allowed the nurse to identify how her way of doing 'procedures' had changed over time and now took place in a way very different from when she had first worked in the unit.

Such discussion highlighted for me how, in working with each nurse, I needed to keep alert to how each nurse positioned me during the observation. Not all nurses were able to position me 'with' them. Some wanted me to be the distant observer, working hard to ignore my presence, others thought I needed information about the science of wound care, and others talked to me and to the patient, and positioned me in what I came to interpret as a privileged 'blurred' position. I came to view what happened to me during each dressing as an indicator of 'comfort' level with my presence, which some nurses came to terms with and others did not. Sometimes, the nurse putting me into the position of 'fly on the wall' became a part of the discussion of the observation record, and came to be a way of identifying their own comfort with their position of nurse practitioner. The effect of my presence showed, as Street has suggested, the problematic nature of visibility in nursing practice.[19]

Many of these nurses were still coming to terms with work on the unit, and when we talked about the dressing afterwards, they would often point out why they had not answered patient questions or had not taken this time to interact with the patient in other ways. Others, more comfortable with their work and with my presence, incorporated me into discussions, at different levels and in differing ways, viewing my needs as different from theirs and different from the patients. Such positioning is evident in the different way that the nurse talked to me and to the patient. In this way, it became apparent to me that nurses and patients who were being observed were actively positioning me, taking account of me. Such effects would imply that Hammersley's critique of ethnographic method has some substance. It would also suggest that desire 'to inform' is continuously problematic (see Bourdieu[15]), and to consider that informants are not 'present', or neutral, in the information they give is to deny the effects of research on 'the researched' and their lives.

Patient and Researcher Presence: Researcher as In Between

Indeed, these interpretations of the observed practices acted, for most nurses, as ways of focusing discussion we had that led to very fruitful insights for us. As I highlighted, the nurse was able to say how, when she read the observation, she wondered if she had not been too hard on the patient at that time. We talked about how difficult it is to choose the 'right' moment to provide some forms of information, and how difficult it was to motivate these patients. This next excerpt highlights what I specifically identify as 'different' in this observation.

> This was the first time that anyone had suggested this to the patient and in some ways he told me that he was taken aback by it. He said that part of not doing anything had come from not being sure as to what he could do and that no-one else had told him this.

On looking back through my field notes I confirmed that no other nurse had informed him of his part in his recovery, or had chosen the dressing time as an opportunity to do this. Many had asked him to wash himself; very few ever said why. But in talking with the patient about what was said, it was also a time for him to share some of the ways he was feeling at this particular time. Because each of the patients who agreed to participate in this study became the focus of my study at that time, each of them 'became' very used to my presence. They also often positioned me as confidante, always it seemed to me as 'nurse' someone they could talk to about what was happening and how they felt, and in some respects as someone outside of the care situation. I do not, however, wish to gloss this situation. Not all patients were as open, or told me everything, but they did position me as an outsider who had a different perspective from the nurses providing them with care.

This was a very difficult position for me to take, one circumscribed and inscribed with ethical dilemmas, which abound in such research. On the one hand, I was positioned as confidante (which may at times place me outside of the nursing position and with the patient), and conversely it was also apparent that patients were always aware that I was a nurse as well. Using my notes in this way opened up very different forms of discussion with patients and nurses, and made evident the different positions open to them in the situation. In talking about this observation, the patient told me of the context of his feelings at the time. He was lonely, homesick and depressed. He was worried about his wife and children and told me that he felt guilty about the way in which the accident had interfered with and endangered his life – a deeply 'personal' response. What became apparent to me from these talks with patients was that their talk signalled a 'resistant positioning and discourse.[16,20] Such talk gave me their positioning, and indeed how complex this was. The patient described a positioning of a 'life on hold', away from his familiar environment, at a moment when he was feeling 'down' and coming to terms with his part in his recovery. It is also obvious that his positioning is fragmented by the incident, by his responsibilities at home, by the uncertainties that surround the entire healing process.

In some ways I was privileged with both sides of the story. However, alerted to the idea of desire, I sometimes wondered whether patients confided in me so that I could act as a bridge. It was always possible that discussion about how they felt at that time were therapeutic in their outcomes. At other times, I believe that the patients used these discussions as interpretive bridges, in the belief that such information would inevitably get back to the nurses. But should I pass such information on? How would this position me, and was what we were talking about to remain in confidence between me and the patient?

Conclusion

This paper has outlined researcher/researched positioning evidenced within one observational record in research into nursing–patient interactions focused on one nursing procedure. What it exposes is how researcher positioning is not static, neither is the position of informant or participant. It also suggests that researching in the clinical context as a nurse means it is difficult to re-move oneself from the research, even when nurses locate you as outside of the event. As author of such notes, it is important to recognize 'author' pos-itions, as well as 'researched' positions, in the discursive framings of such notes. They not only indicate power relations within the text, but also the dynamics in the positionings by all participants in the research.[21] To deny effects of any one of these positions is to disavow the desire for mastery of the field evident when maintaining the 'outsider' researcher positioning of trad-itional ethnography.

While I recognize that this is but one record in a long study, I believe it does provide evidence of how a 'post' positioning challenges the myth of objectivity. Such analysis also renders problematic research that seeks to remove 'the nurse' from research within nursing. As this research focused on a single nursing procedure, much of the day-to-day work within the unit escaped analysis. As Marcus would suggest, in seeking a research focus and by (re)analysis of field notes it becomes evident how much of this record 'remains the surplus of difference beyond, and perhaps because of our circumscription' (p. 567).[17] Marcus warned that research will only provide a partial and partisan 'reality'. In troubling the transparency and congruence of these notes, I would position myself as one who wonders, not colonizes; travels with 'the researched' rather than conquering the field; and recognizes how we all have come to live with, not excavate, the field of nursing.

References

1. Said E. *Representations of the Intellectual.* London: Vintage, 1994.
2. Hammersley M. *What's Wrong with Ethnography: Methodological Explorations.* London: Routledge, 1992.
3. Simon R & Dippo D. On critical ethnographic work. *Anthropology and Educational Quarterly* 1986; **17**: 195–202.
4. Carr W & Kemmis S. *Becoming Critical: Knowing through Action Research.* Victoria: Deakin University Press, 1986.
5. Geertz C. Making experience, authoring selves. In: Turner VW & Bruner EM (eds). *The Anthropology of Experience.* Urbana: University of Illinois, 1986.
6. Clifford J. *The Predicament of Culture.* Cambridge: Harvard University Press, 1988.
7. Clough PT. *The End(s) of Ethnography: From Realism to Social Criticism.* Newbury Park: Sage, 1992.
8. Van Maanen J. *Tales of the Field: On Writing Ethnography.* Chicago: University of Chicago Press, 1988.
9. Clifford J & Marcus GE (eds). *Writing Culture: The poetics and Politics of Ethnography.* Berkeley: University of California Press, 1986.
10. Geertz C. *Local Knowledge: Further Essays in Interpretive Anthropology.* New York: Basic Books, 1983.
11. Pratt ML. Fieldwork in common places. In: Clifford J & Marcus GE (eds). *Writing Culture: The Poetics and Politics of Ethnography.* Berkeley: University of California Press 1986.
12. Tyler S. Post-modern ethnography: From document of the occult to occult document. In: Clifford J & Marcus GE (eds). *Writing Culture: The Poetics and Politics of Ethnography.* Berkeley: University of California Press, 1986.
13. Gore J. What can we do for you? What *can* 'we' do for 'you'? Struggling over empowerment in critical feminist pedagogy. In: Luke C & Gore J (eds). *Feminism and Critical Pedagogy.* New York: Routledge, 1992.
14. Ellsworth E. Why doesn't this feel empowering? Working through the repressive myths of critical pedagogy. In: Luke C & Gore J (eds). *Feminism and Critical Pedagogy.* New York: Routledge, 1992.
15. Bourdieu P. *Outline of a Theory of Practice.* Cambridge: Cambridge University Press, 1977.
16. Cheek J & Rudge T Webs of documentation: the discourse of case notes. *Australian Journal of Communication* 1994; **21** (2): 41–52.

17. Marcus GE What comes (just) after "Post"? The case of ethnography. In: Denzin NK & Lincoln YS (eds). *Qualitative Methods.* New York: Sage, 1994; 563–574.
18. Fairclough N. *Language and Power.* London: Longman, 1989.
19. Street AF *Inside Nursing: A Critical Ethnography of Clinical Nursing Practice.* New York: State University of New York Press, 1992.
20. Buchbinder D. *Masculinities and Identities.* Melbourne: Melbourne University Press, 1994.
21. Bruni N. Reshaping ethnography: contemporary post-positivist possibilities. *Nursing Inquiry* 1995; **2**: 44–52.

Narrative Research

37

How People with Motor Neurone Disease Talk about Living with Their Illness: A Narrative Study

Janice Brown and Julia Addington-Hall

Introduction

L iving with a life-limiting neurological condition such as motor neurone disease (MND) is challenging, frightening and disabling (Krivickas *et al.* 1997, Brown 2003). The diagnosis of MND means that people face progressive physical decline manifested through incremental disability (Hebert *et al.* 2005). In the absence of curative treatments, patients, family carers and professionals must deal with complex and increasing needs for care.

Studies reveal a range of problems that can beset patients with MND, including increasing social isolation, loss of mobility and the ability to communicate (Leigh *et al.* 2003). However, there is little evidence about how people manage these problems (Rigby *et al.* 1999) or how they live with MND (Small & Rhodes 2000, Brown 2003).

Background

Motor Neurone Disease

The biomedical course of MND is becoming better understood (Howard & Orrell 2002, Leigh *et al.* 2003). One pharmacological treatment, riluzole, can prolong survival by 2–4 months (Miller *et al.* 2000), but uncertainty remains

Source: *Journal of Advanced Nursing*, 62(2) (2008): 200–208.

about life expectancy, pattern of muscle weakness and timing of symptoms. Intellect generally remains, intact although cognitive impairment has been reported in approximately 5% of people (Leigh *et al.* 2003). The low global incidence of MND is approximately 2:100,000 (Mandrioli *et al.* 2003, Motor Neurone Disease Association 2007) and, although survival is often cited as between 2 and 5 years (Holmes 2005), this depends on the type of MND. Three principal types have been identified (Beresford 1995): amyotrophic lateral sclerosis (ALS), progressive bulbar palsy (PBP) and progressive muscular atrophy (PMA). More recently, progressive lateral sclerosis (PLS) has been identified (Ince *et al.* 2003). Although each type has a unique presentation, symptoms may merge over time.

We know that newly diagnosed people have specific needs, such as for practical information about the illness and knowledge of their entitlements to services, whereas patients living for longer seek information about treatments, therapies and research (Hughes *et al.* 2005). We also know that there is a need to improve information and communication between healthcare professionals and users (Carter *et al.* 1998, Hughes *et al.* 2005). Brown *et al.* (2006) identifed that patients and families would welcome increased knowledge amongst professionals about MND and the allocatation of a key worker to help manage the complex systems of services. However, Carter *et al.* (1998) found that the responses of professionals caring for people with MND were often negative, particularly in terms of the limited hope they felt able to offer patients. Small and Rhodes (2000) identified the place of uncertainty in living with MND and how denial is one strategy that patients use in dealing with the illness, although Beresford (1995) suggests that continual denial may be more destructive than useful.

The importance of patients and carers in influencing services is central to enhancing care (Small & Rhodes 2000, Department of Health 2005) but information is needed about how people live with MND and how to establish ways of supporting them. Gathering stories from people with MND offers an approach to further develop this understanding. Stories are a crucial and integral part of human life as people are storytellers by nature (Lieblich *et al.* 1998). Hyden (1997, p. 49) considers that narratives are 'one of the most powerful forms for expressing suffering and experiences related to suffering'.

Using a Narrative Approach with Patients

There is evidence of a therapeutic influence from the use of narrative (Heiney 1995, Carlick & Biley 2004) for patients coping with cancer and amongst older people and adults with chronic illness (Chelf *et al.* 2000). Banks-Wallace (1999, p. 21) identifies that storylines 'help people cope with milestones or transitions' as they are often remembered long after facts and figures are forgotten (Kelly 1995), and the listener has time to process the content and reflect on their own situation. It is also known that healthcare professionals use stories as metaphors to help patients achieve their desired goals (Burns 2001), and that patient stories are used by clinical educators to develop medical students' understanding of patients' conditions (Charon *et al.* 1995).

Narratives are also one of the most important media through which we can define and shape our personal and cultural interactions. Skultans (1998) suggests that patient narratives tell two stories: the personal experience of the patient and the deeper cultural narrative. To think, through the telling of one's story, is to 'experience it affecting one's own life' (Frank 1995, p. 23) by integrating the remembered past from the perspective of the present. Through remembering, 'culturally available knowledge becomes situated knowledge, connected to a particular person, context and illness history' (Garro 2000, p. 72).

Theoretical Framework

The theoretical basis for the study reported here was social constructionism (Berger & Luckman 1966), where the assumption is that the telling of personal stories is important for the social construction of the self because selves are created, like culture and identity is revised and responsive to events and situations (Miller 1994). Somers (1994) supports this theoretical view that people construct identities (albeit mutiple and changing) by locating themselves within an exisiting limited repetoire of narratives existing in society and culture.

An approach to narrative analysis consistent with social constructivism is the examination of 'plot' or form of narrative. Frank (1995) draws on an existing repetoire of available 'plots' or storylines in society, such as heroism, so that the individual appears unique but in reality is a social creation. He identifies three narrative types in understanding chronic illness: a 'restitution' storyline reflecting a plot of adventure, how a person may seek how to be healthy again; a 'chaos' storyline reflecting a plot of anarchy in which there is a lost genesis and future; and a 'quest' storyline offering a sense of a suffering hero. Frank considers that the range of narrative types can be told as storylines, alternately and repeatedly across the journey of an illness, by one individual because 'no one actual telling conforms exclusively' (Frank 1995, p. 76). The storylines do not claim to be representative of people's characters or to offer a series of expected stages that someone might travel through; rather, they offer examples of how people tell their stories in different circumstances. Smith and Sparkes (2004) draw on Frank's theory to understand people's stories of living with spinal injury whereas others have examined narratives from an evaluative perspective as in multiple sclerosis (Gergen & Gergen 1983, Robinson 1990) identifying progressive, regressive and stability types of narratives. We do not know the storylines of people living with MND.

The Study

Aim

The aim of the study was to explore patient experiences and how they talk about living and coping with MND.

Design

Narrative case studies were used, the unit of analysis being a patient living in their own home or in a care home.

Participants

There is no UK database of people with MND but the MND Association estimates that they are aware of over 66% of those diagnosed. Patients were informed and invited to join the study through the MND Association's Regional Care Development Advisors (RCDAs), a method of recruitment used successfully in two previous studies (Brown 2003, Brown *et al.* 2006).

The inclusion criteria were a firm diagnosis of MND, ability to communicate at the point of recruitment, willingness to participate and being over 18 years of age.

Regional Care Development Advisors identified potential participants, from across four National Health Services (NHS) primary care trusts and gave out recruitment packs containing a letter of invitation to join the study, an information sheet and a reply slip. Potential participants were invited to return their reply slip to the researcher if they were interested in the study. On receipt of a completed reply slip the researcher contacted the potential participants to answer questions and, if appropriate, to recruit them into the study.

Thirteen participants across four types of MND was achieved (Table 1). It was anticipated that this number would be sufficient to reach data saturation. The age range was 39–85 years. The sample was a good match against national profile of gender, age and type of MND (Beresford 1995, Motor Neurone Disease Association 2007).

Table 1: Type of motor neurone disease (MND)

	Type of MND				
	Amyotrophic lateral sclerosis	Progressive bulbar palsy	Progressive muscular atrophy	Primary lateral sclerosis	Total
Male	5	1	1	2	9
Female	3	1	0	0	4
Total	8	2	1	2	13

Data Collection

Narrative interviews were used to collect the data. Participants were invited to be interviewed at three-monthly intervals over 18 months, resulting in six rounds of data collection.

Interviews addressed the research question 'How do people live and cope through MND?' Each interview was organized into three parts (Wengraf 2001): first, the patient narrative was guided by the question, 'I am interested in learning about how you are living and coping with MND. Please begin wherever you like. I will listen first, I won't interrupt you. I'll just take some notes in case I have any questions when you've finished telling your story'. In part two, the researcher sought further detail about particular issues. Part three involved asking generic questions including, 'What was important to you before your illness and what is important to you now?'.

Ethical Considerations

The study was approved by an NHS ethics committee. Participants were advised in an information sheet that it could be distressing to talk about their illness and of the need to discuss with the researcher potential supporters such as a friend or family member. Written consent was obtained. If a patient was unable to sign because of disability, they were invited to give oral consent in the presence of a witness and this was recorded in writing in the presence of the researcher. The researcher informed the MND Association of the study and they were available to participants via their telephone helpline.

Data Analysis

In narrative research, the researcher is intimately involved in both the process and product of the study (Horsburgh 2003) whereby reflexivity is essential to enhance trustworthiness (Grinyer 2002, Holloway & Freshwater 2007). Achieving reflexivity is 'not a straightforward endeavour' (Dowling 2006, p. 15) and three reflexive strategies were employed (i) questioning the data; (ii) maintaining a field journal and (iii) engagement with a mentor and advisory group. The analysis focused on the form and content of the narratives (Frank 1995). The first of five iterative stages (Figure 1) involved the researcher being immersed in the data from round one.

Questions were asked of the data in stage 2 of the analysis process, such as 'What does the story tell us about how the illness journey is being lived? and 'Are Frank's three narrative types recognizable across the stories?' Echoes of Frank's narrative types were difficult to untangle but, as Reissman (1993, p. 57) observes, the 'focus for analysis often emerges or becomes clearer as I see what respondents say'. Commonality of content across the narratives was

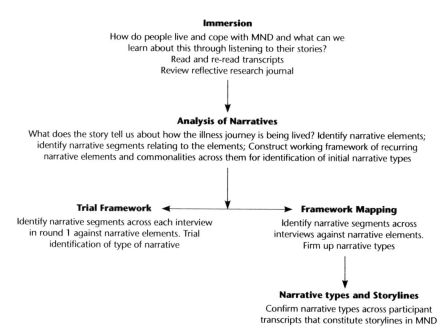

Figure 1: Iterative process for analysis of narratives about motor neurone disease

recognized as all participants told stories about their outlook on life, their attitude to the illness and how they managed changing circumstances; these were labelled narrative elements.

To substantiate these narrative elements, stage three of the analysis process involved identifying associated narrative segments from the transcripts. This process is 'not a technical operation but the stuff of analysis itself, the 'unpacking' of structure that is essential to interpretation' (Reissman 1993, p. 58). These narrative segments were copied verbatim from each transcript and placed in an EXCEL 2007 spreadsheet against the appropriate narrative element. This process led to the construction of the trial framework, an analytic device reflective of the work of Miles and Huberman (1994). This iterative process led to the development of new narrative elements being constructed, such as orientation to time (Table 2), and ultimately the overall framework map.

Scrutiny of all narrative segments within the framework map led to the final stage of analysis, understanding patterns of meaning, or storylines. For example,

Table 2: Narrative elements

Outlook on life
Attitude to the illness
Approach to managing changing circumstances
Orientation to time
Use of humour
Metaphors/descriptions
Approach to helping self

---

narrative segments from patients 1, 2 and 4 had similarities in form, reflecting a positive outlook on life, relating what could still be achieved rather than what was lost. In contrast, narrative segments from other patients (3 and 12) reflected their outlook on life as a fight against the prospect of death.

The incremental process of analysis facilitated dialogue and scrutiny of the process between the researcher (J. B) and mentor (J. A. H), as well the advisory group (two service users, three academics, two clinicians, one MND Association member), stimulating further researcher reflexivity and refinement of the framework, with the researcher recognizing 'In the final analysis, the work is ours. We have to take responsibility for its truths' (Reissman 1993, p. 67).

Findings

Four consistent types of narrative or storylines in MND were identified: sustaining, preserving, enduring and fracturing. Although the complete stories of some participants reflected a duality of narrative type or even all four types, the value of presenting the four narrative types as distinct entities is to appreciate their differences. This is not to detract from acknowledging that all four types can exist alongside each other in one person's story, as strands in a complex life. The names and circumstances have been changed to ensure anonymity.

Sustaining Narrative Storyline

The sustaining storyline is rich with what remains positive in life, expressing an outlook of what can be achieved rather than what may no longer be possible. It is underpinned by hope, albeit knowing that survival may be an ambitious desire.

Ms Green lived with her husband and two young children. She joined the study 5 months after diagnosis, when she was mobile but walking slowly and slightly dragging her right foot. She was able to talk but her words were soft, slow and carefully articulated although radiating the positive:

> I just think, well, I can still walk. I can still move. I can still do these things, so be grateful for that. So that's what I try and do. I mean, I still feel I could be a lot worse off. I mean I know everything's hard work but there's no pain with it…I'm not with drawers of tablets. (Ms Green)

Faced with increasing immobility was particularly hard:

> I hadn't used the wheelchair…I didn't want to because that was sort of accepting that you needed it whereas before that you could pretend you didn't, so I suppose it was a bit of denial, just try and keep as normal as possible as long as we can. (Ms Green)

But keeping up with her family was a keen motivator to use new equipment:

> Going on holiday was quite hard but we did have the wheelchair, so when I think of it we still went to see [all the attractions] and all of that, I can still do all of that, so that's what I try and focus on; the good things and not the bad things. (Ms Green)

She recognized that death might be imminent as her symptoms were progressing aggressively, but she took an objective approach, seeing two aspects at work: survival and managing her symptoms. She wanted to survive, and her approach in this regard was living positively each day, dealing with her symptoms one by one, day at a time. This approach engendered hope and in the life remaining:

> It's sort of a two layer thing. My overall principle of thinking is that I need to be a survivor, but underneath that, my practical side just says well, we can cope with this, this week; we can cope with that, that week. So, I suppose we are a little bit at odds with each other. But the longevity one is more about coping with the whole thing; the other one is more to do with the day to day side and to put them…you're not dealing with the MND, you're dealing with the fact your legs are not working or your arms are not working or I suppose I sort of isolate those things. (Ms Green)

Enduring Narrative Storyline

The enduring storyline tells us about quiet suffering when neither life nor death is the easier option. Enduring was a way to live through an unwelcome and difficult situation.

Mr White was confined to a chair, his arms and hands immobile. He had voluntarily entered a care home to reduce the care demands on his partner and to be in a place of safety. His neck muscles were weak but he used an environmental controller with his chin to control the TV, lights and call bell. He talked quietly but clearly:

> You get fed up with television and I go to bed about 9.30pm, that's my day. I sleep in the chair…Alright, it's not too bad in this chair, but it's not 100% you know. I have a pill; they give me a sleeping pill. But I think you have to put up with a lot of things, it's not going to change is it?…I think you suffer sometimes, you slow down and suffer. You can't keep calling them every five minutes…I just got to put up with it. I know it's hard to say that, I do get emotional about it, I start to cry. (Mr White)

The question, 'What can I do about it?' permeates his story. It is as if he cannot find the words to express his situation and powerlessness:

> I know I keep repeating myself but what can you do? You tell me? If I could jump up and down, I would. Or if I could have an injection for a

year to make myself better I would take it and then die I would, but it's not going to happen. (Mr White)

The consistent message of stoic endurance through his narrative is reinforced by reflection about others whom he considers may be in worse situations than himself:

They say there's not much they can do about it, you have just got to take it. There are a lot of people worse off than me. (Mr White)

One can feel his wait for the inevitability of death, which he almost embraces in making an advance directive:

I've told them, because they have to ask a few questions that if anything happened to me, like if I had a heart attack or anything like that, I don't want to be resuscitated. I don't, I'd rather go...you do sit here sometimes and you think to yourself I wish I could go because what good am I sitting here like this? You tell me? What good am I sitting here just like this? (Mr White)

Preserving Narrative Storyline

The preserving storyline is about fighting death and actively taking opportunities to increase one's chances of survival. It is about seeking hope, and rocks between great optimism and depths of despair.

Mr Cotton had been happily married for over 30 years. He had always been in control of his life and, in the main, that of his family also. At interview, he was fully mobile but with a marked limp in his left leg, and his left hand was quite weak. In reading about MND, he had found a book explaining a survival regime. This resulted in him eradicating neurotoxins from his life and seeking alternative remedies. He banned chemicals from the house, visited a naturalist and took a cocktail of 'alternative' drugs as well as prescribed medication, using all means for a 'cure':

I'm seeking help from alternative therapy. I take lots of supplements and I find they help definitely with the tiredness. I've cut out all dairy products because when I had tests carried out they said I was highly intolerant of dairy...I take water melon seeds for going to bed. (Mr Cotton)

This process was attributed to reading an influential book:

I've read this book...he claims he is actually getting better by avoiding toxins and special nutrition. I am now seeing a (naturalist) and she's treating 5 people with MND and she has got them all stabilized apart from me. I'm her last one so I am just willing to try anything. (Mr Cotton)

This supported his survival story with a ready-made strategy:

> I just think I really try very hard to eliminate all toxins so I won't have anyone use spray deodorant in the house. I use a natural one with no nasties in and my wife does use a roll on now as well, I won't put petrol in the car, my wife gets out to do it...this (book), people newly diagnosed, to read something and you think it's not the end of the world, there are things I can do and I think part of it is that you actually feel 'I am doing something myself to take control of this disease' and I think having positive thoughts and feeling like, you are actually doing something can help, certainly with your frame of mind'. (Mr Cotton)

However, his preservation style led him also not to turn his back on conventional help:

> I eat loads of fruit and veg...and nuts and I try to eat as healthily as possible I take supplements and the only toxins I take are these Rilutek. I am not brave enough to stop taking those but my body doesn't like them. (Mr Cotton)

Fracturing Narrative Storyline

The fracturing narrative tells of loss, breakdown of self, fear of the future, denial of reality and living in a surreal notion of time. The thought of a lost future and having to abandon personal and professional plans is shattering.

Ms Connor had been fit and well all her life, and so when her voice changes were explained by the diagnosis of PBP, there was obvious shock. One month after diagnosis, as she began to tell her story, she had walking, swallowing and voice difficulties. She was able to write and did so aggressively, frustrated by her deteriorating speech. Her story was her expression of angst and confusion, reflecting fear and shock at how her life was spiralling out of control and out of time. She could not even comprehend how she had developed this illness:

> It is now over a month since I was diagnosed with MND and I have not got used to it at all...there is no known cause of this illness, so I can't identify with any reason for getting it me. (Ms Connor)

This double lack of explanation or understanding is told with great angst and disbelief as she talks further about her outlook on life. She uses words like abandon, surreal, unexpected, fear, fall apart:

> I had many plans for my future both personally and as a [professional] and I find it hard just to abandon them...all the aspects of this predicament I have suddenly found myself in are so surreal and unexpected that I just can't fully embrace any of them...I try and remain optimistic and fear that if the day comes when I have to fully embrace this illness, possibly

because of increasing symptoms, then I will totally fall apart. I am trying
to postpone that moment. (Ms Connor)

Her descriptions and use of language remain vivid and filled with descriptions
of trauma:

I feel as if I'm locked inside my head...powerless but a lot of anger, like a
car-crash would be, a lot of negative thoughts...the bleak potential future.
(Ms Connor)

Despite this fractured approach to her narrative, she offers a glimmer of wanting to take some control. She talks enthusiastically about being given things
to do to help herself:

I am taking riluzole tablets which seem the only medication available. It
is obviously possible that some scientist will come up with a genuine cure
one day and I try and believe in that...

I think the physiotherapy will help a lot and I'll be doing [exercises] that
as it's a process I can control. (Ms Connor)

Focusing on what she can do for herself has its downside when the evidence
is poor regarding the only medication, survival rates and projected level of
physical deterioration. This establishes a limit on practical things that can be
performed by her, which leaves her with denial:

Everything was negative...when I read the riluzole website it started with
bad statistics (notes) I obviously know what MND is but ignoring it...I am
not dealing with it...like the physiotherapist has given me exercises and
I will pursue it...all positive things that I can do myself. (Ms Connor)

...it is an instinct to avoid the big picture...in terms of avoiding acceptance
...these are my strategies until things get worse I'll continue this approach.
(Ms Connor)

Discussion

Discussion of Findings

Four types of storyline were identified, in contrast to Frank's (1995) three.
The storylines do not represent people's characters or stages of illness, but
'storylines that can be recognized' (Frank 1995, p. 75). The analysis of narratives can identify plots from disordered experiences (Cronon 1992), with
resultant storylines offering explanation for way(s) of being so patients can
see both 'themselves and their situations from fresh perspectives' (Charmaz
1999, p. 375). This may be supportive of their choices/decisions at certain milestones (Banks-Wallace 1999) or, when oral communication becomes difficult,

storylines could be useful to inform others about their current stance in living with MND. Personal experiences are located in particular times and places (Garro 2000), and so storylines may allow patients to reflect on influences in living with their illness as people's narratives reflect the working parts of their culture as much as the individual's experience. An example of this can be seen in the enduring storyline, where the culture of stoicism or 'British stiff upper lip' can be heard.

Stories can be a source of knowledge (Frank 1995, Smith & Sparkes 2004) to enhance understanding of how people with MND live and cope with this illness and they may assist in building a dynamic patient profile. The fracturing storyline may be particularly challenging and uncomfortable to hear. Professionals may become guarded and unsure about how to help, as it has echoes of a person presenting features of the 'unpopular patient' (Stockwell 1984); however, it also raises the importance of listening and understanding this distress (Frank 1995). Hearing a sustaining narrative offers professionals a window of opportunity to enhance a positive perspective with patients, supporting them to live their life with as much normality as possible. The enduring story is telling us about quiet, deep suffering. Understanding this narrative type presents opportunities to embrace the person socially, to listen to their sadness, to plan time to be with them and to support their sense of self and worth. When one has so much to live for, the preserving narrative is understandable. Although use of alternative medicine is increasing in all industrialized countries there is limited evidence of its use in MND (Wasner *et al.* 2001, Vardeny & Bromberg 2005). Spending money on alternative therapies might create tension in families and amongst professionals although supporting patient decisions might be the key message here – helping a person live in these extreme circumstances by following their lead.

Methodological Considerations

The theoretical contribution of this research offers a transferable approach to capture difference in people's lives, to untangle threads of their complex stories, whatever their cultural setting (Kleinman 1988). This narrative approach has the potential to enhance learning about living and coping with other life-limiting neurological illnesses such as multiple sclerosis, or Parkinson's disease.

Study Limitations

It is not claimed that the four storylines exhaust all possibilities or that they are generalizable as they have been constructed from a small sample size of 13 patients. Narrative methods require time for attention to detail (Reissman 1993) and therefore may be unsuitable for a study with a large number of participants. We did not specifically examine differences amongst the four presentations of MND or explore differences in stage of symptom presentation, which may be influencing factors and merit further examination. Although no patients claimed symptoms of psychological or cognitive impairment, these cannot be ruled out as influencing the narratives.

Conclusion

The evidence base of how people live or manage coping with MND is very sparse. Healthcare professionals need to know how best to help people live with this illness and, while every patient undoubtedly has a unique experience in living through a life-limiting illness such as MND, identifying storylines is a way of highlighting complex threads. Listening to complex stories can be challenging, as the elements of the stories can be intertwined and therefore difficult to appreciate.

The narrative research approach used in this study is one way of finding out from patients what it is to live with this illness. Four narrative types or storylines of living with MND have been identified and there may be more, but they do offer us a beginning to make sense of the unique experience people face in living with MND. The storylines are offered as a way to promote closer attention to people's stories as an organizing thread to support patients, family care-givers, nurses and other healthcare professionals in understanding patient approaches to living with MND.

References

Banks-Wallace J. (1999) Storytelling as a tool for providing, politic care to women. *American Journal of Maternity and Child Nursing* **42**(1), 20–24.

Beresford S. (1995) *Motor Neurone Disease*. Chapman & Hall, London.

Berger P.L. & Luckman T. (1966) *The Social Construction of Reality. A Treatise on the Sociology of Knowledge*. Doubleday & Company, New York.

Brown J.B. (2003) User, carer and professional experiences of care in motor neurone disease. *Primary Research and Development* **4**, 207–217.

Brown J.B., Lattimer V. & Tudball T. (2006) An investigation of patients and providers' views of services for motor neurone disease. *British Journal of Neuroscience Nursing* **1**(5), 249–252.

Burns G.W. (2001) *101 Healing Stories: Using Metaphor in Therapy*. John Wiley, New York.

Carlick A. & Biley F. (2004) Thoughts on the therapeutic use of narrative in the promotion of coping in cancer care. *European Journal of Cancer Care* **13**, 308–317.

Carter H., McKenna C., Macleod R. & Green R. (1998) Health professionals' responses to multiple sclerosis and motor neurone disease. *Palliative Medicine* **12**, 383–394.

Charmaz K. (1999) Stories of suffering: subjective tales and research narratives. *Qualitative Health Research* **9**(3), 362–382.

Charon R., Trautmann B.J., Connelly J.E., Hawkins A.H., Hunter K.M., Jones A.H., Montello M. & Poirer S. (1995) Literature and medicine: contributions to medical practice. *Annals* **122**, 618–619.

Chelf J.H., Deshler A.M.B., Hillman S.M.S. & Durazo-Arvizu R. (2000) Storytelling: a strategy for living and coping with cancer. *Cancer Nursing* **21**(2), 1–5.

Cronon W. (1992) A place for stories: nature, history and narrative. *Journal of American History* **78**, 1347–1376.

Department of Health (2005) *National Service Framework for Long-Term Conditions.* Department of Health, London.

Dowling M. (2006) Approaches to reflexivity in qualitative research. *Nurse Researcher* **13**(3), 7–21.

Frank A. (1995) *The Wounded Storyteller.* University of Chicago Press, London.

Garro L. (2000) Cultural knowledge as a resource in illness narratives. In *2000 Narrative and the Cultural Construction of Illness and Healing* (Mattingly C. & Garro L., eds), University of California Press, London, pp. 70–87.

Gergen K. & Gergen M. (1983) Narratives of the self. In *Studies in Social Identity* (Sabin T. & Scheibe K., eds), Praeger, New York, pp. 254–273.

Grinyer A. (2002) *Cancer in Young Adults Through Parents' Eyes*. Open University Press, Buckingham.

Heiney S.P. (1995) The healing power of story. *Oncology Nursing forum* **22**(6), 899–904.

Hebert R.S., Lacomis D., Easter B.A., Frick V. & Shear M.K. (2005) Grief support for informal caregivers of patients with ALS: a national survey. *Neurology* **64**, 137–138.

Holloway I. & Freshwater D. (2007) *Narrative Research in Nursing.* Blackwell Publishing, London.

Holmes T. (2005) Motor neurone disease and the NSF for long-term neurological conditions. *Primary Health Care* **15**(9), 27–31.

Horsburgh D. (2003) Evaluation of qualitative research. *Journal of Clinical Nursing* **12**(2), 307–312.

Howard R.S. & Orrell R.W. (2002) Management of motor neurone disease. *Postgraduate Medical Journal* **78**, 736–741.

Hughes R.A., Sinha A., Higginson I. Down K. & Leigh P.N. (2005) Living with motor neurone disease: lives, experiences of services and suggestions for change. *Health and Social Care in the Community* **13**(1), 64–74.

Hyden L.C. (1997) Illness and narrative. *Sociology of Health and Illness* **19**(1), 48–69.

Ince P.G., Evans J., Knopp M., Forster G., Hamdalla H.H.M., Wharton S.B. & Shaw P.J. (2003) Corticospinal tract degeneration in the progressive muscular variant of ALS. *Neurology* **60**, 1252–1258.

Kelly B. (1995) Storytelling: a way of connecting. *Nursingconnections* **8**(4), 5–11.

Kleinman A. (1988) *The Illness Narratives.* Basic Books, USA.

Krivickas L.S., Shockely L. & Mitsumoto H. (1997) Home care of patients with amyotrophic lateral sclerosis (ALS). *Journal of Neurological Sciences* **152** (Suppl. 1), S82-S82.

Leigh P.N., Abrahams S., Al-Chalai A., Ampong M.A., Goldstein L.H., Johnson J., Lyall R., Moxham J., Mustafa N., Rio A., Shaw C. & Willey E. (2003) The management of motor neurone disease. *Journal of Neurological and Neurosurgical Psychiatry* **74**(Suppl. IV), iv32–iv47.

Lieblich A., Tuval Maschiach R. & Zilber T. (1998) *Narrative Research, Reading, Analysis and Interpretations.* Sage, Thousand Oaks, CA.

Mandrioli J., Faglioni P., Merekki E. & Sola P. (2003) The epidemiology of ALS in Modena, Italy. *Neurology* **60**(4), 683–689.

Miles M.B. & Huberman M.A. (1994) *Qualitative Data Analysis.* Sage Publications, London.

Miller P. (1994) Narrative practices: their role in socialisation and self construction. In *The Remembering Self* (Neisser U. & Fivush R., eds), Cambridge University Press, Cambridge, pp. 158–179.

Miller R.G., Mitchell J.D., Lyon M. & Moore D. H. (2000) Riluzole for amyotrophic lateral sclerosis (ALS)/motor neuron disease (MND). *Cochrane Database Systematic Reviews*, 2000 Issue 1 Art. No: CD001447, doi: 10.1002/14651858.CD001447.pub2.

Motor Neurone Disease Association (2007) *Information Sheet No. 6. MND Statistics.* MND Association, Northampton. Retrieved from http://www.mndassociation.org on 25 July 2007.

Reissman C.K. (1993) *Narrative Analysis.* Sage Publications, London.

Rigby S.A., Thornton E.W., Tedman S., Burchardt C.A., Young C.A. & Dougan C. (1999) Quality of life assessment in MND: development of social withdrawal scale. *Journal of the Neurological Sciences* **169**(1–2), 26–34.

Robinson I. (1990) Personal narratives, social careers and medical courses: analysing life trajectories in autobiographies of people with multiple sclerosis. *Social Science and Medicine* **30**(11), 1173–1186.

Skultans V. (1998) Anthropology and narrative. In *Narrative Based Medicine: in Dialogue and Discourse in Clinical Practice* (Greenlagh T. & Hurwitz B., eds), BMJ Publications, London, pp. 225–233.

Small N. & Rhodes P. (2000) *Too Ill to Talk? User Involvement in Palliative Care.* Routledge, London.

Smith B. & Sparkes A. (2004) Men, sport and spinal cord injury: an analysis of metaphors and narrative types. *Disability and Society, 2004* **19**, 613–626.

Somers M. (1994) The narrative constitution of identity: a relational and network approach. *Theory and Society* **23**, 605–649.

Stockwell F. (1984) *The Unpopular Patient.* Croom Helm, London.

Vardeny O. & Bromberg M.B. (2005) The use of herbal supplements and alternative therapies by patients with amyotrophic lateral sclerosis. *Journal of Herbal Pharmacotherapy* **5**(3), 23–31.

Wasner M., Klier H. & Borasio G.D. (2001) The use of alternative medicine by patients with amyotrophic lateral sclerosis. *Journal of the Neurological Sciences* **191**(1–2), 151–154.

Wengraf T. (2001) *Qualitative Research Interviewing: Biographic Narrative and Semi-Structured Method.* Sage Publications, London.

38

Telling Stories: Narrative Approaches in Qualitative Research

Margarete Sandelowski

O ne mark of the turn away from positivism and toward interpretation in the behavioral and social sciences has been a renewed attention to the human "impulse to narrate" (White, 1980, p. 5). Mourning the devaluation of narratives as sources of knowledge, and emphasizing the moral force, healing power, and emancipatory thrust of stories, scholars across the disciplines have (re)discovered the narrative nature of human beings (Banks, 1982; Bell, 1988; Brody, 1987; Heilbrun, 1988; Polkinghorne, 1988). Many scholars now view physicians and patients, analysts and analysands, fieldworkers and natives, and researchers and subjects as partners engaged in the distinctively "historic and hermeneutic" (Banks, 1982, p. 23) activity of storytelling. Patients, analysands, natives, and subjects recount the events of their lives and narrate them into temporal order and meaning and physicians, analysts, fieldworkers, and researchers, in turn, narrate their versions of those lives in their clinical case studies, research reports and scientific treatises. Such diverse phenomena as ethnography (E. Bruner, 1986), psychoanalysis (Spence, 1982, 1987), the life course (Cohler, 1982), the life history (Peacock, 1984), the research interview (Mishler, 1986), the physician-patient relationship (Brody, 1987), developmental theories (Gergen & Gergen, 1986), and every-day explanations (Gergen, 1988) have been viewed as having traditions, forms and structures exemplifying the narrative, as opposed to the logico-scientific, mode of thought (J. Bruner, 1986).

Scientists under the influence of such interpretive traditions as phenom-enology, hermeneutics, symbolic interactionism, and feminist and cultural

Source: *Image: Journal of Nursing Scholarship*, 23(3) (1991): 161–166.

criticism have developed a "literary consciousness" (Marcus, 1986, p. 262), assuming standpoints and employing techniques once distinctively associated with literary analysis and criticism. Newly preoccupied with forms of expression, literary devices, rhetorical conventions, and the reading and writing of texts of experience (including bodies, lives, and literature), scholars now see the story in the study, the tale in the theory, the parable in the principle, and the drama in the life (Bordo, 1990; Clifford & Marcus, 1986; Rosaldo, 1989; Ruby, 1982; Sacks, 1987; Suleiman, 1986; Turner & Bruner, 1986). Scientific texts, for example, have been viewed as Kuhnian tales where theories are presumed to be largely governed by prevailing plots and aesthetic forms (E. Bruner, 1986; Gergen & Gergen, 1986). Such literary devices and narrative conventions as the use of the third person and passive voice in typical science reports and the severing of method from results and from interpretation are deemed "anti-narrative" strategies that separate authors from their texts and mask the narrativity of science (Myerhoff & Ruby, 1982, p. 22). The study of narratives has linked the sciences with history, literature and everyday life to reflect the increasing reflexivity that characterizes contemporary inquiry and furthers the postmodern deconstruction of the already tenuous boundaries among disciplines and realms of meaning (Ruby, 1982).

This (re)conceptualization of human beings as narrators and of their products as texts to be interpreted constitutes a potentially critical moment for nursing scholars (especially those engaged in qualitative inquiry) because it reveals, and suggests solutions for, analytic problems that have typically been disguised in conventional theory-and-method debates about objectivity and validity. These analytic problems involve the ambiguous nature of truth, the metaphoric nature of language in communicating a putatively objective reality, the temporality and liminality of human beings' interpretation of their lives, the historical and sociocultural constraints against which individuals labor to impart information about themselves to other individuals who, in turn, labor to listen, and, most significantly, the inherently contradictory project of making something scientific out of everything biographical (Barthes, 1982a; Geertz, 1988).

Narrative approaches to the study of lives reveal the extent to which these problems have been conditioned by empirical rather than narrative or biographical standards of truth and by a preoccupation with obtaining information at the expense of understanding expression. Anthropologist James Peacock, for example, observed that the narrative patterning in life history is important in its own right, but has been ignored and "cannibalized to feed analyses at other levels" (1984, p. 96). Narrative analyses of texts force scholars to attend first to what is placed immediately before them – stories – before transforming them into descriptions and theories of the lives they represent. Narrative analyses reveal the discontinuities between story and experience and focus on discourse: on the tellings themselves and the devices individuals use to make meaning in stories. By contrast, analytic techniques, such as content analysis and constant comparison (as typically used in nursing research) that emphasize informational content, assume a close correspondence between a telling and the experience that is told and ignore such features of talk as asides and the storied placement (as opposed to actual sequencing) of events. Narrative as an interactive and interpretive product is the focus even before it becomes subject to the researcher's purposes. The interview and the research report need to be rescued from efforts to standardize and scientize them and be reclaimed as occasions for storytelling (Denzin, 1989a; Mishler, 1986). Because lives are understood as and shaped by narratives, narrative approaches to inquiry parallel the ways individuals inquire about experience (Cohler, 1982) and, in a sense, naturalize (or remove some of the artifice from) the research process.

Like other scholars practiced in the empirical realm but drawn to the aesthetic and synoptic visions of literature and history by virtue of their human subject matter, we nursing scholars remain largely "literary innocents," (Geertz, 1988, p. 24) unschooled in the techniques of the historian and biographer, and only marginally concerned with the reflexivity and silences of talk (Barthes, 1982;). Recent nursing publications have addressed the dilemmas of discourse (Dickson, 1990; Hays, 1989) and nurses conducting qualitative studies typically create conditions in which stories are told; yet, we have not explored directly the storied nature of human interpretation and placed it at the center of our analyses. Accordingly, in this paper I consider narrative as a framework for: a) understanding the human being as subject of nursing inquiry; b) conceptualizing the interview; and c) analyzing and interpreting interview data. Although narrative knowing assumes that all the parties in inquiry – research subjects, researchers, and readers of research – are narrators and places them in a hermeneutic circle of interpretation, I focus here on issues distinctively related to research respondents as narrators and on the interpretive possibilities for nursing in their narrations. I begin with a necessarily abbreviated overview of narrative knowing.

In Search of Stories

A prevailing conceptualization of narrative is that it is one of many modes of transforming knowing into telling (Mishler, 1986). Competing views of narrative are that it is the paradigmatic mode in which experience is shared and that experience itself is storied, or it has a narrative pattern. Human beings are "immersed in narrative," telling themselves stories in a "virtually uninterrupted monologue" (Polkinghorne, 1988, p. 160) and tirelessly listening to and recognizing in their own stories the: stories of others. Literary scholar Roland Barthes (1982b) noted the "prodigious variety of genres" constituting narratives that are present in language, image, gesture and myth, painting and conversation. Narratives assume many forms. They are heard, seen and read;

they are told, performed, painted, sculpted and written. They are international, trans-historical and trans-cultural: "simply there, like life itself (p. 252).

Narrativists across the disciplines have many views of what a telling must consist of to be labeled as narrative, variously emphasizing such factors as rhythm and pacing, time and place, human agency, categories of narrators and audiences, complicating action and plot (Bal, 1985; Chatman, 1978; Polkinghorne, 1988; Toolan, 1988). Literary critic Seymour Chatman (1978), for example, viewed narratives as having both content and expression that are manifested in different media, such as the novel, film or painting. Narratives are composed of a story or fabula, comprised of actions, happenings, characters, settings, discourse or plot – the way the story is communicated. The same story elements may accordingly, be differently plotted, resulting in a variety of narratives. (Nursing theories might be viewed as different narratives produced by different emplotments of nurse, patient, environment and health). Sociolinguist William Labov (1972) viewed a complete oral narrative as composed of an abstract, or what the store is about; an orientation, or the who, when, where and what of the story; some complicating action, or the then-what-happend?; an evaluation, or the so-what?; a resolution, or the what-finally-happend?; and a coda, or a signal that the story is over and a return to the present (A conventional scientific research report, a clinical case study may be viewed as oral or written narratives).

Generally, narratives are understood as stories that include a temporal ordering of events and an effort to make something out of those events: to render, or to signify, the experiences of persons-in-flux in a personally and culturally coherent, plausible manner. Narration is a threshold activity in that it captures a narrator's interpretation of a link among elements of the past, present and future at a liminal place and fleeting moment in time (Churchill & Churchill, 1982). Narrators are socially positioned to tell stories at given biographical and historical moments and under the influence of prevailing cultural conventions surrounding storytelling, the social context of narration and the audience for a telling (Burner, 1984; Polanyi, 1985; Rosaldo, 1989). For example, Westerners expect stories to have beginnings, middles and ends that are meaningfully related to each other. What in one culture constitutes a story may in another constitute a lie (Toolan, 1988). What to one person constitutes a good story to live by (for example, the traditional marriage-and-children narrative for women) may to another person constitute a story that must be resisted (Heilbrun, 1988; Personal Narratives Group, 1989). Not surprisingly, the narrative conventions and audiences in everyday conversations differ from those in formal research or clinical interviews. Moreover, the relationship between teller and listener is generally asymmetrical in the conventional research or clinical interview situation, with the interviewer-listener typically dominant and often directing and even preventing or interrupting respondent-tellers' narrative efforts (Agar & Hobbs, 1982; Fisher, 1988; Fisher & Todd, 1983; Mishler, 1984, 1986; Todd, 1989).

In tellings, events are selected and then given cohesion, meaning and direction; they are made to flow and are given a sense of linearity and even inevitability. The problem of telling is illuminated when it is understood as the necessity of communicating the seeing-things-together as one-thing-after-another (Polkinghorne, 1988; Rosaldo, 1989). Literary theorist Frank Kermode observed how advantageous it was to find in life the simplicity of narrative order; to be able to say that when one thing happened, another thing happened. The mind is put to rest by the illusion of sequence and order, the appearance of causality and the look of necessity (1967, p. 127). Narratives (like scientific theories) tidy things up – things that in real life may (or even ought to) be left lying awkwardly around (Humm, 1989, p. 52). Narration, therefore, constitutes a kind of: a) causal thinking, in that stories are efforts to explore questions of human agency and explain lives; b) historical (as opposed to scientific) understanding that events cannot be explained except in retrospect; c) moral enterprise, in that stories are used to justify and serve as models for lives; and a kind of d) political undertaking, in that individuals often struggle to create new narratives to protest a perceived storylessness in the old ones (Freeman, 1984; Heilbrun, 1988; Robinson & Hawpe, 1986, Rosaldo, 1989).

The imposition of a narrative order on life illuminates the differences among what anthropologist Edward Bruner (1984) called a life-as-lived (what actually happened), a life-as-experienced (the images, feelings, desires, thoughts, and meanings known to the person whose life it is), and a life-as-told (a narrative). Persons would have to be letter-perfect copies of their culture, with no discrepancies among outer behavior, inner state, and, most importantly, how they chose to characterize these behaviors and states in stories, for there to be an ideal correspondence among their three lives. A life history, or self-story, or any personal account is still a story, a representation of a life at a given moment rather than the life itself. Moreover, these representations do not simply represent, but rather (re)construct lives in every act of telling for, at the very least, the outcome of any one telling is necessarily a re-telling.

Narrative Techniques

Narratives have been studied from a variety of perspectives. Mishler (1986) summarized analyses of spoken narratives as emphasizing: a) textual matters, or the syntactic and semantic devices internally connecting parts of the text; b) ideational matters, or the referential meaning of what is said; and c) interpersonal matters, or the role relationships between teller and listener as reflected in speech. Narrative analyses have incorporated sociolinguistic, ethnoethodological and phenomenological techniques (Agar & Hobbs, 1982; Paget, 1982; Swartz & Swartz, 1987).

Narrative research can also be categorized as descriptive and explanatory (Polkinghorne, 1988). In descriptive narrative research, the researcher may

seek to describe; a) individual and group narratives of life stories or particular life episodes; b) the conditions under which one storyline, or emplotment
and signification of events, prevails over, coheres with, or conflicts with other
storylines; c) the relationship between individual stories and the available
cultural stock of stories; and d) the function that certain life episodes
serves in individuals' emplotment of their lives. In explanatory narrative
research, the researcher seeks to render an accounting via narrative of why
something happened.

Several narrative studies suggest approaches that can be developed for
nursing inquiry. Susan Bell (1988) analyzed three stories told in the course of
an interview with a DES daughter to show how she became a political woman.
Faye Ginsburg (1989) emphasized the narrative devices pro-choice and pro-
life activists used to frame their lives. Marianne Paget (1982) interpreted
the meaning of one story of a medical error, attending to dialect, expressive
phonology and structure. These studies illustrate how lives can be understood,
revealed and transformed in *stories* and *by the very act of storytelling*. Moreover,
they demonstrate that no single method of transcription is adequate to
every analytic task and that any transcription is necessarily incomplete. A
transcription of a speech event is based on some (often implicit) theory of language, speech and social interaction and, therefore, serves different analytic
purposes (Atkinson, 1988; Mishler, 1986). For example, verbatim transcripts
with strict notations of such features of talk as pauses, repetitions, false starts
and asides are necessary for many kinds of narrative analyses based on the
assumption of language as a structure, but not for constant comparison in
the service of generating grounded theory or for content analyses in the service of instrument development where language is assumed to be a transparent vehicle for communicating information.

Analysts can look for narrative forms in naturally occurring accounts
and graph individuals' story lines, labeling life events by age and an interpretation of the respondents' evaluation of those events. Respondents can
also be asked to graph their own story lines, itemizing relevant (varying with
the purpose of inquiry) life events, when they occurred and their evaluative
responses (happy/unhappy, high/low point). In one study using this storyline technique, the Gergens (1988) found that the most common narrative
form used by college students in depicting the first 20 years of their lives was
the comedy. Interestingly, this form approximated the typical middle-class
American cultural myth of childhood as happy, of adolescence as a time of
conflict and of the college years as happy again. This finding affirmed the
argument that life stories are communal or cultural products with their forms
often constrained by the narrative storylines available to communicate them.
In addition, the Gergens (1988) found that although respondents agreed that
adolescence was a low lime, the varied in the selection of events contributing
to these low points. Again, emphasizing the communal nature of narrative
forms, they provocatively suggested that the respondents might have been

more influenced by the prevailing cultural narrative about what adolescent life is and *must have been* than by any specific life event *per se*.

Using such narrative models, researchers can gain insight into the way human beings understand and enact their lives through stories. For example, in my own interviews with infertile couples, I have noticed that they variously portray themselves as romantic questers who get close to but are continually thwarted from achieving fertility (the often-cited rollercoaster effect), as tragic and ironic heroes fatefully unaware of and forever marked by their infertility, or as somewhat comic travelers on the road of trials to parenthood who ultimately prevail after many reversals. These infertility stories are recognizable to me as a listener, reader and writer of infertility stories, and as a member of a pronatalist culture that pities couples unable to conceive, views the achievement of pregnancy as the best resolution to infertility and values persistence in the pursuit of goals until success is achieved.

In contrast, one of the respondent couples (especially the wife) protested the familiar cultural narrative that married couples and, most particularly, women, want children of their own, that infertility is tragic and adoption is a second-best way to become a parent. This couple's story stood out from the others because infertility never functioned as a factor moving them away from a goal (biological parenthood), but rather as one moving them toward a goal (alternatively presented as voluntary childlessness or adoptive parenthood). This couples' narrative was characterized by a we-are-different trope; they viewed themselves as different from other infertile couples in always being more attracted to adoption than pregnancy as a means of achieving parenthood, in having experienced ambivalence toward having children at all, and in feeling less anxious about having to wait for a child to adopt than other infertile and adopting couples. Moreover, their characterization of themselves as different rang true when they mentioned that friends had told them that infertility had happened to the right couple because of their low investment in pregnancy. Significantly, this couple's story revealed their recognition of, but protest against, typical infertility stories in which infertility is plotted as a negative event.

In searching for emplotments, researchers look for the ways respondents (re)sort life events to create differently formed narratives, for a story once told as a tragedy can become a romance or comedy in another telling. Narrative forms reveal individuals' construction of past and future life events at given moments in time. Analysts can look for model and variant narrative forms in individuals experiencing common events (pregnancy, illness, hospitalization). Reversals in story lines and the steepness of up-and-down slopes can be indicators of the intensity and drama with which events are experienced as well as illuminate critical moments in which changes in health and well-being are likely to occur. For example, infertile couples often experience the achievement of pregnancy as a sudden reversal and, consequently, suffer from shock, disorientation and a sense of disbelief that may delay acceptance of pregnancy. In addition, infertile couples may experience the period of pregnancy as a move to happier times, to being on-track with other pregnant couples or as troubled as the preconceptional period. In the former instance, pregnancy constitutes a reversal to good times; in the latter instance, pregnancy constitutes turmoil as usual.

Descriptive narrative research can also reveal how respondents explain their situations. For example, employing a narrative framework based on Arthur Kleinman's (1980, 1988) conceptualization of explanatory models and Gareth Williams' (1984) configuration of narrative reconstruction, we described how infertile couples used two critical referents – the presence or absence of a child, and the timing of these presences or absences in relation to infertility – to construct explanations of infertility that resolved its medical and cultural paradoxes. (Sandelowski, Holditch-Davis, and Harris 1990). The narrative framework offered a satisfactory solution to the analytic problem of capturing the momentary and liminal nature of these couples' explanations.

In contrast to narrative research that aims to describe the nature and function of stories, the goal of narrative explanation is to provide an intelligible, comprehensive and verisimilar *narrative* rendering of why something happened that is well grounded and constitutes a supportable emplotment of events (actions and intentions). Explanatory narrative research, (exemplified in history, investigative journalism and psychoanalytic therapy, but typically not used in the sciences), is retrospective and retrodictive in that: a) certain events in the past are interpreted as hanging together by being narrated into a story with a beginning, middle, and end; and b) a story must be ended before it can be explained. A life event is not explainable while it is happening; only when it is over can it become the subject of narration. The researcher is interested in cause – in presenting an explanation of an end or outcome – by locating those critical moments of human action and intention when the story could have ended differently. Employing a what-if strategy', the researcher looks for what has happened and imagines what has not happened by asking such questions as: what if this particular action had not been taken?; what if this particular motivation had not been operative? Would the outcome have changed (Polkinghorne, 1988)? For example, an important question in the study of infertility is why some couples quickly terminate medical treatment for infertility while other couples remain in treatment for years without achieving conception. Explanatory narrative research suggests an alternative to statistical techniques for establishing cause and reclaims the concept of cause from formal science. Moreover, narrative explanations exhibit rather than demonstrate causal connections by clarifying the significance of events (including perceptions, motivations and actual occurrences) in relation to a preselected end (Polkinghorne, 1988). Such explanations may ultimately be useful in making predictions (a typically scientific aim), but the larger objective of narrative explanation is not so much to foretell as to tell and re-tell: to provide an insight only possible when looking back (Freeman, 1984).

Although analyses of narratives in oral accounts elicited in the course of interviews is new and needs much development and refinement for nursing projects, they are potentially very useful for grabbing fleeting configurations of wholes, for capturing the continuity and change in the phenomena nurses researchers most often study and for dramatically engaging informants with a project in which they are already engaged by virtue of being human: storytelling. Moreover, the method contributes to the phenomenological mission of nursing inquiry: the understanding of lives in health, illness, and transition.

In Search of True Stories

I regret the replacement of Literature by Science as Clio's closest ally. Research has been substituted for imagination; the True has fallen victim to the Actual (Trevanian, 1983, p. 134).

In the narrative context, the concept of truth (like the concept of cause) is reclaimed from logical positivism (Polkinghorne, 1988). Narrative truth is distinguished from other kinds of formal science truths by its emphasis on the life-like, intelligible and plausible story. Stories typically reflect a coherence (as opposed to correspondence) theory of truth in that the narrator strives for narrative probability – a story that makes sense; narrative fidelity – a story consistent with past experiences or other stories; and aesthetic finality – a story with satisfactory closure and representational appeal (Brody, 1987; Spence, 1982). Narrators, in a "remembering moment," (Spence, 1982, p. 31) strive to achieve the most internally consistent interpretation of the past-in-the-present, the experienced present and the anticipated-in-the-present future. Tellings are remembrances, retrospections and constructions about the past in a fleeting present moment soon to be past (Freeman, 1984, p. 4). Located in a hermeneutic circle of (re)interpretation, narratives with common story elements can be reasonably expected to change from telling to telling, making the idea of empirically validating them for consistency or stability completely alien to the concept of narrative truth. Misguided efforts to verify findings (for example, the use of test-retest and interrater reliability kinds of measures) suggest a misplaced preoccupation with empirical rather than narrative standards of truth and a profound lack of understanding of the temporal and liminal nature and vital meaning-making functions of storytelling. Extending Jerome Bruner's (1986) observation, what preoccupies the storyteller and audience (here, the subject and researcher) is not how to know truth, but rather how experience is endowed with meaning.

If the concept of narrative effaces the distinctions between story and study and literature and science, it also illuminates the artificial distinction between truth and fiction. Anthropologist Clifford Geertz (1988) noted the longstanding Western confusion of the imagined with the imaginary, the fictional with the false, and the making-things-out with making-things-up (p. 140). Sociologist Norman Denzin (1989a, 1989b) observed that a life story is a fictional (often literary) production, something made up out of experience. He defined (auto) biographical truth as agreement within a community of minds with events believed to have occurred (facts) and with how these events were experienced by interacting individuals (facticities). Fictions are not opposed to truths in the narrative context, but rather they are truths within the stories that contain them. Narratives are truthful fictions, but fiction is itself linked to interpretation in that all interpretation (even scientific explanation) involves human fabrication: the making out of what happened and the making up of what something means. As writer Annie Dillard (1982) observed, all interpretations (meaning all mental activity) "miss their mark or invent it, make it up. Humanity has but one product, and that is fiction" (p. 148), with various fictional enterprises (whether stories or theories) having different rules for their fabrication.

Toward a New Narrative in Qualitative Analysis

A decision to view respondents in qualitative research as narrators and interview data as stories poses new problems but also provides new opportunities for nursing research. Narrative approaches move us to develop some of the analytic sensitivities and skills of the literary critic and historian. A narrative framework affords nursing scholars a special access to the human experience of time, order, and change, and it obligates us to listen to the human impulse to tell tales.

References

Agar, M., & Hobbs, J. R. (1982). Interpreting discourse: Coherence and the analysis of ethnographic interviews. *Discourse Processes*, 5, 1–32.

Atkinson, P. (1988). Review of Mishler, E. (1984). The discourse of medicine. *Culture, Medicine and Psychiatry*, 12, 249–256. Norwood, NJ: Ablex.

Bal, M. (1985). Introduction to the theory of narrative. Toronto: University of Toronto Press.

Banks, S. A. (1982). Once upon a time: Interpretation in literature and medicine. *Literature and Medicine*, 1, 23–27.

Barthes, R, (1982a). Authors and writers. In S. Sontag (Ed.). *A Barthes reader* (pp. 185–193). New York: Hill & Wang.

Barthes, R. (1982b). Introduction to the structural analysis of narratives. In S. Sontag (Ed.), *A Barthes reader* (pp. 251–295). New York: Hill & Wang.

Bell, S. E. (1988). Becoming a political woman: The reconstruction and interpretation of experience through stories. In A. D. Todd, & S. Fisher (Eds.), *Gender and discourse: The power of talk* (pp. 97–123). Norwood, New Jersey: Ablex.

Bordo, S. (1990). Rending the slender body. In M. Jacobus. E. F. Keller, & S. Shuttleworth (Eds.), *Body/Politics: Women and the discourses of science* (pp. 83–112). New York: Routledge.

Brody, H. (1987). *Stories of sickness.* New Haven: Yale University Press.

Bruner, E. M. (1984). Introduction: The opening up of anthropology. In S. Plattner & E. M. Bruner (Eds.), *Text, play and story: The construction and reconstruction of self and society* (pp. 1–16). Washington, DC: American Ethnological Society.

Bruner, E. M. (1986). Ethnography as narrative. In V. W. Turner & E. M. Bruner (Eds.), *The anthropology of experience* (pp. 139–155). Urbana: University of Illinois Press.

Bruner, J. (1986). *Actual minds, possible worlds.* Cambridge, Massachusetts: Harward University Press.

Chatman, S. (1978). *Story and discourse: Narrative structure in fiction and film.* Ithaca, NY: Cornell University Press.

Churchill, L. R., & Churchill, S. W. (1982). Storytelling in medical arenas: The art of self-determination. *Literature and Medicine*, 1, 73–79.

Clifford, J., & Marcus, G. E. (1986). *Writing culture: The poetics and politics of ethnography.* Berkeley: University of California Press.

Cohler, B.J. (1982). Personal narrative and life course. *Life-Span Development and Behavior,* 4, 203–211.

Denzin, N. K. (1989a). *Interpretive biography,* Newbury Park, California: Sage.

Denzin, N. K. (1989b). *Interpretive interactionism.* Newbury Park, California: Sage.

Dickson, C. L. (1990). A feminist post structuralist analysis of the knowledge of menopause. *Advances in Nursing Science,* 12, 15–31.

Dillard, A. (1982). *Living by fiction.* New York: Harper & Row.

Fisher, S. (1938). *In the patient's best interest: Women and the politics of medical decisions.* New Brunswick, NJ: Rutgers University Press.

Fisher, S., & Todd, A. D. (1983). *The social organization of doctor-patient communication.* Washington, DC: Center for Applied Linguistics.

Freeman, M. (1984). History, narrative, and life-span developmental knowledge. *Human Development*, 27, 1–19.

Geertz, C. (1988). *Works and lives: The anthropologist as author.* Stanford, CA: Stanford University Press.

Gergen, M. M. (1988). Narrative structures in social explanation. In C. Antaki (Ed.), *Analyzing everyday explanation: A casebook of methods* (pp. 94–112). London: Sage.

Gergen, M. M., & Gergen, K.J. (1984). The social construction of narrative accounts. In K.J. Gergen & M. M. Gergen (Eds.), *Historical social psychology* (pp. 173–189). Hilldale, NJ: Lawrence Erlbaum Associates.

Gergen, K. J., & Gergen, M. M. (1986). Narrative form and the construction of psychological science. In T. R. Sarbin (Ed.), *Narrative psychology: The storied nature of human conduct* (pp. 22–44), NY: Praeger.

Ginsburg, F. (1989). Dissonance and harmony: The symbolic function of abortion in activists' life stories. In The Personal Narratives Group (Ed.), *Interpreting women's lives: Feminist theory and personal narratives* (pp. 59–84). Bloomington, IN: Indiana University Press.

Hays, J. C. (1989). Voices in the record. *Image: Journal of Nursing Scholarship*, 21, 200–204.

Heilbrun, C. G. (1988). *Writing a woman's life.* New York: Ballantine.

Humm, P. (1989). Waiting for a child. In R. D. Klein (Ed.), *Infertility: Women speak out about their experiences of reproductive medicine* (pp. 51–58). London: Pandora Press.

Kermode, F. (1967). *The sense of an ending: Studies in the theory of fiction.* NY: Oxford University Press.

Kleinman, A. (1980). *Patients and healers in the context of culture: An exploration of the borderland between anthropology, medicine, and psychiatry.* Berkeley, CA: University of California Press.

Kleinman, A. (1988). *The illness narratives: Suffering, healing and the human condition.* New York: Basic Books.

Labov, W. (Ed.) (1972). *Language in the inner city: Studies in the Black English vernacular.* Philadelphia: University of Pennsylvania Press.

Marcus, G.E. (1986). Afterword: Ethnographic writing and anthropological careers. In J. Clifford & G.E. Marcus (Eds.), *Writing culture: The poetics and politics of field work* (pp. 262–266). Berkeley, California: University of California Press.

Mishler, E. G. (1984) *The Discourse of medicine: Dialectics of medical interviews.* Norwood, NJ: Ablex.

Mishler, E.G.(1986). *Research interviewing: Context and narrative.* Cambridge, MA: Harvard University Press.

Myerhoff, B., & Ruby, J. (1982), Introduction. In J. Ruby (Ed.), *A crack in the mirror: Reflexive perspectives in anthropology* (pp. 1–35). Philadelphia: University of Pennsylvania Press.

Paget, M. A. (1982). Your son is cured now: You may take him home. *Culture, medicine and psychiatry,* 6, 237–259.

Peacock, J. L. (1984). Religion and life history: An exploration in cultural psychology. In S. Planner & E. M. Bruner (Eds.), *Text, play and story: The construction and reconstruction of self and society* (pp. 94–116). Washington, DC: American Ethnological Society.

Personal Narratives Group (Eds.). (1939). *Interpreting women's lives: Feminist theory and personal narratives.* Bloomington, IN: Indiana University Press.

Polanyi, L. (1985). *Telling the American story: A structural and cultural analysis of conversational storytelling.* Norwood, NJ: Ablex.

Polkinghorne, D. E. (1988). *Narrative knowing and the human sciences.* Albany, NY: State University of New York Press.

Robinson, J. A., & Hawpe, L. (1936). Narrative thinking as a heuristic process. In T. R. Sarbin (Ed.), *Narrative psychology: The storied nature of human conduct* (pp. 111–125). NY: Praeger.

Rosaldo, R.(1989). *Culture and truth: The remaking of social analysis.* Boston: Beacon Press.

Ruby, J. (ed.). (1982). *A crack in the mirror: Reflexive perspectives in anthropology.* Philadelphia: University of Pennsylvania Press.

Sacks, O. (1987). *The man who mistook his wife for a hat and other clinical tales.* New York: Harper & Row.

Sandelowski, M., Holditch-Davis, D., & Harris, B. G. (1900). Living the life: Explanations of infertility. *Sociology of Health and Illness,* 12, 195–215.

Sarbin, T. R. (Ed.). *Narrative psychology: The storied nature of human conduct.* NY: Praeger.

Spence, D. P. (1982). *Narrative truth and historical truth: Meaning and interpretation in psychoanalysis.* NY: Norton.

Spence, D. P. (1987). *The Freudian metaphor: Toward paradigm change in psychoanalysis.* NY: Norton.

Suleiman, S. R, (1986). (Re)Writing the body: The politics and poetics of female eroticism. In S. R. Suleiman (Ed.), *The female body in Western culture: Contemporary perspectives* (pp. 7–29). Cambridge, MA: Harvard University Press.

Swartz, S., & Swartz, L. (1987). Talk about talk.: Metacommentary and context in the analysis of psychotic discourse. *Culture, Medicine and Psychiatry,* 11, 395–416.

Todd, A. D. (1989). *Intimate adversaries: Cultural conflict between doctors and women patients.* Philadelphia: University of Pennsylvania Press.

Toolan, M.J. (1988). *Narrative: A critical linguistic introduction.* London: Routledge.

Trevanian. (1983). *The summer of Katya.* New York: Ballantine.

Turner, V.W., & Bruner, E. M. (1086). *The anthropology of experience.* Urbana, II: University of Illinois Press.

White, H. (1980). The value of narrativity in the representation of reality. *Critical Inquiry,* 7, 5–27.

Williams, G. (1984). The genesis of chronic illness: Narrative re-construction. *Sociology of Health and Illness,* 6, 2, 175–200.

39

Narrative Methods in Quality Improvement Research

T. Greenhalgh, J. Russell and D. Swinglehurst

Q*SHC* and *BMJ* distinguish research reports presented as IMRAD – Introduction, Methods, Results and Discussion)[1] from quality improvement reports (presented as COMPASEN – Context, Outline of problem, Measures, Process, Analysis, Strategy for change, Effects of change, and Next steps).[2] In their taxonomy, *research* is seen as systematic and focused enquiry seeking truths that are transferable beyond the setting in which they were generated, while *quality improvement* is seen as real time, real world work undertaken by teams who deliver services.

Quality improvement research – that is, applied research aimed at informing change that improves policy and practice – has emerged as a tradition in its own right, embracing a broad range of methods including randomised controlled trials, cross-case comparisons, in-depth case study, and action research. The question of when quality improvement initiatives should be published as new knowledge in academic journals (and under what circumstances they should be subjected to the stringent ethical and data protection standards that now govern research) remains a contentious issue,[3,4] especially when the study involves the use of narrative (a term which, in this paper, we use interchangeably with "story").

Source: *Quality & Safety in Health Care*, 14(6) (2005): 443–449.

What is Narrative?

Bruner distinguishes two forms of human cognition: logico-scientific ("science of the concrete") and narrative ("science of the imagination").[5] Logico-scientific reasoning seeks to understand specific phenomena as examples of general laws, while narrative reasoning seeks to understand them in terms of human experience and purpose.[6,7] Conventional research relies mostly on the former.

Stories do not convince by their objective truth but by their emotional impact on the reader – achieved through such literary features as aesthetic appeal (the story is seen as touching, humorous, ironic, for example), metaphor (one thing is made more meaningful or vivid through subjective comparison with something else), and moral order (actors are constructed as heroes who get their just rewards and villains who deserve come-uppance).[7,8]

In one of the great works of literary analysis, *Poetics*, Aristotle suggested that a story (narrative) has three key characteristics: an unfolding of events and actions over time; employment (the rhetorical juxtaposition of these events and actions to evoke meaning, motive, and causality); and trouble (*peripeteia* – the unexpected in the form of surprise, "twist in the plot", and so on).[8] Burke later proposed that story is about *purposeful* action in the face of adversity and risk, and comprises five key elements: the act (what is done); the scene (the context in which it is done); the agent or actor (who does it); the agency (how it is done); and the purpose (why it is done).[9] Box 1 lists some unique advantages of narrative in relation to quality improvement research.

In this article (building on earlier taxonomies[7,10]), we discuss four approaches to using narrative, in quality improvement research (Table 1):

- narrative interview;
- naturalistic story gathering;
- organisational case study; and
- narrative dimensions of collective sense-making.

For each we discuss the rationale, method, approach to data analysis, strengths and limitations. Readers unfamiliar with qualitative research might also find a general introductory text helpful.[11]

Approach 1: Narrative Interview

Rationale

Personal stories are readily collected and can provide a vivid window to the healthcare system within which people's illness experiences are embedded. The study of end of life care based on the collection of the narratives of people dying from lung cancer or heart failure by Murray *et al*[12] is a good example.

Box 1: Ten unique selling points of stories in quality improvement research (compiled from various sources[7,14,17,20,43,48])

---

(1) Stories are *perspectival*. They are told subjectively from the viewpoint of the narrator, thus drawing attention to the individual rather than the institution.

(2) Stories *make sense of experience*. The structuring devices of time and plot retrospectively align events and actions so as to modify mental schemas.

(3) Stories are *non-linear*. They convey multiple and complex truths, depicting events as emerging from the interplay of actions, relationships and environments.

(4) Stories are *embedded in a context*. A particular story about what went on in an organisation is nested within an over-arching meta-narrative of "what tends to go on around here".

(5) Stories have an *ethical dimension*. They depict both acts and omissions, reflecting society's expectations about what a "good doctor" or "good daughter" should have done in such circumstances.

(6) Stories *bridge the gap* between the formal codified space of an organisation (roles, job descriptions, and lines of accountability) and informal uncodified space (relationships, feelings, "unwritten rules", and subcultures).

(7) Stories offer insights into what *might have been* (what Bruner calls "subjunctivization"[17]). The imaginative reconstruction of the end of a story allows us to consider different options for change.

(8) Stories are *action-oriented*, depicting what people did (and what happened to them), and also igniting and shaping their future action.

(9) Stories are *inherently subversive* since (in Bruner's terminology) they embrace the tension between the canonical (i.e. an organisation's standard routines and procedures) and the unexpected (i.e. new ways of thinking and working).

(10) Leadership is related to storytelling. *"Leaders are people who tell good stories, and about whom good stories are told".*[43]

Method

In narrative interview the researcher invites participants to "tell me what happened" and allows them to speak uninterrupted until the story ends. The key structuring devices are *chronology* (linking events in time) and *emplotment* (use of metaphors, imagery and rhetorical devices to imply causality and agency). The interview may be semi-structured (driven by a series of questions set out in advance) or unstructured (conducted in a more emergent, conversational style). In either case, prompts should only be used to preserve the flow of the story (hence "how did you feel at that point?" or "what happened next?"). The researcher might invite ideas for change in the form of a different ending to the story – as in "if you went through that experience again, what would make it easier for you?". Indeed, the prompt itself might be presented in the form of a short narrative fragment (vignette) and the respondent invited to continue the story. For a detailed methodology of narrative interviewing see Wengraf[13] or Riessman.[14]

Table 1: Approaches to the use of narrative in quality improvement research

Approach	Operational definition	Unit of analysis and analytical approach	Main research methods	Intended output of research	Example
Narrative interview	Researcher collects the stories of service users and/or the people involved in the quality improvement initiative	Individual narrative, analysed for structure, coherence, and meaning in a particular social context	Unstructured or semi-structured interview	Insights into individual experiences in the hands of the organisation/system	Patients' experiences of dying of heart failure or lung cancer[12]
Naturalistic story gathering	Researcher becomes a field worker immersed in the organisation so as to collect "real" stories in informal space and interpret them in context	Organisational subgroup, e.g. junior nurses. Analysed for subtleties in individuals' and groups' different interpretations of the same event/action over time	Ethnography	Thick description of organisational culture and how it influences particular behaviours and choices of individuals	Nurses' experience of introduction of computerised records (involved both formal interviews and informal story-gathering)[49]
Organisational case study	Researcher presents an account of the quality improvement initiative in the form of a detailed story	"The case" (perhaps the organisation), analysed for complex and dynamic influences on key events and processes	Multiple Qualitative and quantitative methods e.g. interviews, questionnaires, documentary analysis	Detailed description of "the case" as a context for events, plus chronological account of particular events as they unfolded during the study	Impact of learning facilitators on organisational change[34]
Collective sense-making	Researcher joins quality improvement team and works with them to develop a shared perspective on the problem and its causes, and to plan and implement action	Change team analysed for development and enaction of shared meanings/ purpose	Action research	Action intended to change practice ("organisational drama")	Action research study of quality improvement in a "failing" hospital trust[45]

Note: In practice, many empirical studies, contain elements of more than one of these (e.g. the organisational case study that includes narrative interviews as one data source.

Analysis of Data

Narrative interviews are, of course, qualitative data, and on one level can be approached using any mainstream method for analysing text. But narrative analysis per se takes the story as a whole, rather than segments of text, as its focus. Muller[7] describes five overlapping stages of narrative analysis: entering the text (reading and preliminary coding to gain familiarity), interpreting (finding connections in the data through successive readings and reflection), verifying (searching the text and other sources for alternative explanations and confirmatory and disconfirming data), representing (writing up an account of what has been learned), and illustrating (selecting representative quotes).

These analytical stages can be approached through one of several disciplinary lenses. All share what Muller calls "the focus on the broad contours of the story" – that is, the context in which it is told, its structure, the dynamics of how the plot unfolds, and any patterns that emerge from multiple stories about the same event. Riessman, for example, suggests that narratives can by analysed conversationally (as teller-listener dialogue), performatively (as drama), or politically (the unfolding of events is seen as constrained by prevailing social and institutional norms).[15] Frank uses a literary framework to analyse the stories of people with serious illness.[16] Their narratives, he suggests, fall into three basic categories: "restitution", "quest", and "chaos", corresponding to the literary genres of adventure, [coping with] tragedy, and nonsense. The narrator constructs their experiences respectively as restorative, heroic, or absurd using devices such as metaphor, exaggeration, understatement, and humour.

Strengths and Limitations

The main strength of the narrative interview is its inherent subjectivity. The story is irreducibly perspectival. A frequent theme in classical literature (consider *Great Expectations* or *The Grapes of Wrath*) is the struggle of society's underdogs against social injustice or institutional incompetence. Perhaps for this reason, the narrative interview 'comes into its own when considering a quality improvement, initiative from the perspective of disadvantaged groups such as the socially excluded, the seriously ill, and the very old.[17]

But the perspectival nature of stories is potentially a major limitation when they are used as research data. Furthermore, a story is an interaction – an artistic and rhetorical performance for an audience who (actively or passively) shapes the telling. The narrative interview has been described as *"practical production, the meaning of which is accomplished at the intersection of the interaction of interwiewer and respondent".*[18] A different interviewer on a different day will never be able to collect the "same" story from a respondent.

The challenge of narrative research is not to "control for" the inherent subjectivity, inconsistency, and emotionality of stories but to capture these phenomena as data and interpret them appropriately. Gabriel[19] offers some sound methodological advice: *"It is the researcher's task not merely to celebrate the story or the narrative but to seek to use it as a vehicle for accessing deeper truths than the truths, half-truths and fictions of undigested personal experience."*

The process of "accessing deeper truths" is not straightforward, and narrative research should not be equaled with privileging the judgment of the researcher over that of the informant. The validity of the research process rests heavily on evidence of the researcher's reflexive awareness. Aristotle's definition of good literature is that it has a powerful emotional impact on the reader."[8] The researcher must acknowledge and engage with this emotional dimension – thus turning sympathy, joy, revulsion, and even "mixed emotions" into research data. As in all qualitative research, there should also be a transparent account of how the researcher decided what aspects of the story to include and exclude as data, and how inferences were made.

Incidentally, the need to systematically and repeatedly interrogate the "truth" of narratives collected in a research study is one reason why it is generally poor practice to use stories supplied for one purpose (for example, in a clinical encounter) for research. It would also be unethical. A more in-depth discussion of these and other issues of methodological rigour in narrative research can be found elsewhere in the literature.[15,20,21]

Approach 2: Naturalistic Story Gathering

Rationale

As Table 1 shows, stories told informally may be especially valuable for accessing that elusive composite of shared values and meaning systems that can make or break a quality improvement initiative – namely, organisational culture. Through the interplay and exchange of stories, members of an organisation interpret, contextualise and collaboratively reframe the events they hold in common. Clifford Geertz[22] states: *"Believing, with Max Weber, that man is an animal suspended in webs of significance he himself has spun, I take culture to be those webs, and the analysis of it to be therefore not an experimental science in search of law but an interpretive one in search of meaning"* (page 5).

This semiotic (meaning based) view of culture is strongly echoed by three leading organisational anthropologists. Czarniawska[10] states that *"Modern institutions ... run on fictions, and the task of the scholar is to study how these fictions are created and sustained"* (page 10). Gabriel[20] highlights that stories exchanged by people in organisations have multiple functions in the creation of meaning: they variously inform, entertain, warn, advise, justify, explain, reassure, console, educate, sustain and transmit ideas or values, and draw moral lessons. Boje[23] has observed that informal stories in organisations are generally multi-authored (with different members alternating the role of teller and listener): highly reflexive (that is, the past is continually re-created and re-interpreted in the light of the present); dialogical (that is, the narrative is co-constructed through a dynamic interaction between each teller and listener); and often allusory and fragmented (emerging "in bits" rather than as fully formed narratives with a fixed cast of characters).

Method

The subtle complexities of organisational culture will be inaccessible to the researcher who arrives with a tape recorder and only collects narrative interviews as in Approach 1. Naturalistic enquiry, in which researchers undergo "immersion in the field" to study actors in their own environment, relatively free of intervention or control, offers scope to produce what Geertz has called "thick description" – that is, multilayered interpretation of social actions in context.[22] The main data source for such enquiry is the stories and story fragments exchanged in informal interaction with staff. The researcher must, of course, be selective in deciding which of the hundreds of stories heard during the course of the field work 10 capture as data, and also in assigning the status of "story" to what might be no more than a sentence, and (as with ethnography in general) the naïve or incompetent researcher, will lack the skill and sensitivity to select appropriately. For more detail on these methodological challenges in organisational research, see Boje's recent book.[24]

In one variant of the naturalistic approach, the researcher is appointed from within the quality improvement team rather than from an external research team (an example of autoethnography). In another variant, known as applied ethnography, the researcher explicitly feeds their ethnographic findings back into the organisation in order to effect change.[25]

Analysis

The principles of narrative analysis set out in Approach 1 above are also pertinent to the analysis of stories gathered in naturalistic settings. Close analysis of the stories as texts will not, of course, be possible if they have been recorded second-order as retrospective field notes (as is usual practice in ethnography). However, collecting and interpreting particular stories within a wider ethnographic study of the organisation gives the researcher a rich context within which to interpret their significance. Atkinson (cited in Hosburgh[26]) has strongly criticised the conventional narrative interview as characterised by "... *an extraordinary absence of social context, social action, and social interaction [and]... remarkably little sense of how narratives are forged in face-to-face interaction or how they are elicited in given social contexts*".[27] In other words, Atkinson sees a very positive trade-off between the accuracy with which the text of a narrative is recorded and the richness (and hence validity) of the context in which it is captured. For a more detailed methodology of ethnography in general, see Geertz,[22] and for organisational ethnography, see Gabriel[20] or Boje.[24]

Strengths and Limitations

A naturalistic approach enables the collection and comparison of multiple stories about a single issue or event. "Trouble" within the organisation will generate stories from different actors, and each person's story will change with repeated tellings. Not only is the "real" version of events an unhelpful concept, but the very plasticity of stories is the key to what Gabriel calls the "organisational dreamworld" – with multiple narratives interacting and challenging one another.[20] Gabriel's own field work has highlighted the contrast between organisations' official version of their own story ("well oiled machine, cutting edge technology") and the subversive metaphors used by the members ("the [pompous, incompetent] management, nothing works round here").[20]

The limitations of naturalistic story gathering are both practical and theoretical. "Prolonged immersion in the field" holds little currency with today's cost conscious research funders and, in any case, quality improvement initiatives may move too quickly. Being an "insider" to the quality improvement initiative has both advantages (in-depth knowledge and understanding of issues, rich social networks, mutual trust, timeliness, a longitudinal perspective, ability to effect change and integrate research with development) and disadvantages (lack of critical distance, a specific role in the organisation, prejudices arising from past personal experience, lack of knowledge of wider context). These issues are discussed further by Winter *et al.*[28]

Approach 3: Organisational Case Study

Rationale

Case study research considers a social system ("case") in context and explores it in sufficient detail to illuminate relationships and processes and provide insights into *why* particular events unfold as they do.[29,30] Like ethnography (with which it overlaps considerably), case study involves detailed reflexive field work leading to rich authentic description.

Method

Case study requires the prospective in-depth investigation of an organisation, team, or inter-agency initiative using multiple methods – typically, a combination of formal interviews, focus groups, participant observation, and collection of contemporaneous materials (minutes of meetings, emails, memos, etc). We must distinguish case study research, which can take years to produce, from the much more common quality improvement case *report* in which one or more members of a team tell a personal story about their initiative and its impact.

Constructing a case study requires considerable judgment and skill. The elements of the case must be iteratively defined through a sequence of sampling (to identify somewhere to start), progressive focusing (to refine and systematically explore what has been sampled), theorising (about interactions within the arbitrarily defined case and across the boundary with the world beyond it), analysing (testing how well the data fit the theory), and interpreting (deriving meaning from the data).[29,30]

Analysis

Organisations are complex, containing much social action (and a good bit of trouble) so, in practice, most organisational case studies get analysed and written up in a story-like way. An organisational case study is generally based on a large, heterogeneous, dynamic and complex collection of empirical data, each component of which will first need to be analysed separately – for example, quantitative data statistically; qualitative data thematically – before being woven into a higher order interpretation of the whole picture and how and why it has changed through time.

"Storying" the case – that is, constructing a chronological emplotted account of the key actions and events – is a way of selecting which data to focus on and which to omit. It is also a way of drawing meaning from different data sources and making causal links between aspects of the case, either tentatively (as hypotheses to be tested in further research) or more firmly as lessons or conclusions (if the links are particularly strong and plausible). In practice, organisational case studies tend to be the product of several researchers working together over months or years, and the task of processing, interpreting and integrating the data into a coherent story is achieved through interaction between team members – especially the repeated exchange and negotiation of stories.

Stake[30] draws on Van Maanen[31] to suggest four approaches to "storying" that researchers may use to present in-depth case studies:

- realist tales: a direct, matter-of-fact portrait, a chronological or biographical development of the case;
- confessional tales: the researcher's personal account of coming to know the case and the challenges they faced;
- impressionist tales: a sequential description of several major components of the case, "*personalised accounts of fleeting moments of fieldwork case in dramatic form*"; and
- illustrative tales: the use of vignettes (storied episodes) to illustrate particular aspects of the case.

In all these approaches a good case study researcher, like a good storyteller, will use literary devices to place emphasis and convey surprises and ambiguities, and will "zoom in" judiciously to analyse the behaviour of individuals within (and as influenced by) the wider system. Once again, an important criterion for judging the rigour of a case study is evidence of the researchers' reflexive awareness and the transparency of their inferences from the data.

Strengths and Limitations

Case study has been described as "strong in reality" – that is, as having high potential for validity within the confines of the case itself.[30] But researchers who have been raised on the conventional hierarchy of evidence (with randomised controlled trials at the top and anecdote at the bottom) often find it hard to identify much value in case study research. The central epistemological question might be put: to what extent does case study trade external validity (i.e. direct transferability to other contexts) for internal coherence and richness, and (conversely) to what extent will a detailed and systematic analysis of one unique "case" give us robust, transferable lessons for elsewhere?

This question is much debated amongst case study theorist (see, for example, a recent compilation[32]). Yin[29] takes a conventional scientific view that a case is only meaningful as a member of a sociological family of cases which provide the analytical framework to understand it ("previously developed theory is used as a template with which to compare the empirical results of case studies"). Stake,[30] in contrast, argues from an interpretive perspective that the case is meaningful in its own right (the "sample of one" or what he calls "the intrinsic study of the valued particular").

May, quoted in Simons,[33] describes how his understanding of trees was changed forever when he saw a painting by Cézanne. The tree in the painting was not statistically representative of trees in general, nor did it contain features present in every tree. Nevertheless, the qualities that Cézanne had illuminated in his *particular* tree enabled the author to see every subsequent tree through new eyes. Simons argues that the hallmark of a good case study is this metaphorical (rather than scientific) generalisability.

Thor *et al*[34] describe a five year case study of an ambitious quality improvement initiative in an acute hospital, based on "learning facilitators" who helped a total of 93 project teams. The researchers attributed the success of the facilitators to allowing each clinical team to remain in charge of their ideas and adopting a supporting role that comprised (a) providing feedback on ideas and progress; (b) helping with demanding (and sometimes menial) tasks; (c) developing specialist skill and experience in quality improvement; and (d) taking responsibility for small practicalities such as refreshments for meetings. Arguably, the validity of this case does not rest on (nor would it be enhanced by) the presence of a "control group" or "comparative cases": it rests on the authenticity of the observations and interpretations about what happened in *this* case. Of course, we cannot extrapolate these findings to every quality improvement project (for example, we cannot say that providing cookies at meetings will always improve the quality of decisions). But we can learn a general lesson from a facilitation approach characterised by "mucking in" and taking account of specific contextual features (in this case, that meetings were often held over mealtimes).

Another potential limitation of in-depth case study is that, because of the detailed contextual information necessary to understand the case, organisations (and the individuals within them) may be identifiable. Elwyn *et al*[35] have described a way of fictionalising organisational case studies by first abstracting the key themes from a sample of cases – for example, high user expectations, lack of cash, external policy mandates, and so on – and then writing a new story that includes all these key themes.

Approach 4: Using Narrative in Collective Sense-Making

Rationale

An alternative conception of narrative research is developing (and enacting) shared meanings rather than collecting or writing stories.[36] Contemporary theories of organisational development centre on the construction, acquisition, transfer and use of knowledge, and on the need for the members of an organisation to make sense of change efforts by assimilating them into their cognitive schemas.[37] Organisational members are active "framers", cognitively making sense of the events, processes, objects and issues that comprise (say) a quality improvement initiative and fining it into their current cognitive schemas. When the initiative (or the goals that justify it) are perceived as new, the individual may retain an outdated schema of the organisation rather than discarding or modifying it. The result is cognitive inertia – that is, the tendency to remain with the status quo and resist changes that lie "outside the frame".[38]

To be successfully assimilated by staff (and service users), a proposed change must make sense in a way that relates to previous understanding and experience – and this is where story comes in. People caught up in a change initiative (or who are trying to "stay afloat" in a changing environment) engage in a continuous stream of experience and action which generates a succession of equivocal situations.[39] They then *retrospectively impose* a structure or schema to make these situations sensible. In other words, the act of sense-making is itself the construction of a narrative, requiring elements to be selected out, highlighted as significant or surprising, juxtaposed with one another (and with the existing cognitive schema), given meaning, and so on.[40,41] For a taxonomy of such interpretive approaches, see Czarniawska.[10]

The notion of narrative as sense-making fits closely with a rapidly expanding "knowledge based" tradition within organisational research (including Stage's work on the learning organisation[42]). In this tradition, "management" is seen not as a technical process of keeping the cogs oiled and maintaining throughput, but as the effective creation and circulation of knowledge. Leadership is conceptualised not as "command and control" but as providing the opportunities and facilitation needed for people to build and exchange knowledge.[43] In a change effort the leader's role is to pull a team together around a shared story of innovation, improvement, and action. In practice, this means initialing and leading discussions around the *meaning* of any proposed changes.

Method

A good example of this research approach is Paul Bate's story of a quality improvement initiative in a "failing" UK NHS hospital trust.[44] Change was achieved through an action research design (defined as "*a mutual learning process within which people work together to discover what the issues are, why they exist, and how they might be addressed*") in which members of the organisation met periodically for facilitated discussion, reflection, and action planning.[45] A striking aspect of the change effort in this study was the perception that all the members of the change team, from the chief executive to the cleaner, felt that they were all pulling together in a common ethical endeavour about which they had strong (and positive) personal feelings. The conventional narrative of organisational change, Bate argues, is couched in "*the vocabulary of coercion, competition, tyranny, hegemony control, subjection, engineering, manipulation, domination, subordination, resistance, opposition, diversity, negotiation, obedience and compliance*". The more contemporary "knowledge creation" approach uses different vocabulary: "*cooperation, convergence, coherence, integration and consensus*", for which the development of a shared story can prove the critical mechanism.[45] In emphasising the critical role of enacting stories as a vehicle for collective action, Bate cites the commentary by Kling[46] on social movements:

"Social movements are constituted by the stories people tell to themselves and to one another. They reflect the deepest ways in which people understand who they are and to whom they are connected ... They are constructed from the interweaving of personal and social biographies – from the narratives people rehearse to themselves about the nature of their lives ... The construction of collective action therefore, is inseparable from the construction of personal biography from the ways, that is, we experience the imprecation of our individual and social selves".

Strengths and Limitations

One great strength of the sense-making approach is its action orientation. Collective sense-making of past and present events feeds into creative team-driven action – less narrative, more organisational drama, Buckler and Zein[47] emphasise the critical role of informal stories in organisational innovativeness and change. Stories, they claim, are inherently subversive. They create the backdrop for new visions and embody "permission to break the rules". In an old fashioned machine bureaucracy, behaviours and events that go beyond the existing structures and systems are implicitly (and often explicitly) "wrong". But, by presenting "innovation and change in story form, its agents can be imbued with positive virtues such as courage, tenacity and creativity ("Mrs Patel from the records department went in and told them straight"). Rule breakers become hero[in]es and the change effort a moral epic, enabling members of the organisation to reject the rules and routines more confidently. By using the enacted story as the vehicle for change, a current of subversion can be run through a previously indifferent organisation.

The main limitation of collective sense-making is that it is a highly specialised and intensive approach, of which there are as yet few rigorously conducted examples in the literature.

Conclusions

The richness and flexibility of the story form make it an enticing addition to the researcher's toolkit in the hard to research world of quality improvement. This paper has attempted to classify the different theoretical positions that might underpin a narrative approach to quality improvement research, and to provide some practical advice for those who seek to use these methods in empirical work.

The slippery nature of narrative truth means that we must be wary of so-called "narrative research" that is nothing of the sort. Box 2 lists a provisional checklist of questions to ask when considering whether stories elicited, interpreted, analysed, or constructed in relation to a quality improvement initiative should count as research at all, and to assess the rigour of such research.

Box 2: When should a narrative be classified as research in quality improvement initiatives?

The following questions, used alongside relevant critical appraisal checklists, should inform this complex judgement:

- Did the investigator(s) collect, interpret, collate or present the stor(ies) with the intention of answering a clear and focussed research question?
- Did the investigator(s) use a recognisable methodological approach (such as narrative interview, detailed ethnographic fieldwork, multi-method case study, or action research)?
- Was the approach applied rigorously and transparently? Consider aspects such as sampling frame, choice of instruments or tools, method of data collection, method of analysis, and so on.
- Did the investigator(s) demonstrate reflexive awareness in all aspects of the research process and the researcher role?
- Was there an identifiable unit of analysis (e.g. the person, the incident, the team, the organisation, the patient journey)?
- Was there a competent and transparent attempt to analyse empirically collected data using a recognised theoretical framework? In other words, did the researchers go beyond "letting the stories speak for themselves"?

References

1. Davidoff F, Batalden P. Toward stronger evidence on quality improvement. Draft publication guidelines: the beginning of a consensus project, *Qual Saf Health Care* 2005;**14**:319–25.
2. Moss F, Thomson R, A new structure for quality improvement reports. *Qual Health Care* 1999;**8**:76.
3. Lynn J. When does quality improvement count as research? Human subject protection and theories of knowledge. *Qual Saf Health Care* 2004;**14**:67–70.
4. Casarett D, Karlawish JH, Sugarman J. Determining when quality improvement initiatives should be considered research: proposed criteria and potential implications. *JAMA* 2000;**283**:2275–80.
5. Bruner J, *Actual minds, possible words*. Cambridge: Harvard University Press, 1986.
6. Polkinghorne DE, *Narrative knowing and the human sciences*. Albany: State University of NY Press, 1988.
7. Muller J, Narrative approaches to qualitative research in primary care in Crabtree BF, Miller WL, eds. *Doing qualitative research* 2nd ed. London Sage Publications, 1999:221–38.
8. Aristotle *Poetics*. Translated by Malcolm Heath. London: Penguin, 1996:540.
9. Burke K. *A grammar of motive*. Berkeley: University of California Press, 1945.
10. Czarniawska B, *A narrative approach to organization studies*. Qualitative Research Methods Series 43. London: Sage Publications, 1998.
11. Atkinson P, Coffey A, Delamont S. *Key themes in qualitative research: continuities and changes*. London: AltaMira, 2003.
12. Murray SA, Boyd K, Kendall M, *et al* Dying of lung cancer or cardiac failure: a community-based, prospective qualitative interview study of patients and their carers. *BMJ* 2002; **325**:929–32.
13. Wengraf T. *Qualitative research interviewing: biographic, narrative and semi-structured methods*. London: Sage Publications, 2001.

14. Riessman CK, *Narrative analysis*. Newbury Park, CA: Sage Publications, 1993.
15. Riessman CK, Analysis of personal narratives. In: Gubrium JF, Holstem JA, eds. Handbook of qualitative research. London: Sage Publications, 2001.
16. Frank A, Just listening narrative and deep illness. *Families Systems Health* 1998; **16**:197–216.
17. Bruner J, *Acts of meaning*. Cambridge: Harvard University Press, 1990.
18. Fontana A, Frey J. From structured questions to negotiated text. In: Denzin M. Lincoln P., eds. *Handbook of qualitative research*. 2nd ed. London: Sage Publications, 2003.
19. Gabriel Y. The voice of experience and the voice of the expert – can they speak to each other? In: Hurwitz B, Greenhalgh T, Skultans V, eds. *Narrative research in health and illness*. London: BMJ Publications, 2004.
20. Gabriel Y, *Storytelling in organisations: facts, fictions and fantasies*. Oxford: Oxford University Press, 2000.
21. Gubrium JF, Holstein JA, Narrative practice and the coherence of personal stories. *Social Q* 1998;**39**:163–87.
22. Geertz C, *The interpretation of cultures*. New York: Basic books, 1973.
23. Boje DM. The storytelling organization: a study of story performance in an office-supply firm. *Admin Sci Q* 1991;**36**:106–26.
24. Boje D. *Narrative methods for organizational and communication research*, London: Sage Publications, 2001.
25. Chambers X. Applied ethnography, in: Denzin M, Lincoln P. eds. *Handbook of qualitative research*. London: Sage Publications, 2003.
26. Hosburgh D. Evaluation of qualitative research. *J Clin Nurs* 2003;**12**:307–12.
27. Atkinson P. Narrative turn or blind alley? *Qualitative Health Res* 1997;**7**:325–44.
28. Winter R, Munn Giddings C. *A handbook for action research in health and social care*. London: Routledge, 2001.
29. Yin RK. *Case study research: design and methods*, 2nd ed. London: Sage Publications, 1994.
30. Stake R. *The art of case study research*, London: Sage, 1995.
31. Van Maanen J. *Tales of the field: on writing ethnography*, Chicago: University of Chicago Press, 1988.
32. Gomm R, Hammersley M, Foster P. *Case study method*. London: Sage Publications, 2000.
33. Simons H. The paradox of case study. *Cambridge J Educ* 1996;**26**:225–40.
34. Thor J, Whittlov K, Herrlin B, *et al*. Learning helpers: how they facilitated improvement and improved facilitation. Lessons from a hospital-wide quality improvement initiative. *Qual Manage Healthc* 2004;**30**:60–74.
35. Elwyn G, Hocking H, Burtonwood A, *et al*. Learning to plan? A critical fiction about the facilitation of professional and practice development plans in general practice. *J Interprofessional Care* 2002;**16**:349–58.
36. Mattingly C. *Healing dramas and clinical plots: the narrative structure of experience*. New York: Cambridge University Press, 1998.
37. Fiske ST, Neuberg SL. A continuum of impression formation, from category-based to individuating processes. *Advon Exp Soc Psychol* 1990;**23**:1–74.
38. Bartunek JM. Changing interpretative schemes and organizational restructuring: the example of a religious order. *Admin Sci Q* 1984;**19**:355–72.
39. Weick KE. *Sensemaking in organizations*. Thousand Oaks, CA: Sage, 1995.
40. Brown JS, Duguid KP. *The social life of information*. Boston, MA: Harvard University Press, 2000.
41. Boland RJ, Tenkasi RV, Te'eni D. Designing information technology to support distributed cognition. *Organization Sci* 1994;**5**:456–75.
42. Senge PM. *The fifth discipline – the art and practice of the learning organisation*. New York: Random House Business Books, 1993.

43. Gardner H. *Leading minds: an anatomy of leadership*. London: Harper Collins, 1995.
44. Bate P. Synthesizing research and practice: using the action research approach in health care settings. *Soc Policy Admin* 2000;**34**:478–93.
45. Bate SP. The role of stories and storytelling in organisational change efforts: a field study of an emerging 'community of practice within the UK National Health Service. In: Hurwitz B, Greenhalgh T, Skultans V, eds. *Narrative research in health and illness*. London: BMJ Publications, 2004.
46. Kling N, Anderson N. *Innovation and change in organisations*. London: Routledge, 1995.
47. Buckler SA, Zein C. The spirituality of innovation: learning from stories. *J Product Innovation Manage* 1996;**13**:391–405.
48. Ricoeur P. *Time and narrative*, Volume 1. Chicago, University of Chicago Press, 1984.
49. Timmons S. How does professional culture influence the success or failure of IT implementation in health services? In: Ashburner L, ed. *Organisational behaviour and organisational studies in health care: reflections on the future*. Basingstoke: Palgrave, 2001:218–31.

40

One Voice, Different Tunes: Issues Raised by Dual Analysis of a Segment of Qualitative Data

Jan Savage

Introduction

This paper considers the relationship between qualitative data, the way it is analysed and the findings that emerge, particularly in the context of post-modernist debates about the meaning of texts, or rather where meaning resides. Texts can be understood as anything articulated as language (Culler 1983). It has been argued that texts do not carry a single or unified meaning imposed by the text's author, but that the plurality of meanings in a text become fused by the reader (Barthes 1977). Clearly this understanding of text raises important issues of intentionality, authenticity and interpretive authority for researchers that have relevance throughout the research process. This paper, however, is particularly concerned with data analysis and its relationship to the plurality of meanings that may be found in textual data. It reports on the outcome of the same analyst using two different forms of data analysis (thematic and narrative analysis) to explore the same segment of data, following in the steps of Coffey & Atkinson (1996). These different approaches were chosen on the basis that they treat text in very different ways. Thematic analysis is generally associated with a realist approach in which it is assumed that there will be some fit between the outcome of data analysis and some external or overarching reality. In contrast, a narrative approach is more concerned with understanding how people use cultural resources

Source: *Journal of Advanced Nursing*, 31(6) (2000): 1493–1500.

to construct stories I that describe locally produced, and more ambiguous, realities (Silverstone 2000). This exercise is therefore not an attempt at triangulation, which involves:

> ... the comparison of data relating to the same phenomenon but deriving from different phases of the fieldwork, ... or, as in respondent validation, the accounts of different participants (including the ethnographer) involved in the setting. (Hammersley & Atkinson 1983 p. 198)

Instead, the concern is with re-exploring the *same* segment of data using different approaches to see if different sets of meanings emerge and, if so, to consider what this difference means.

Analysis, Interpretation and 'Truth'

Wolcott (1994) makes a useful distinction between the research activities of description, analysis and interpretation, while also being careful to emphasize that they are not mutually exclusive ways of exploring data. With description, Wolcott suggests, the data are treated as fact and allowed to speak for themselves: description answers the question of 'What is going on here?'. With analysis, the role of the researcher extends beyond a purely descriptive account to the systematic elucidation of key factors and the relationships between these, or how things work. Interpretation, he argues, goes beyond the degree of certainty often assumed with analysis, and represents an attempt to reach an understanding about meaning, particularly in relation to context: interpretation attempts to deal with the question of 'What is to be made of it all?' (Wolcott 1994 p. 12). Taking Wolcott's distinctions as a springboard, this paper is partly concerned with the relationship between thematic analysis as a systematic trawl for key factors and the interpretation of narrative as an attempt to establish meaning. However, a concern with interpretation immediately locates the discussion in a larger debate about social inquiry and 'whether its truths are invented or found, fictional or factual' (Jackson 1989 p. 171).

It is only recently that social scientists have begun to reflect critically on the way that they produce texts and the way that these are read (Coffey & Atkinson 1996). This decade has seen both the rise of post-modernism[1] and advocacy of the 'interpretive turn', both of which have led to widespread repudiation of empirical approaches (Morris 1997). There has thus been a shift in this field from the pursuit of objectivity in which the researcher is portrayed as an impartial observer who produces an authoritative and unified account, towards greater subjectivity, more reflexive authorship and experiments with forms of writing that give expression to a broader range of voices or perspectives (Clifford 1988, Atkinson 1990). For some post-modernists, the text takes on a huge significance, so much so that they argue there is no knowledge of the world except through language: outside of the text, there is nothing (Derrida 1976).

More generally, interest in texts has focused on the sets of relations that bring them into production: in other words 'who speaks? who writes? when and where? with or to whom? under what institutional and historical constraints?' (Clifford 1986 p. 13, Smith 1994). This has led to accounts of fieldwork that are acutely self-conscious of the researcher's role in the generation of data (see, for example, Okely & Callaway 1992). As a result, the transformation of data into text is widely regarded as a product of particular social encounters, and closer to 'persuasive fiction' (Atkinson 1990 p. 26) rather than the pre-sentation of 'facts' which exist independently of such social relations, as empiricists might suggest.

Post-modernist approaches in particular have 'recognized the multiplicity of voices, views, and methods present in any representation or analysis of any aspect of reality, including the reality of health care' (Cheek 1999 p. 385). There are those (see the debate between Lucas (1997) and Burnard (1997) for example) who suggest that the same informant may provide different accounts of the same event at different times and to different people, or that people may mean more than one thing when they speak (Nijhof 1997 p. 173). Others (such as Bloch 1998) warn against confusing what people say with what they know, on the premise that different kinds of knowledge may be organized in different ways, with each kind of knowledge having a specific relationship to language.

To explain this point, Bloch (1998) gives the example of a well-known experiment in which volunteers are shown an office, with typical office furniture and equipment, but with two bananas on one of the desks. When asked to recall what they saw later, volunteers almost always refer to the bananas first, before listing the more typical office equipment. According to Bloch this demonstrates how we pay attention to the uncommon, presumably because this might require a more considered response from us than the mundane or familiar. In addition, he suggests, it indicates that interpreting the scene of 'furniture and bananas' depends on a particular form of knowledge, or schema. This schema enables us not only to recognize a particular space as 'an office' because it has certain features, such as word processors, but it enables us to recognize other offices that have new configurations of these features. Bloch's point is that although volunteers in the study talked about the bananas and not about the various elements of the office, this did not mean that they had remembered one and forgotten the other: 'in a sense, it could be said that they remembered those [office] things too well but not in an explicit, verbalized way' (Bloch 1998 p. 45). Thus, he argues, 'knowing' involves different kinds of activities, and different relationships to language.

This example of furniture and bananas may be pedestrian in nature, yet it shows the complexity of an apparently simple speech act of description, and can readily be transposed to other contexts (such as the way that nurses may describe a patient's condition to other health professionals, omitting what is known 'too well'). It draws attention to the silences in what people say, that they may speak more, for example, about the atypical, and less about what is assumed to be shared knowledge: there is therefore a need to acknowledge the different emphases and modulations, indeed the spoken and the unspoken 'voices' of a single speaker.

Such debates, which raise questions about the nature of meaning (see Hobart 1982, Burnard 1997) and particularly whether meaning is inherent within data or merely imposed upon data by the researcher, have implications for approaches to analysis. For example, should certain types of analysis only be used for data arising from particular ideological approaches, with thematic analysis, for instance, limited to research grounded in empiricist or realist traditions, or is this too prescriptive? Can we accept that there is nothing in what informants say other than what the reader chooses to read into it, or is this a nihilistic and patronising premise? Or is an alternative way possible that avoids the straight-jacket imposed by accepting different paradigms as discrete and polarized?

There are recent indications of greater openness and flexibility in applying different research approaches and methods of analysis to access the multiple voices or perspectives within a group (Morse 1999, Cheek 1999). Nevertheless, there has been little attention to whether, or how, methods of data analysis can cope with the 'multivocality' – that is, the varied perspectives and inflections (for example, the silence regarding what is assumed to be shared knowledge) – that may be present in the data from any one individual.

This paper describes an attempt to explore the multivocality of one speaker using an approach outlined by Coffey & Atkinson (1996). They argue the need for 'multiple practices, methods and possibilities of analysis', suggesting that it is possible to treat the same data more than once, using different perspectives: as they put it 'analytically speaking, there is more than one way to skin a cat' (Coffey & Atkinson 1996 p. 20). They are careful to state, however, that the alternative perspectives that might be generated by different techniques cannot be aggregated, as some suggest,[2] to form a unified, more complete picture, or be converged to reach a single conclusion. To suggest this would be to imply that it is possible to gain an increasingly accurate representation of a single and homogenous social world. Rather, Coffey and Atkinson argue that using different analytical procedures may be helpful in teasing out different layers of understanding represented in the data, and allow the construction of different, and even contrary, versions of the social world.

The Data

The data chosen to be subjected to alternative forms of analysis are derived from an interview with an experienced nurse, 'Ann'. This interview was one of a series with nurses asking them to describe their previous day on duty as part of a study concerning the nature of nursing culture, and looking at the role of nursing culture in relation to staff retention and patient care. The study was a focused ethnography of a mixed HIV/acute medical ward in a large teaching hospital. The methods employed were those of non-participant observation of everyday life on the ward, group interviews with nursing staff, a survey of the nursing staff and a series of one-to-one interviews with nurses and medical colleagues. (For fuller details of this study see Savage 1998.)

One of the most notable features associated with this ward was the emphasis placed by all nurses on their collective support needs, as demonstrated by the way they had initiated a regular, facilitated support group that augmented the informal support available from colleagues on an *ad hoc* basis. It is the value nurses placed on support that appears to be particularly relevant in the account provided by Ann, who describes the dilemma she experiences when asked to 'keep an eye on' colleagues beyond her own ward.

The segment of data explored here comes from the very beginning of the interview with Ann in which she provides an account of her last shift. As there is insufficient space to present Ann's story verbatim, it is summarized as follows.

The day Ann described had been atypical for her. Due to the absence of more senior staff, she had been asked for the first time in years to carry the bleep for the medical unit. This meant that she was expected to give support to nurses in other clinical areas (for example, helping them to check drugs, or to help them to make professional or ethical decisions) in addition to supporting members of her own team and carrying out her own clinical caseload. Her own ward leader, Irene, was on holiday, and after Ann had been relieved of the bleep at midday, she was then asked to stand in for Irene and organize support for another clinical area (Latimer Ward) where the ward leader and a number of other nurses were off sick. It was not clear how long Ann would be required to act in this capacity.

Her response to these demands was partly one of frustration at having to fit in these additional duties on top of her own clinical caseload. Ann gave a picture on the one hand of having to cope with broad and unfixed responsibilities beyond the ward, while faced with the necessity of completing her own clinical duties according to fixed deadlines. She was also unhappy about having to work in areas that were unfamiliar to her, being concerned that, in the case of an emergency, she would not know where the necessary equipment was stored. Ann was unfamiliar with the staff on the other ward, beyond knowing that some were newly appointed. She was therefore unsure of their competence, and the kind of help that they might need from her.

Thematic Analysis

The segment of transcript from Ann's interview summarized above was subjected first to 'thematic' analysis, a term open to a wide range of interpretations. Its use here, however, refers to a relatively simple process of coding, clustering codes to develop concepts or categories from the coding, and developing themes from these concepts or categories that help to explain the phenomena under investigation (Coffey & Atkinson 1996). Thematic analysis was chosen in preference to other approaches consistent with a realist perspective, such as content analysis, partly because, depending on the way coding is employed, it allows the consideration of process and meaning, and thus shares some similarities with narrative analysis.

Codes, according to Miles & Huberman (1994 p. 56), are 'tags or labels for assigning units of meaning to the descriptive or inferential information compiled during a study'. If coding is kept to a general level, it can be understood as a way of reducing the data with a view to identifying a simple conceptual schema and enabling the retrieval of elements of the data that can be brought together under the same codes. However, coding is often a mixture of data reduction and data complication – a way of expanding the data, to develop new questions and interpretative ideas, in which, according to Wolcott's (1994) distinctions, the focus shifts from analysis (the identification of key factors) to interpretation. According to Coffey & Atkinson (1996), qualitative coding is *primarily* a way of interacting with and thinking about data, in which the process of reflection involved in coding is more important than the procedure chosen.

A number of codes emerged with the thematic analysis of Ann's story. Figure 1 shows how these codes eventually were grouped together through a cyclical process of:

- dividing the data into units of meaning;
- thinking of the appropriate codes to represent each unit's meaning; and
- considering the relationship between the codes and the data segment overall, together with how the codes might be meaningfully clustered together.

This essentially subjective process led to the development of provisional, overarching categories, namely: 'knowledge and place' and 'boundaries and role (knowledge, time and place)'; and sub-categories of 'nature of role' and 'extent of responsibility'.

Findings from Provisional Thematic Analysis

The category of *'knowledge and place'* encapsulates references made by Ann about the way that she felt less confidant when she worked in an unfamiliar environment, and the importance of knowing the layout of a ward (and the storage of emergency equipment, for example) to function efficiently.

The other category, *'boundaries of role (knowledge, time and place)'* refers to the limits of Ann's role and her uncertainty concerning these on this particular day: she was unclear about how long, at least in the medium term,

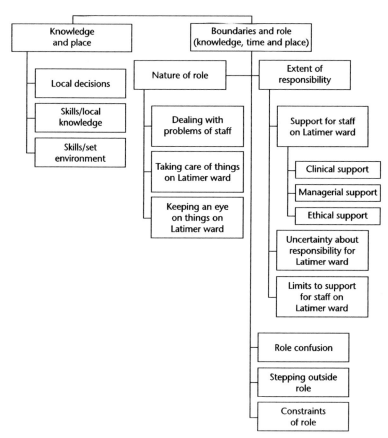

Figure 1: First thematic analysis

that she was supposed to offer support; she was aware of the constraints that limited her fulfilment of the role as she understood it (as demonstrated in the earlier quote about her association of sound practice with a known environment). This category also includes reference to the way that Ann used to enjoy broader responsibilities in the past when she was a night sister, with the suggestion that besides carrying a clinical caseload in addition to the bleep, staying on one ward for a long time had made shouldering this wider role more difficult.

Within this category, the sub-category 'nature of role' brings together elements of the role that Ann juggled with when carrying the bleep or supporting colleagues on Latimer ward. This included recognition of the problems that staff might face (such as problems with drug administration), and the maintenance of some element of 'supervision' of staff on the other ward for the foreseeable future.

The sub-category of 'extent of responsibility' refers to Ann's commitment to support staff on Latimer Ward, but also her uncertainty about how much time this would take. It further includes a recognition of the limits to what

Ann (and members of her team) could offer given, for example, their lack of knowledge of levels of competence on this other ward. Within this sub-category lies another sub-area, '*nature of support*' that incorporates the different types of support Ann was called on to provide: helping to make decisions about whether informed consent had been given; helping with clinical matters such as drug administration; and giving managerial or administrative support, such as advising when to call in agency staff.

In summary, what emerges most strongly from this form of analysis are provisional themes of place, time, role and knowledge, and the relationship between these. What appears to lie at the heart of Ann's account is the co-dependency of these themes and how this inter-reliance helps to explain the difficulties she experienced on the day in question.

This, of course, is not a conventional thematic analysis which would nor-mally entail amalgamating codes from across the data set, that is, from across the accounts of all informants, to produce categories and themes (Grbich 1999). However, thematic analysis of this isolated segment of data is useful as a way of thinking about the data and allowing some broad comparison between this approach and that of narrative analysis.

Narrative Analysis

Narrative has been viewed as perhaps the primary mechanism by which human understanding of experience is registered (Brock & Kleiber 1994). Interest in narrative has risen with the emergence of postmodernism and its incredulity towards the meta-narratives, largely those of the Enlightenment, under-pinning scientific theory and knowledge (Lyotard 1984). Such scepticism led to a shift towards everyday knowledge based on very different kinds of testimony, such as technical or ethical statements (Lash 1990). In response, many social researchers have come to deny the feasibility of gaining direct access to 'reality', turning instead to local narrative and 'messy texts' which are inevitably open-ended, multivoiced and in which no particular interpretation is given precedence (Denzin 1997).

Analysis of local narrative can be understood as 'doing research with first-person accounts of experiences' (Coffey & Atkinson 1996). Although much narrative analysis in health care research appears concerned with under-standing the experience of illness and suffering (see, for example, Kleinman 1988, Charmaz 1999), there are other applications. Narratives are recognized as offering ways of going beyond description to exploring aspirations and moral imperatives: as May & Fleming (1997 p. 1098) have put it, narratives are 'constitutive of self and professional identity'. There has been recent interest in reviving the tradition of narrative in the teaching and practice of medicine (Greenhalgh & Hurwitz 1999) and the usefulness of narrative approaches is increasingly recognized in nursing research (Sandelowski 1991, May & Fleming 1997, Anderson 1998).

Just as there are different types of narrative, there are many types of narrative analysis, some of which are much more formal than others (Manning & Cullum-Swan 1994). However, as Denzin (1997 p. 128) points out, 'these strategies falter the moment when the recorded or analysed text is taken to be an accurate (visual) representation of the worlds and voices studied'. The form of narrative analysis considered here is one that is loosely formulated, almost intuitive, and broadly follows the example of Coffey & Atkinson (1996) who in turn draw on the work of Labov (1982), stressing the importance of structure as much as content.

Labov developed an evaluation approach to narrative, arguing that narratives have formal structural properties related to their social functions. These properties or structural units can be defined in terms of *the abstract* (what the story is about); *the orientation* (providing information about the context, actors, and so on); *the complication* (what happened); *the evaluation* (an appraisal), *the result* (what finally happened); and *the coda* (the signing off). These units occur in recurrent patterns that can be identified and used to interpret each segment of narrative, although not all the elements will necessarily occur in any one narrative, occur in order, or occur just once. According to Coffey & Atkinson (1996), thinking about stories within data in this way, identifying such structural units, enables creative thinking about data and their interpretation and it is this exploration of structure that underlies the narrative analysis described here.

Table 1 shows how the narrative can be understood in terms of its structural elements, as defined by Labov. Looking at the data as narrative, the abstract highlights that the story concerns an atypical day. The orientation indicates that it begins to be atypical from the point at which Ann is asked to carry the bleep, although the story is not entirely or essentially concerned with the changes carrying the bleep introduces. This is demonstrated by the way that the main part of the account, the 'complication', continues after the return of the bleep, and with Ann being asked to take responsibility for Latimer ward. The evaluative part of the narrative, the part which highlights the point of the story, appears to be summarized in the sentence 'What are we supposed to do with our colleagues and things like that?'.

The narrative can therefore be understood as essentially concerned with the nature of the relationship between nurses who are ostensibly peers, and the concern Ann expresses as to whether she can support nurses on Latimer Ward appropriately. The evaluation indicates that the experience of taking responsibility for nurses beyond her own ward has made Ann question the appropriateness of this role and prompted her to look more closely at how she supports colleagues on her own ward. The coda closes the story by reiterating that this was an atypical day. Significantly what has emerged

Table 1: Narrative analysis

Element	Potential question	Narrative
Abstract (makes proposition that will be exemplified)	What is this about?	'Yesterday was very atypical'
Orientation (establishes situation, time, context)	Who, what, where, when?	Anne was asked to take the bleep. Anxious and angry – feels unprepared but accepts bleep
Complication (the major account of events, problems and how these were made sense of by narrator)	Then what happened?	*Event (1) Carrying the bleep* Dealt with range of professional/ethical issues on behalf of staff beyond own ward Torn between responsibilities as bleep carrier and those as senior staff nurse on own ward with clinical workload
Break in complication		*Event (2) Covering the other ward* Asked to cover sister ward due to staff absence for indefinite period Identifies practical support needed (e.g. drugs) Unsure of competence of staff
Evaluation (highlights point of narrative)	So what?	Episode made Ann look at own practice with own team, and wonder about responsibility to little known colleagues on other ward: 'What are we supposed to do with our colleagues and things like that?'
Results (describing outcome)	What finally happened?	'We are going to keep an eye on things, . . . hope the senior nurses are keeping an eye on things as well'
Coda (indicating closure)	What finally happened?[finish]	'So, yesterday started off really atypical'

using this approach is Ann's moral dilemma about how to support staff whose competence and needs are unknown to her, and that this was not a typical day – ways of understanding the data that were less apparent with the first, thematic approach to analysis.

Discussion

Before comparing the two analytical approaches, a number of limitations to this exercise need to be acknowledged. There are, of course, considerable problems in concentrating on only one segment of data rather than an entire data set. Not least, the brevity of this kind of paper means that these data have to be considered out of context, dissociated both from a detailed understanding of the nurse's working environment and from similar data provided by her colleague's accounts. In the 'thematic' analysis, an attempt has been made to cluster codes and concepts that emerged from within one data segment and not across a data set. The decisions made, such as how to break the text into units of meaning, and what tags or codes to assign to such units, are provisional and unrefined. What can be claimed as a result of this exercise is therefore tentative both in terms of producing an analysis of the data, and in terms of addressing the broader, epistemological issues raised at the beginning of this paper.

Looking first at the outcome of narrative analysis, what emerges from Ann's account is the glimpse of the moral concerns that appear to lie at the heart of Ann's approach to her work and her relationship with other nurses. Her story indicates distress on her part that she will be unable to support and supervize nurses on the other ward as she does not know their levels of competence. At the same time, if this is an atypical day, it provides an indication of what is typical. Thus, indirectly, the narrative suggests something about Ann's everyday practice concerning colleagues on her ward and the support she feels able to offer colleagues. This interpretation of Ann's story is the result of searching for the story's structural properties, and retaining a holistic approach to the data.

In contrast, the thematic analysis fragmented the data. Instead of an overall story with a core motif, the data were sorted into codes, in much the way that a pack of cards might be dealt to different players, with each code initially being treated as if it carried as much weight as any other. This approach facilitated a different kind of understanding, that was more concerned with the relationship between time, space, role and knowledge, and gave less emphasis to the moral dimension of Ann's relationships with other nurses.

The findings from both forms of analysis overlap in the sense that they are both concerned with issues regarding professional identity, and with the way that such identity is linked to a number of domains such as space and knowledge. However, I would not go so far as suggesting that they result in 'different approximations of a single truth' (Coffey & Atkinson 1996): ostensibly there is more than one 'truth' here – there is, for example, a professional imperative (concerned with working within Ann's own sphere of competence) and also a moral imperative (her responsibility to others who are vulnerable). Yet the different analyses do not lead to radically different interpretations – instead they offer different emphases on meaning.

Significantly, when Ann read a draft of this paper, the different interpretations were equally meaningful to her. This question returns us to the first part of the paper which made reference to issues of interpretation and assumptions about the extent to which meaning is implicit or imposed by researchers and readers, and how these assumptions are associated with different traditions or epistemological positions, such as those of realism and post-modernism. These traditions are seemingly opposed (Morris 1997) and yet, as Jackson (1989) argues, might be more usefully understood as dialectical or mutually informing. To make his point (and inspired by the work of Kurt Vonnigut), Jackson draws an analogy between the discourse of social science and the children's pastime known as cat's cradle. He reminds us of the way that a cat's cradle – a single, closed loop of string which is woven into a series of loose shapes – can suggest a range of phenomena such as buildings, animals, people – and as such, is a structure suspended between the poles of reality and make-believe. The discourse of social inquiry, he suggests, can be likened to such string figures; it is 'a game we play with words, the thread of an argument whose connection with reality is always oblique and tenuous (1989 p. 187). As such, he argues, truth is indeterminate: it is in the spaces as much as in the structure of discourse, in fiction as much as in fact.

Conclusion

In the post-modern context, data analysis as a method of discovering a single and definitive set of meanings in a set of data becomes problematic, even when these derive from a single source. In this article I suggest that the use of more than one analytical method by the same researcher may be a useful (if limited) response to this dilemma. Rather than attempting to pin down one objective reality, re-analysis using different approaches, and even bringing together different paradigms, may offer a way of opening up the process of interpretation, reweaving meanings (as with Jackson's analogy of the cat's cradle) and glimpsing different kinds of 'truths'.

Notes

1. According to Cheek (1999 p. 386), post-modern approaches are 'a way of thinking about the world that shapes the type of research that is done and the types of analyses that are made', but there is no universally accepted definition of 'postmodern'. Instead, there are a range of theoretical approaches which emphasize that reality is manifold, and there is no single way to view, interpret or characterize that reality. 'Post-modern approaches provide a challenge to the view that it is possible to represent any aspect of reality in its entirety, speak for others, make truth claims, and attain universal essential understandings. In doing so, post-modern approaches challenge the way that reality has come to be represented' (Cheek 1999 p. 385).
2. See, for example, Bazeley (1999) and Miles and Huberman (Chapter 3, 1994) on combining quantitative and qualitative approaches.

References

Anderson G. (1998) Creating moral space in prenatal genetic services. *Qualitative Health Research* **8**, 168–187.

Atkinson P. (1990) *The Ethnographic Imagination: Textual Constructions of Reality*. Routledge, London.

Barthes R. (1977) *Image, Music, Text*. Hill and Wang, New York.

Bazeley P. (1999) The *bricoleur* with a computer: piecing together qualitative and quantitative data. *Qualitative Health Research* **9**, 279–287.

Bloch M. (1998) *How We Think They Think: Anthropological Approaches to Cognition, Memory and Literacy*. Westview Press, Boulder, Colorado.

Brock S. & Kleiber D. (1994) Narrative in medicine: the stories of elite college athletes' career-ending injuries. *Qualitative Health Research* **4**, 411–430.

Burnard P. (1997) Qualitative data analysis: a response to Lucas's article. *Social Sciences in Health* **3**, 254–258.

Charmaz C. (1999) Stories of suffering: subjective tales and research narratives. *Qualitative Health Research* **9**, 362–382.

Cheek J. (1999) Influencing practice or simply esoteric? Researching health care using post-modern approaches. *Qualitative Health Research* **9**, 383–392.

Clifford J. (1986) Introduction: partial truths. In *Writing Culture: the Poetics and Politics of Ethnography* (Clifford J. & Marcus G. eds), University of California Press, Berkeley, pp. 1–26.

Clifford J. (1988) *The Predicament of Culture: Twentieth Century Ethnography, Literature and Art.* Harvard University Press, Cambridge, Massachusetts.

Coffey A. & Atkinson P. (1996) *Making Sense of Qualitative Data: Complementary Research Strategies.* Sage, Thousand Oaks, California.

Culler J. (1983) *On Deconstruction: Theory and Criticism After Structuralism.* Routledge and Kegan Paul, London.

Derrida J. (1976) *Of Grammatology* (Spivak G. trans.). John Hopkins University Press, Baltimore.

Denzin N. (1997) *Interpretive Ethnography: Ethnographic Practices for the 21st Century.* Sage, Thousand Oaks, California.

Grbich C. (1999) *Qualitative Research in Health: An Introduction.* Sage, London.

Greenhalgh T. & Hurwitz B. (1999) Narrative based medicine: narrative medicine in an evidence-based world. *British Medical Journal* **30**, 323–325.

Hammersley M. & Atkinson P. (1983) *Ethnography: Principles in Practice.* Tavistock, London.

Hobart M. (1982) Meaning or moaning? An ethnographic note on a little-understood tribe. In *Semantic Anthropology* (Parkin D. ed.), Academic Press, London, pp. 39–63.

Jackson M. (1989) *Paths Towards a Clearing: Radical Empiricism and Ethnographic Inquiry,* Indiana University Press, Bloomington.

Kleinman A. (1988) *The Illness Narratives: Suffering, Healing and the Human Condition.* Basic Books, New York.

Labov W. (1982) Speech actions and reactions in personal narratives. In *Analysing Discourse: Text and Talk* (Tannen D. ed.), Georgetown University Press, Washington, District of Columbia, pp. 219–247.

Lash S. (1990) *Sociology of Postmodernism.* Routledge, London.

Lucas J. (1997) Making sense of interviews: the narrative dimension. *Social Sciences in Health* **3**, 113–126.

Lyotard J.-F. (1984) *The Post-Modern Condition: A Report on Knowledge* (Bennington G. & Massumi B., trans.). University of Minnesota Press, Minneapolis.

Manning P. & Cullum-Swan B. (1994) Narrative, content and semiotic analysis. In *Handbook of Qualitative Research* (Denzin N. & Lincoln Y. eds), Sage, Thousand Oaks, California, pp. 463–478.

May C. & Fleming C. (1997) The professional imagination: narrative and the symbolic boundaries between medicine and nursing. *Journal of Advanced Nursing* **25**, 1094–1100.

Miles M. & Huberman M. (1994) *Qualitative Data Analysis: An Expanded Sourcebook* 2nd edn. Sage, Thousand Oaks, California.

Morris B. (1997) In defence of realism and truth: critical reflections on the anthropological followers of Heidegger. *Critique of Anthropology* **17**, 313–340.

Morse J. (1999) The role of data. *Qualitative Health Research* **9**, 291–293.

Nijhof G. (1997) Response work: approaching answers to open interviews as readings. *Qualitative Inquiry* **3**, 169–187.

Okely J. & Callaway H. (1992) *Anthropology and Autobiography* Routledge, London.

Sandelowski M. (1991) Telling stories: narrative approaches in qualitative research. *Image: Journal of Nursing Scholarship* **23**, 161–166.

Savage J. (1998) *The Role of Nursing Culture in the Practice of Nursing: A Focused Ethnographic Study*. Royal College of Nursing, Oxford.

Silverman D. (2000) *Doing Qualitative Research: A Practical Handbook*. Sage, London.

Smith D. (1994) *Texts, Facts and Femininity: Exploring the Relations of Ruling*, Routledge, London.

Wolcott H. (1994) *Transforming Qualitative Data: Description, Analysis and Interpretation*. Sage, Thousand Oaks, California.

41

Telling a Story, Writing a Narrative: Terminology in Health Care

John Wiltshire

The purpose of this paper is simple. It is to make a distinction between the terms 'story' and 'narrative' as they are employed in the contexts of health care. These terms are widely used both in publications addressed to medical practitioners and to nurses and other health care providers, and are often key arms of a progressive and 'humanistic' reassessment of the nature of both nursing and health care more generally. It will be argued that to make a distinction between these terms is useful because it highlights certain ideological and cultural issues. It is helpful to make a distinction between a verbal account of illness, produced in dialogue with, and elicited by, a nurse or other health care professional, and a narrative written and initiated by the patient in his or her own right. Therapeutic claims may be based on both forms but they are different, and this difference, as well as the therapeutic importance of narrative forms, needs to be clarified.

It is clear that interest in the 'story' is widespread in health care.[1] Increasingly, doctors and nurses are instructed to elicit 'the patient's story' and to give that due weight in assessing the patient's condition and treatment. Increasingly too, nurses see their own practices and professional commitments in terms of story and narrative. Narrative and story are implicitly, sometimes explicitly, held up as an alternative model of practice to science and modes of reasoning taking the physical or biological sciences as a model. Within this tradition, for instance, R. Parker has argued powerfully for a correlation between telling the story of a patient and a 'relational' ethic of health care, an ethic she opposes to the 'rational' bias of the dominant bioethical model.[2] Using the term in a

Source: *Nursing Inquiry*, 2(2) (1995): 75–82.

rather different way, Anne Boykin and Savina O. Schoenhofer propose that 'story' can give direct access to key dimensions of the ontology of nursing, proposed as 'the nursing situation'. 'In bringing the nursing situation to life through the use of story', they write, 'students of nursing are enabled to participate in the lived experience, and to create within the nursing situation'.[3] Betty Carey Best, a sociologist, has emphasized the 'storywork' that takes place in family care conferences, as nurses and other workers in a hospice collaboratively build stories about their patients that are meaningful and are therefore grounds for action.[4]

This emphasis on 'story' in some recent nursing literature reflects developments in the more general field of health care. Arthur Kleinman argued some time ago for the importance of eliciting 'the patient's explanatory model' of illness and for giving this equal weight with the clinician's model of disease.[5] Increasingly, Kleinman has emphasized narrative – both the spoken accounts by patients and by doctors – as an essential tool in the understanding of suffering as a human experience.[6] From another orientation, S. Kay Toombs, a phenomenologist, outlining the differing perspectives of patient and physician in her *The Meaning of Illness*, argues that narrative is an important instrument for understanding the experience of the patient, providing a 'window' into that experience and thereby enabling the health care worker to transcend his or her necessarily limited perspectives and insight into illness. 'In providing a lifeworld description of bodily disruption', Toombs writes, 'the clinical narrative deepens the physician's understanding of the lived experience of illness. Such narratives disclose what it is like to suffer from, say, multiple sclerosis, heart disease, arthritis...'.[7]

Toombs, like other writers, uses 'story' and 'narrative' synonymously and interchangeably. This is true, for example, of another significant contribution, Kathryn Montgomery Hunter's *Doctors' Stories: The Narrative Structure of Medical Knowledge*.[8] Here the emphasis is not on the patient's story, but on the role that 'story-telling activities' play within medical practice, bridging the gap, in Hunter's analysis, between the textbooks and the individual patient, who never precisely exemplifies what the textbooks say. Hunter's book valuably outlines the various roles that narrative plays in the daily activities of a large hospital, from case presentations to rounds, though (not untypically) she disregards nursing staff in her analysis. Kleinman's *The Illness Narratives*, on the other hand, is concerned primarily with the words of patients, elicited by the doctor, and with the therapeutic role that speaking of one's illness to an 'empathic witness' can play. At the same time, since these words are presented by the physician and re-narrated in his own words, and within an ongoing argument constructed by him, the title of his book suggests a certain ambiguity: are the 'narratives' concerned the patient's or the doctor's? The possibilities of 'story' within health-care have received perhaps their strongest, and certainly their most popular, demonstration in Oliver Sacks' 'clinical tales' (as for example in *The Man Who Mistook His Wife For a Hat*[9]) which have become famous for their emphasis on the importance of listening to the patient and for their representation of his or her experience. But here the same issue arises: the 'clinical' tale may refer to the doctor's narrative form, or to the 'raw material' of the patient's words. In effect it allows us to assume that both are the same, that the patient's language may unproblematically and straightforwardly become the language of the health care provider.[10]

This recent attention to narrative within medicine is, of course, to be welcomed. These instances are concerned with the narrative as it focuses on the patient: emphasizing 'story' is a way of highlighting that more is involved in the activities of caring for patients than the administration and titration of drugs, the management of intravenous lines or the measuring of biological phenomena. It is a means of calling attention to those aspects of the patient's symptomatology that cannot be encompassed within biomedical frameworks.[11] How is the body in pain,[12] the suffering, the lived body[13] to be represented and addressed within an epistemology that divides the body from the mind and segments its professional attention in the same fashion? Narrative heralds a way in which body and psyche may be conceptually reunited.

The emphasis on story in much current work in nursing is perhaps powered by additional urgencies. It promises to give formal shape to nursing's sense of distinct group identity. Discussing the 'crisis of representation' of nursing in a recent issue of *Nursing Inquiry*, Kim Walker calls for a new 'regime of truth' that can withstand that of science, which is eminently representable through its technological manifestations – 'the sphygmomanometer, the pulse oximeter ... the intravenous pump', whereas nursing as caring is not. 'Science', he writes, 'insidiously permeates our understanding of who we are, who we can be as nurses, with its own understandings.'[14] Narrative, it would seem, is an obvious mode in which such a 'regime of truth' within nursing can be articulated. It serves as a rallying point for a critique of the more narrowly scientistic or positivistic conceptions of the body, of medicine and of health care, which dominate the field. Narrative can demonstrate, as no other form can, what we mean when we speak of nursing as caring.

Even more fundamentally, a focus on narrative emphasizes nursing's intellectual affinities with a group of theorists who have been vocal in their critique of the positivist and 'Enlightenment' assumptions – that truth, and power over nature will unfold progressively as the result of the utilization of humanity's rational faculties – which continue to underpin most medical practice, medical research, and much of medicine's bioethical reflection. Nurses find in an intellectual culture that disputes these assumptions a heartening corroboration of their own practice knowledge, and perhaps of their own scepticism towards some of medicine's more imperialistic claims. What is sometimes called the 'counter-Enlightenment'[15] provides a welcome alternative tradition and source of validation. Drawing on such theorists as Jean-Pierre Lyotard,[16] who argues for narrative as an alternative mode of knowledge to science, and Jerome Bruner,[17] who demonstrates that narrative is a universal mode of cognition, narrative is currently enjoying unprecedented prestige as an avenue through which substantive meaning, or at least working knowledge, can be developed.

Many writers who emphasize the modality of narrative also argue that *all* 'truth' is 'constructed' and therefore local and contingent. There is not one knowledge, but a variety of competing 'knowledges' each of which is developed within a specific cultural, professional or institutional framework.[18] Emphasizing the 'fictive', provisional and discursive aspects of all 'knowledge production', they draw on such sources as Kuhn's work on scientific paradigms[19] and Foucault[20] to dispute the outright truth claims of science. If 'science and its techniques and technologies of power – its representations – is able to weave itself further and further into the fabric of the culture of nursing', as Walker[13] suggests, postmodern theorists argue in return that narrative is necessarily already woven into the fabric of 'science'. In this broad, sweeping (and I would argue, weak) sense, science itself turns into a 'story'.

A recent issue of the journal *Literature and Medicine* 'Narrative and Medical Knowledge' edited by Kathryn Montgomery Hunter, reflects these recent developments in the field. One article, for example, presents pairs of narratives written by patients and anaesthesia residents.[21] Yet simply because narrative arouses so much current interest, functions so readily as a focus for anti-positivist analyses of medical interactions, it is ripe for appropriation. An article by a medical ethicist and physician, Howard Brody,[22] arguing for the significance of the joint construction of narrative as a model of communicative interaction in the clinical encounter, raises the question of terminology – and hence of meaning – acutely. Titled 'My story is broken; can you help me fix it?' Brody's article presents a patient who fears that his persistent cough may be a symptom of pneumonia, from which his aunt has recently died. The doctor, after examination, reassures the patient and tells him that the cough is 'probably related to postnasal drip'. This is called the 'new narrative' and also a 'story': [i]f the best way to get over a cough caused by postnasal drip is to use a vaporiser and to drink more fluids, an ideal story of the illness will show how these measures actually play a role in producing an improvement in the symptoms (p. 86).[22]

Why is the word 'explanation', or even 'account', not more accurate here than 'story'? Is it not used because 'story' and 'narrative' tend to imply a democracy of equals – everyone can tell a story – while 'explanation' suggests that the doctor actually has more knowledge than his client? The matter is further confused when narrative is said to provide richer, more useful 'data' (p. 81).[22] When, towards the end of his article, Brody writes that 'Scientific medicine has made great strides ... by focusing instead on quite different stories, at the organic, cellular and molecular level' (p. 91)[22] the term is being used in a loose way where it almost certainly means nothing more than 'account'. The words 'narrative' and 'story' here are being employed in the weak sense, with a breadth that has almost, I believe, deprived them of usefulness, and may well make them vulnerable to hostile dismissal from a scientist's point of view. There is no meaningful sense in which the result of a controlled trial, for instance, that shows that breast-conserving therapy for early stage breast cancer is safe and effective, can be called a 'story'. To do so is, at the least, to conflate one genre or order of knowledge with another.

It is important then, if narrative and story are to become a genuine focus for nursing inquiry, that the meaning of each of these concepts is adequately defined and delimited. It should not be assumed that a narrative form gives direct and unproblematic access either to the patient's condition, or to the nurse's practice knowledge. One cannot think of a narrative simply as a transparent window opening onto new epistemological realms of material and understanding. Windows have frames, and window panes refract and reflect. In other words, narratives display the narrating subject as much as the narrated objects. The position of the writer, the patient, the doctor, or nurse, will slant the narrative one way or another. Narratives are themselves complex formations that involve many dimensions of experience in their making – ethical choice, interpersonal dialogue and aesthetic instinct among them. As a consequence, the reading of narratives is as much a skill as the interpretation of any other complex mode of representation, whether these take the form of X-ray photographs, laboratory results or diagnostic reports.

There are reasons for mistrust when the new school of medical human-ities claims to tell patients' stories.[10] Whether such presentations are not a reconstructed version of medical benevolism, a new form of the professional acting on behalf of the patient, 'in the patient's best interests' will not be considered in this paper. And when such eminent writers as I have cited use 'story' and narrative interchangeably, one might be forgiven for thinking that an attempt to separate the terms would be pointless. Yet it may be helpful in this context to remember first of all what it is that 'story' and narrative contain that 'data' or 'explanation' do not. 'He's been very depressed. They asked for a psychiatry consult and they gave him some tablets. Those tablets won't work for two to three weeks. But they're sending him home tomorrow any-way' (Wiltshire, unpubl. data). This fragment of a report given by a nurse at handover has no particular distinction as a story, although it constitutes a story because the nurse does not simply recite a series of events. Stories are about persons and about relationships – here of the patient to the psychiatrist but also to the story-teller, the narrator, the nurse. Because they involve consequences for the person, there is always an ethical element to the story. Something occurs within a story, that might conceivably have occurred otherwise: in this case, anti-depressives might not have been given, or the patient might have been kept in the ward till his condition improved. 'Those tablets won't work for two to three weeks' interposed as a judgement-laden statement, effectively creates the story as a miniature moral drama. Judgements whether explicit or implied, as in this instance, are always present in the making and telling of a story.

Thus to invoke 'story' as a modality of medical interaction is already to embed 'data' within a fluid social context and ethical matrix. But to separate out story from narrative may provide a further means to enhance these terms' usefulness. A simple, but helpful, distinction can be made between patient 'stories' as these are told to, or reported by, doctors and nurses, and 'narratives' whether these are by patients or by health care providers. In the first place such a distinction would allow one to see that a story does not unproblematically, and as it were invisibly, become a narrative. To become a narrative, a story must be conceptualized, restressed and completed. A narrative is conceptually more sophisticated and structured than a story.

Narrative is from the Latin *narrativus*. Story is middle English, but ultimately derived from the Latin word *historia*. Nevertheless in its contemporary usage 'story' is commonly used in more informal contexts than 'narrative' and quite often contains an element of provisionality. 'That's *her* story', like the 'story-teller' of children's speech, insinuates doubt about the narrative's authenticity. (Consider also the newspaper 'story'). The distinction is often, in effect, between the spoken and the written word. There is something impermanent, perishable and exploratory about a story. Stories are not always, of course, spoken, though the 'short story', the 'tale of detection', the yarn, terms that refer to literary forms, represent a sophisticated and specialized usage. Within the health care context stories are almost always less finished, less formal and less deliberated than the narrative. (The nurse at handover I have quoted would not think of herself as telling a story.)

From this distinction some others follow. Stories and tales are casual, informal, contingent. Narratives are premeditated, organized, more formal and have a structure that is their own. When a patient writes a narrative it implies that she or he envisages in, or ascribes a structure to, certain events. Here, both stories and narratives need to be distinguished from chronicles. A narrative history, argues Hayden White, must not only register events 'within the chronological framework of their original occurrence but narrated as well, that is to say, revealed as possessing a structure, an order of meaning that they do not possess as mere sequence'.[23] Chronicles record an unco-ordinated sequence of (usually) external events over historical time: narratives organize what Bruner has called 'the rich and messy domain of human interaction'[24] into structure. Organizing events into a narrative structure seems in effect to be the same process as the drawing out of 'meaning' among them.

If we apply these distinctions to the health care setting, some interesting results arise. Is the medical record a narrative or a chronicle? On this definition, the medical and nursing notes are a chronicle, not a narrative of the patient, though they may well contain islands of narrative material and sometimes together, more or less adventitiously, amount to a coherent interpretation of the patient's history.[25] The patient who is asked to give his or her account of the meaning of their illness, what they associate with the symptoms etc., can be said, without forcing the word, to be telling their story. The nurse who in the handover, tells her colleagues about her experiences with a patient can be said to tell a story. But when we describe the communal production of meanings within the handover, the negotiated and conscious process of nurses, as some thing undertaken socially as part of a knowledge-making process, we are right, I suggest, to call it a 'collective narrative'.[26] The term narrative – though it refers to spoken and informal discourse as in this instance – reflects the professional and conceptual processes through which the original material (the story, or stories) have been put. (Often, of course, this does not happen, just as the medical record remains at the level of the chronicle.) Similarly, when doctors speak anecdotally to each other about an interesting case, they are telling stories. But when one writes a 'case history' that combines temporal sequence with the consequences of an intervention and its outcome, this is a form of narrative.

The real point of this distinction is that narratives should contain a reflective or theoretical component. It may not be overt, but the shaping and organization of a narrative would usually reflect and transmit the consequences of a meditative or generalizing process of thought. Narratives do not exist as Bruner writes,

> in some real world, waiting there patiently and eternally to be veridically mirrored in a text. The act of constructing a narrative, moreover, is considerably more than selecting events either from real life, from memory, or from fantasy and then placing them in an appropriate order. The events themselves need to be *constituted* in the light of the overall narrative (p. 8).[22]

To construct a narrative is to make an intervention into a field conceptualized (whether fully consciously or not is insignificant) as problematic. It is to address issues, though these are not addressed directly, but through the selection and arrangement of material. Here is an example, transcribed more or less verbatim, from a nursing handover given in a cardio-vascular unit:

> Bed 15. This is a young 57 year old man with a history of diabetes and a six centimeter triple A, which will need further surgery at some time ... But he also was found to have a mass surrounding the thymus gland, and surrounding the lung, so they've actually sent some specimens for further cytopathology and they're due soon. Initially his recovery from the bypass surgery has been extremely good, ... so we're just coasting him through.
>
> He's concerned, and he's aware, that there was some sort of mass in there. His wife's aware, and they've been discussing it just over the bed today and they feel like they're not sure he's having a flat day because of that or because of the heart surgery, they've been told that he'd have flat days. When I told Doctor X he thought the patient didn't know, thought that it'd be a few days down the track, and they'd talk about it. So he's just wondering... (Wiltshire, unpubl. data).

At previous handovers this patient's condition was represented in a check-list recital of different forms of physiological data, with the information about the suspected mass or tumour appended as just another piece of informa-tion. Here the nurse has perceived the moral drama of the patient's situation, and has defined it as not just a drama for the patient and his wife, but for the whole enterprise of nursing and health care. In doing so the nurse has consciously positioned herself as a narrator, enabled by virtue of this status to select and arrange the material and to participate, by means of implicit reflection, on the information and events being described. Narrative is thus, as in this instance, a reflective practice whereas story is not. And because it is a reflective practice, narrative is connected, as story is not, with authority. 'The narrator' is automatically endowed with power, with control over the material he or she presents, a power that flows to her or him through the position as organizer of the material.

The story told by the patient and elicited by the doctor or nurse, is different from that story's reproduction in print and in formal representations of vari-ous kinds by the nurse or doctor. In moving from 'story' to 'narrative' it has be-come part of a reflective, self-conscious and interventionary process. In other words, to construct a narrative requires abstract thought. Perhaps this is not the same as the thought that is required to formulate a research question, to set up laboratory procedures to investigate it, and to organize the resulting data into meaningful results. But to articulate, or more likely – as I have argued – to write a narrative requires intellectual commitment and energy. Moreover the construction of a narrative necessarily involves meditation upon social and ethical issues. (Sometimes, of course, these thought processes are unconscious to the narrator and it is the task of criticism to bring them to light.)

If one recognizes, for example, that patients write narratives, this has political – medico-political – implications. Patients do not simply construct stories, with or without the collaboration of physicians and nurses. If we allow that they are capable of making narratives, then we allow them a principle of organization, an independent centre of knowledge and consciousness. Moreover, the power to organize and reflect upon experience need not depend at all upon the knowledge, expertise and benevolent facilitation of the health care provider. This means that we allow a plurality of knowledges, of meanings around illness and disease. The patient who writes a narrative, just like the hospice workers or the nurses who together have been shown to construct a narrative, may be said to have undertaken a reflective and inte-grational process.

There is a related term that must be discussed here: 'voice'. Along with story and narrative, it is presently in vogue, though this time its antecedents are not with 'postmodern' theorists but with the Russian literary critic and philosopher, Mikhail Bakhtin.[27] Sometimes 'voice' is used synonymously for 'story': and at other times it means 'professional knowledge or orientation'. Articles have appeared about 'the voices of the medical record',[28] for example, and 'the nurses' voice'.[29] The Western tradition since Plato's *Dialogues* has tended to disparage writing as an alienated, lifeless form of expression, and to celebrate the living voice, as a means through which direct access to the 'self' or to subjectivity can be gained. The voice is pure, single, independent; it issues from one throat. When one calls a writing a 'voice' one, then, is enlisting the residual power of this tradition to give power to the group or individual concerned. The term 'voice' tends to carry with it, unconsciously, the assumption that the group has a natural authenticity, is identical to itself, uncontaminated by the language and values of other, usually more dominant, groups.

But, as Jacques Derrida[30] insists, the meanings given by the living voice depend upon a process of differentiation between signs, in this case sound signs, as much as writing does. Speech can, no more than writing, be said to be a transparent medium of subjective experience. The term 'voice' lays claim to this by its own, independent, natural authority. But in fact no language is like this, and no voice is unproblematically free from or, uncontaminated by, the terms, values, concepts of others. When the term 'voice' is used in reference to what is, in practice, writing, we have a rhetorical trope whose complicated elision of these points is quite different from the supposed innocent directness that it is simultaneously claiming. 'Voice' thus collaborates with 'story' in valorizing that which is unpremeditated and apparently unmediated, but the term is in fact involved in quite complicated contestations and valorizations of meaning. It carries much the same meaning as 'representation' in the political sense, but without the separation between origin and signifier that 'representation' always insists upon.

I have suggested some cautions and reservations about the use of the three terms, voice, story and narrative. Nevertheless, it is clear that these modalities will continue to play an important role both in nursing as an everyday practice, as in handover communications, and in the development of nursing theory. There is something urgent and central about narrative and its relation to health care that remains to be addressed. If the voice of the nurse demands to be heard, if story and narrative seem inevitable vehicles for the knowledge and experience that rise out of the life-world of nursing, we need to understand why. I suggested earlier that there is always a hidden ethical kernel to the story. It is this moral aspect which is bound up with the way in which story-telling and the more reflective narrative can function therapeutically.

What then accounts for the centrality of narrative and story to the life-world of medicine and health care? What would be the drive that would lead one to believe that narrative representation is the form in which some knowledge crucial to nursing must be represented? What is the ethical significance of doctors', nurses' and patients' narratives? Three aspects of narrative communication may be distinguished. The first is what one may call, to use a psychoanalytic term, abreaction. Telling a story, as everyone knows, is a means of giving vent to feelings of anger, resentment, guilt, perhaps even of horror, that would otherwise simmer away destructively inside. Telling – bringing into the public domain – helps the individual's own psychological or moral equilibrium. Second, such externalizing is almost always prompted by scandal. By this I mean some particular testing, irresolvable, trying, niggling, painful occurrence, particularly an occurrence difficult to reconcile with one's professional training and standards. A patient incessantly demands pain-killing drugs but eats like a horse, so the nurse does not contact the doctor to see whether the dosage can be increased. Later it is discovered by computer-tomography scan that the patient has acute pancreatitis. The nurse wonders in what way she has failed in her professional duty. Such episodes, which are the unremarkable, everyday stuff of nursing practice, put under stress the ethical values of the individual, and create difficult, anxiety-producing moral divisions. To recite the events and display the problem is a way of dealing with the dilemma. It is as if the moral problem were the node or seed that necessarily forces itself into narrative growth.

Third, telling a story or, more significantly, writing it out as a narrative, permits a corrective emotional experience. The writer is able to rehearse the experiential material and organize, or structure it, so that it now represents, in some form or other, an emotionally and morally coherent series of events. When intellect develops this material, something productive is occurring. It can make something – may be a point, a contribution to professional debate, a drama – out of draining and emotionally distressing occurrences. Experiences that were disempowering to the self can be recuperated, become projects of health-making, when that self is the power holding the pen or organizing the screen. Only this will explain the insistence on the literal 'truth' of their stories that so marks the narratives of patients and care-givers; an emphasis so much at odds with the insistence on the fictionality of all discourse, and especially of autobiographical discourse, of the culture at large. The truth claim is bound up with the wish to intervene in the real world, bound up, that is to say, with the productive desire.

Narrative is, then, not merely a means of discharge and crude catharsis, as story sometimes may be, but is far more complex psychologically. To compose a narrative is itself an index of composure; of physical, ethical and psychological integration, if not ease. It may certainly involve dragging or impelling into the light of language's symbolic order urges and emotions that belong to more atavistic, non-verbal parts of the self.[31] Composition is an activity of recuperation and recovery. And one should not forget that narrative can also be a means of celebration and commemoration. Narrative makes more permanent, more contemplative those moments when the patient or nurse has felt themselves present at, and participating in, some of the great moments of life.

This article then, has been a plea for clarity. Many writers who concentrate on 'story', 'narrative' and 'voice' do so as part of an argument against the biological and mechanistic conceptions of medicine. They argue, after Bruner and others, that narrative is as useful a way of approaching the world of health care and is as useful a tool, as useful data, as more 'scientific' approaches. But these claims will carry little weight if the crucial terms are employed so loosely within the field. 'Story' is informal, provisional and exploratory. 'Voice' means the distinct epistemology of a social, professional and political group. 'Narrative' should mean the consciously formulated, premeditated and coherent account of a medical experience, whether one of illness or of care. When defined in this way, 'narrative' involves recognition of its author as capable, self-defining, and intellectually able. If used of patients' written accounts, it begins to restore the patient to an equivalent position to that of the health care practitioner. 'Nursing narratives' would mean not merely anecdotal, casual accounts, but involve a blending of theoretical with empirical or experiential materials. It is this capacity to connect theory with experience, to foreground the relationship between daily practice and knowledge, that makes narrative a vital tool for the future of nursing inquiry.

References

1. King NPM & Stanford AF. Patient stories, doctor stories and true stories: a cautionary reading. *Literature and Medicine* 1992; **11**: 185–199.
2. Parker R. Nurses' stories: the search for a relational ethic of care. *Advances in Nursing Science* 1990; **13**: 31–40.
3. Boykin A & Schoenhofer SO. Story as link between nursing practice, ontology epistemology. *Image: Journal of Nursing Scholarship* 1991; **23**: 245–248.
4. Best PC. Making Hospice Work: Collaborative Story-Telling in Family-Care Conferences, *Literature and Medicine* 1994; **13**: 93–123.
5. Kleinman A. *Social Origins of Distress and Disease, Depression, Neurasthenia and Pain in Modern China*. New Haven and London: Yale University Press, 1986.
6. Kleinman A & Kleinman J. Suffering and its professional transformation: towards an ethnography of interpersonal experience. *Culture, Medicine and Psychiatry* 1991; **15**: 275–301.
7. Toombs SK. *The Meaning of Illness: A Phenomenological Account Of The Different Perspectives Of Physician and Patient*. Dordrecht: Kluwer Academic, 1992; p. 105.
8. Hunter KM. *Doctors' stories: the narrative structure of medical knowledge*. Princeton, New Jersey: Princeton University Press, 1991.
9. Sacks O. *The Man who Mistook his Wife for a Hat*. London: Picador, 1986.
10. Wiltshire J. Beyond the ouija board: dialogue and heteroglossia in the medical narrative. *Literature and Medicine* 1994; **13**: 209–226.
11. Reiser SJ. Technology and the use of the senses in twentieth-century medicine. In: Bynum WF & Porter R (eds). *Medicine and the five senses*. Cambridge: Cambridge University Press, 1993; pp. 262–273.
12. Scarry E. *The Body in Pain: the Making and Unmaking of the World*. New York: Oxford University Press, 1985.
13. Leder D. A Tale of Two Bodies: the Cartesian Corpse and the Lived Body. In: Leder D (ed.) *The Body in Medical Thought and Practice*. Dordrecht: Kluwer Academic, 1992; pp. 17–36.
14. Walker K. Confronting 'reality': Nursing, science and the micro-politics of representation. *Nursing Inquiry* 1994; **1**: 46–56.

15. Harpham GG. So ... What is Enlightenment? An inquisition into Modernity. *Critical Inquiry* 1994; **20**: 524–556.
16. Lyotard J-P. *The Postmodern Condition: A Report on Knowledge*. Manchester: Manchester University Press, 1984.
17. Bruner J. *Actual Minds, Possible Worlds*. Cambridge, Massachusetts: Harvard University Press, 1986.
18. Lovibond S. Feminism and Postmodernism. In: Thomas Docherty (ed.) *Postmodernism, a Reader*. Hemel Hempstead: Harvester Wheatsheaf, 1993; pp. 390–414.
19. Kuhn TS. *The Structure of Scientific Revolutions* 2nd edn. Chicago: University of Chicago Press, 1970.
20. Foucault M. *The Order of Things; An Archeology of the Human Sciences*. New York: Vintage Books, 1970.
21. Shafer A & Fish MP. A call for narrative: the patient's story and anesthesia training. *Literature and Medicine* 1994; **14**: 124–142.
22. Brody H. 'My story is broken; can you help me fix it?' Medical Ethics and the Joint Construction of Narrative. *Literature and Medicine* 1994; **1**: 79–92.
23. White H. *The Content of the Form: Narrative Discourse and Historical Representation*. Baltimore: Johns Hopkins University Press, 1987; p. 5.
24. Bruner J. The narrative construction of reality. *Critical Inquiry* 1991; **18**: 1–21.
25. Donnelly WS. Righting the medical record: transforming chronicle into story. *JAMA* 1988; **260**: 823–825.
26. Parker J, Gardner G & Wiltshire J. Handover: the collective narrative of nursing practice. *Australian Journal of Advanced Nursing* 1992; **9**: 31–37.
27. Bakhtin MM. *The Dialogic Imagination*. Holquist M (ed.) Austin: University of Texas Press, 1981.
28. Poirier S & Brauner DJ. The voices of the medical record. *Theoretical Medicine* 1990; **11**: 29–39.
29. Parker JM & Gardner G. The silence and silencing of the nurse's voice: a reading of patient progress notes. *Australian Journal of Advanced Nursing* 1992; **9**: 3–9.
30. Derrida J. *Writing and Difference* translated Alan Bass. London: Routledge and Kegan Paul, 1981.
31. McDougall J. *Theatres of the Body; A Psychoanalytic Approach to Psychosomatic Illness*. London: Free Association, 1989.

42

Narrative Turn or Blind Alley?

Paul Atkinson

I n the course of this article, I want to address some key issues in the use of narrative analysis for the contemporary sociology and anthropology of medicine. I seek to establish a series of key issues. They are outlined as follows:

1. An appreciation of narrative forms and functions represents one of the most significant analytic perspectives for contemporary qualitative research on health and medicine.
2. Recent enthusiasm for narrative work has sometimes been based on inappropriate assumptions and reflects unwarranted methodological and theoretical commitments.
3. Narrative analyses, like other formal analytic procedures, need to be built into systematic, principled investigations and should not be treated as single solutions to the multiple problems of social analysis.

For the most part, it will be necessary for me to assert these issues rather than to demonstrate them fully. My detailed comments will be focused primarily on my third point. Using major published works in the field, I shall try to show how authors have made inconsistent and inappropriate claims for narrative approaches. My general point is not to argue against narrative analysis in the social sciences in general or in qualitative health research in particular. Rather, I want to suggest that the particular application of narrative perspectives to be found in some influential publications is inappropriate.

Source: *Qualitative Health Research*, 7(3) (1997): 325–344.

Narrative Analysis

It would be wrong to single out any one approach to qualitative analysis as enjoying particular popularity and esteem. During the past 15 years or so, qualitative methods of all sorts have gained increasing currency, in practice and in methodological literature. Nevertheless, narrative analysis has gained a particularly strong position within that methodological canon, and some strong claims have been entered on its behalf. I suspect that such claims, and their recent rise in popularity, reflect more general and longer-standing interests and commitments among English-speaking social scientists, those from the United States in particular. First, then, I want to explore some of the sources of that popularity.

To begin with, I suspect that although narrative per se may be a recent enthusiasm, it may be a new guise for much older preoccupations. American social science, and its popularizers, have long been obsessed with "the life." It hardly needs recapitulating here that the early days of empirical sociology in the Chicago School witnessed a celebration of the "life history" and the "life document." The life was portrayed as the unit of analysis par excellence. The famous life-history studies, such as Shaw's *The Jack-Roller* (1930), embody that methodological and analytic spirit. More popular manifestations of social investigation have also capitalized on the life and the representation of individual character. One thinks of popular writers such as Joseph Mitchell, whose *New Yorker* reportage of characters in the city are now collected and republished as *Up in the Old Hotel* (Mitchell, 1993). One thinks, too, of fiction peopled by urban characters: Maupin's *Tales of the City* (1989) sequence or Runyon's (1975) picaresque stories of Broadway. Whether they stress the exotic or the ordinary, they celebrate the individual. The speaking voice, the subject of recorded or reported speech, is represented as a unique and privileged locus of character and experience. The same can be said of those areas of American fiction in which realism and social commentary are confluent. In particular, one might instance Farrell's sociologically inspired *Bildungsroman* in the *Studs Lonigan* trilogy (Farrell, 1988; cf. Cappetti, 1993).

These long-standing cultural emphases on the individual character are supplemented by increasing contemporary preoccupations with the revelation of personal experience through confession and therapeutic discourse. These are in turn predicated on the assumption that an interior self, that is, anterior to external evaluation, can be accessed via the interview. The contemporary culture of the interview permeates many popular representations of self and character. The interview is not only celebrated among media commentators and pundits. It is also endorsed by many aspects of contemporary social science. The very notion of the in-depth interview often carries with it connotations that the surface of the respondent can be probed, and that the personal, private aspects of "experience" can be rendered visible through dialogue (see Holstein & Gubrium, 1995).

Not all researchers subscribe to this fallacy, of course. The most sensitive of treatments recognize that narratives, such as life histories, are no less conventional than any other form of data. They recognize that memory, experience, time, and biography are constituted through conventional acts of narrating. They recognize, for instance, that the relationship between a life and a life history is far from simple. A vulgar realism, which assumes narratives to be transparent, is no longer tenable in most quarters, it would seem.

Nevertheless, a close reading of much of the contemporary literature also suggests that even sophisticated treatments of the topic imply a *recuperative* role for narrative research. The justifications are various: the desire to give voice to otherwise muted groups, the desire to do justice to the personal experiences of narrating subjects, the contrast between narrating subjectivity and other modes of constructing experience. In place of vulgar realism, we often find a sentimental and romantic version. I shall return to this latter approach in due course.

For the moment, I want to suggest that the popularity of narrative data and narrative analysis is a mixed blessing. On one hand, it may reflect a sophisticated appreciation of one contribution to qualitative inquiry, reflecting the "narrative turn" to be found across the human and cultural disciplines. On the other hand, it may also represent an implicit attempt to reverse recent tendencies in those selfsame disciplines: an attempt to reintroduce the person as an autonomous speaking (narrating) subject.

Irrespective of the current fashion for narrative analysis, there can be little doubt of the centrality of narrative – and other forms of oral performance – to the culture of medicine. Notwithstanding the significance of written texts, including the medical case record, the operative report, the medical journal paper, and so on, the oral transmission of medical knowledge and medical opinion is powerful. There are numerous occasions within the modern clinic when narrative performances are required of medical practitioners.

For the purposes of this discussion, I focus on the general domain of my own research – the social production and reproduction of clinical medicine in elite hospital settings. I shall not recapitulate the full range of my own interests here. Suffice it to say that when one pays close attention to interactional forms of collegial discourse or the forms of medical instruction, then one cannot help but be struck by the many kinds of narratives that doctors recount to one another – or of the many rhetorical devices, more broadly defined, that are routinely employed in the production and exchange of plausible accounts of work and its outcomes. Indeed, I have suggested, with my characteristic cynicism, that in the modern clinic the patient is but a pretext for a round of orations, narratives, and disputations.

The late modern clinic, with its ultracomplex division of labor, draws on and engages a large number of techniques and technologies. The patient and her or his illness is translated into a multiplicity of measurements and representations. The sites of such representations are numerous, in laboratories and diagnostic specialisms. Yet, these technologized representations are by no means the whole story. Indeed, the whole story is precisely what counts. Dispersed in time and space in the clinic are numerous tellings of the patient. "Telling the case" is a powerful mechanism for the enactment of professional work.

Just as hospital doctors migrate through what Fox (1992) has called the "circuits of hygiene," they also circulate through the "circuits of discourse" (Atkinson, 1995). There is a repetitive "round" of "rounds" and other meetings. Formal occasions, such as grand rounds or morbidity and mortality reviews, are among the major occasions during which the tellings of medical work are enacted. At daily working rounds, and in the multiplicity of daily collegial contacts, cases are narrated. There is a generalized exchange of narratives. One can think, indeed, in terms of a kind of economy in which the stories of medical work are the tokens.

Value is derived from various attributes. As in many exchange systems, rarity has intrinsic value. Medical narratives of the unusual and the outre are highly prized and circulate widely. Likewise, narratives that are suspenseful have particular value. These qualities derive from narrative qualities in themselves. They reflect the cultural evaluation of what can be narrated and how that can be narrated. Like many other social settings, medical narrative gains social worth for its teller if it instructs its audience and provides them with novelty and entertainment.

By the same token, social worth reflects back on narrativity. Professional status is a major determinant of status as a potential or actual narrator. Senior physicians have reserved rights to tell particular kinds of stories, for instance. They have the right to tell personal stories of professional experience and can claim the floor to do so before an audience of peers and juniors. Juniors can rarely claim the floor to tell personal anecdotes about their patients and their professional experience. The value of memory and the value of narrative are closely correlated, of course, and are clearly demarcated by the hierarchy of professional position and authority. I have described in more detail before (Atkinson, 1995) how physicians engage in anecdote and recollection as devices for the expression of medical maxims and advice. As I and other authors, such as Bosk (1979), have demonstrated, such accounts are powerful forms through which socialization takes place – and through which professional values are enacted and endorsed – and may be symbolic means of sanctioning inappropriate or mistaken medical work.

Physicians themselves become surrogate narrators of others' work. In making presentations to other professionals, they encode within their narrative forms the work and responsibilities of others in the hospital; they also recapitulate the narratives of their patients. They make cases out of the narrative work of others and out of their own narrative performances. Physicians' narratives are densely and subtly coded for the credibility of others' work and opinions, for their own degree of trust in the results of investigations, for the differential diagnosis, and so on. This is rhetorical work, and the oral performances of hospital physicians are integral to the daily round of the clinic. The "gaze" of the clinic refers not merely to direct observation of the patient's body and reading the semiology of disease (Foucault, 1973). The clinical gaze is embodied, often ritualized, through the rhetorical forms of narration. In an unjustly neglected work, Hunter (1991) offers an excellent review of the significance of narrative forms and occasions in the culture of medicine. She makes clear that narrative work is fundamental to the everyday accomplishment of medical knowledge and of medical work. Although lacking in sustained analysis of actual discourse, Hunter firmly locates spoken performance at the heart of clinical culture.

I have begun with the narratives of the clinical gaze deliberately to reverse the usual emphasis. The narratives of the patient's illness usually receive greater attention from contemporary analysts. It is emphasized that illness is itself narrated not only through the history, elicited on successive occasions by health professionals but also through personal narratives of illness and suffering. Indeed, the intersection of narratives, lay and professional, encapsulates a great deal of the transformation of patients into cases and the cultural production of biomedical reality.

Illness and the Exaggeration of Narrative

Although it may readily be demonstrated, then, that a great deal of medical work is enacted through narrative forms and that the spectacle of the clinic is narrated as well as embodied, there are, I believe, dangers in inflated claims made for the significance of narrative and medical understanding. To be precise, a number of commentators have clearly attached particular values to narrative and have used the perspective for purposes of advocacy. These seem to me to be illegitimate extrapolations.

The general issue can be illustrated from the specific field of medical anthropology. In their studies of medical interviews, both Kleinman (1988) and Mishler (1984) advocate the analysis of narrative form but portray it as a vehicle for a neoromantic construction of the social actor. The speaking subject reappears under the auspices of storytelling, whereas everyday life is represented as "storied" reality. The interview or the social encounter (such as the medical interview) is the arena in which such a narrative performance of authentic biographical experience can be realized. Equally, for these commentators, such encounters – including the interview – can inhibit the revelation of the self. The narrative unfolding of the self and a life's history may thus be represented as a potentially unique site of authenticity. According to such sociological proponents of *Homo sentimentalis*, the ideal of such a self-revelation is to be contrasted with the realities of everyday professional or social science practice.

The exemplar of such a perspective is to be found in Kleinman's *The Illness Narratives* (1988), in which he explores "how chronic illness is lived and responded to by real people" (p. xii). It is an appreciation grounded in part in a phenomenological sensibility, emphasizing the meaningfulness of the life-world. Kleinman's position is partly summarized as follows:

> Patients order their experience of illness – what it means to them and to significant others – as personal narratives. The illness narrative is a story the patient tells, and significant others retell, to give credence to the distinctive events and long-term course of suffering. The plot lines, core metaphors, and rhetorical devices that structure the illness narrative are drawn from cultural and personal models for arranging experiences in meaningful ways and for effectively communicating those meanings. (p. 49)

Although Kleinman here alludes to a formal analysis of narrative forms and conventions, in practice he stresses the role of narrative in the expression of meaningful, personal experience. His interest in the biographical is stronger than any concern for the formal. The personal narrative of suffering, Kleinman repeatedly suggests, provides a unique mode of access to the personal life of the patient and his or her illness. The subtitle of his book, *Suffering, Healing and the Human Condition*, helps to convey the flavor of much of his work in this vein. The patient is portrayed, in Kleinman's reconstructions, as the hero or heroine of his or her personal narrative. Through narrative, experience and meaning are rendered whole. This essentially humane view of narrative and illness experience is emphasized in Kleinman's insistence on the place of *empathic listening* in the practice of medicine. Kleinman rather misleadingly likens this to the work of ethnography. It is misleading insofar as it implies that the work of ethnography is to produce empathic, experiential accounts of social actors and their worlds. In Kleinman's view, the clinician and the ethnographer are seen to be engaged in similar tasks of understanding and interpretation: The clinical encounter and the clinical investigation are described as a miniethnography. Describing features of this clinical ethnography, Kleinman (1988) writes:

> The first level of the mini-ethnography reconstructs the patient's illness narrative. The interpretation of that story's four types of meanings – symptom symbols, culturally marked disorder, personal and interpersonal significance, and patient and family explanatory models – thickens the account and deepens the clinician's understanding of the experience of suffering. Analysis of the narrative's content clarifies what is at stake for the patient and family. Deconstruction of the structure of the illness account – the rhetorical devices and plot outlines used by the patient to assemble particular events into a more or less integrated story line – can reveal hidden concerns that the patient has not verbalized. (p. 233)

This is clearly not a naive perspective. Kleinman's (1988) attention to narrative and rhetorical form as well as content indicates once again an orientation to the properties of illness narratives as constructions. Nevertheless, the more general tenor of Kleinman's remarks here, and elsewhere in his book, indicates a faith in the revelatory power of the narrative. The interpreter of the narrative may thus gain access to "hidden concerns" and may arrive at a "deep" understanding of the "experiences" of suffering. In other words, there is more than a hint that narrative provides an especially – perhaps uniquely – valid way of understanding the patient and her or his biographically grounded experience. The narrative mode, it seems, from this perspective somehow preserves and guarantees the integrity of the life and the experiences of the lifeworld. This may be thought to be an unduly negative characterization of Kleinman's contribution, and authors such as Fox (1993) certainly find a more sympathetic and more sophisticated version of his work (pp. 111–113), but Fox concludes that "Kleinman's actor is a modern one, of the romantic sort – suffering the existential angst of suffering and mortality" (p. 111).

Incidentally, it seems to me that insofar as Kleinman's (1988) general approach can be said to owe anything to a phenomenological perspective, his work exemplifies a misappropriation of phenomenological sociology or anthropology as well. The phenomenological emphasis on meaning construction, and the primacy of the lifeworld of mundane experience (the *Lebenswelt*), is an exercise in epistemology. Phenomenologists and social scientists inspired by the phenomenological movement, such as Schutz (1967), recognize the centrality of the "natural attitude" and its associated mode of knowing. Everyday understanding – commonness – must be the starting point for sociological analysis because it is the means whereby social actors construct their ordinary reality. Interpretative social science is not just about the second-order typifications produced by sociologists but the first-order typifications and interpretations produced by everyday social actors. The phenomenologist recognizes that there are different provinces of meaning, with different modes of experience and different ways of knowing. He or she makes that recognition, however, not to privilege one domain over another but to celebrate the world of everyday common sense by negating specialized provinces of meaning. But this is just what authors like Kleinman are in danger of doing. They conflate different connotations of experience. On one hand, it is incontrovertible that all phenomena are the product of experience and are rendered meaningful by acts of interpretation or definition. All definitions of health and illness, therefore, are given by acts of interpretation. They are all aspects of experience. On the other hand, Kleinman obviously wants to privilege certain ways of experiencing over others. He wants us to believe that the narrative self-knowledge and the narrative self-revelation of the patient are inherently more valid and more authentic modes of knowing or experiencing than other modes of interpretation.

A very similar view is to be found in Mishler's (1984, 1986) analyses of medical consultations and of the research interview itself. In a general vein similar to Kleinman's (1988), based on more formal analyses of medical encounters, Mishler contrasts two "voices": the voice of the lifeworld and the voice of medicine. In the course of routine diagnostic encounters between patients and medical practitioners, Mishler argues, these voices interrupt one another. The voice of medicine articulates the patient's condition in a decontextualized discourse and represents it in a reductionist manner; it is essentially the voice of biomedical understanding. The voice of medicine contrasts with the voice of the lifeworld. This latter mode of construction constructs the patient's troubles in a narrative format, grounded in the everyday lifeworld and the biographical details of the individual patient.

The narrative voice is thus valorized in Mishler's (1984) treatment of medical encounters, in just the same way that Kleinman (1988) celebrates the narratives of suffering. Mishler's analysis is, therefore, suffused with the implication that the narrative mode of the lifeworld is more authentic – by virtue of its biographical warrant – than the decontextualized discourse of biomedicine. Such a view is explicated in Mishler's (1986) extended treatment of the research interview. Here, by way of a slight digression through narratives and interviews in medicine, we return to the culture of the interview in social research. Mishler's combination of humane values in psychiatric and medical practice and his analytic interest in spoken discourse combine in a discussion of research interviewing. Mishler grounds his commentary in a critique of conventional interviewing for the purposes of sample surveys and other exercises in data collection. He provides a thorough review of narrative analysis in arguing that interview talk is properly to be understood in terms of speech events and the collaborative production of meaning. His use of formal narrative analysis, drawing on authors like Propp and Labov, indicates the importance of socially shared conventions. Formal analysis, after all, reminds us once more that the gesture is social, not the unique attribute of an individual social actor. In the last analysis, however, Mishler (1986) clearly wishes to promote a more romantic view of the person. He stresses a critical approach to social research that – in contrast to standardized research strategies – empowers the respondent. His own language, moreover, has a therapeutic flavor. He describes his own alternative proposals as being "concerned primarily with the impact of different forms of practice on respondents' modes of understanding themselves and the world, or the possibility of their acting in their own interests" (p. 118). In the same vein, Mishler (1986) writes:

> My intent is to shift attention away from investigators' "problems," such as technical issues of reliability and validity, to respondents' problems, specifically, their efforts to construct coherent and reasonable worlds of meaning and to make sense of their experiences. (p. 118)

These emphases on empowerment and the promotion of respondents' insight into their own problems, experiences, and interests reveal preoccupations that go beyond the purely methodological. The interview and the celebration of personal narratives take on an almost therapeutic and emancipatory aspect. An apparently methodological issue is transformed into an ethical concern for the integrity of the person and the biographically grounded experience. Narrative is celebrated as the revelation of the personal and the interview as the research device for its authentic elicitation. Ironically, a social-constructivist discourse, focused on narrative structures, is made to serve a Romantic agenda. I am not entirely dismissive of the ethical agendas proposed by Mishler (1984, 1986), Kleinman (1988), and authors in the same vein. The empowerment of patients and others in their encounters with professionals, and the obligation of the powerful to attend to the voices of everyday life, are clearly important. It is my contention, however, that such commitments do not in themselves provide foundations for an adequate methodology. Indeed, the implication of my argument is that such authors' practical and ethical concerns can lead them to miss the significance of narrative and biographical work.

It is at junctures like these, then, that we can detect the dangers of narrative being misused. It starts to transcend the realm of analytic methodology and becomes a surrogate form of liberal humanism and a romantic celebration of the individual subject. In the hands of a Kleinman (1988), it seems to me, we do not find a commitment to understanding the forms of social life or even the forms of narrative. For Kleinman is at heart a storyteller rather than a story analyst, and his goals are therapeutic rather than analytic. Moreover, his analysis dissolves the social. Ironically, for an anthropologist, he strips out the shared forms of social life – the organizing principles of shared culture – to look for something else. He wants to find the personal and the private. Far from examining the everyday work of social actors, Kleinman wants to reconstitute individual subjects. In other words, Kleinman's is a profoundly Romantic program. The same tendency may be found elsewhere. Indeed, I have focused on Kleinman (1988) and Mishler (1984, 1986) (whose analyses have significant differences as well as key similarities) only because they are such eloquent and distinguished representatives of this particular persuasion. But I want to suggest that the tendency is flawed and misleading. For we are in danger of recreating a new, individualized homunculus that escapes sociological or anthropological comprehension. We may have abandoned forever (though others have not) the model social actor driven solely by self-interest or the rational actor of classical economics. We should not reintroduce a new variant – the isolated actor who experiences and narrates as a matter of private and privileged experience.

A similar desire for redemption through narrative is to be found running through a third major text on illness narratives. *The Wounded Storyteller* (Frank, 1995) is a sustained and significant attempt to comprehend the dialectic between voice, body, illness, and narrative. Frank (1995) takes a somewhat different tack from Kleinman (1988) and Mishler (1984, 1986), but displays some of the same underlying assumptions. He focuses on the conditions and characteristics of illness stories, seeking to relate them to postmodern notions of self and identity.

Frank (1995) suggests that serious illness calls forth stories in two ways. First, stories "have to *repair* the damage that illness has done to the ill person's sense of where she is in life, and where she may be going. Stories are a way of re-drawing maps and finding new destinations" (p. 53). Second, "stories of the illness have to be told to medical workers, health bureaucrats, employers and work associates, family and friends" (pp. 53–54). The sick person is, in Frank's treatment, a "narrative wreck." Disease interrupts, and the sick person recreates narrative consistency through self-stories: "The way out of the narrative wreckage is telling stories" (p. 55). Frank draws on a variety of published sources for many stories of ill people, as well as his own biography and his engagement with ill people. The published materials predominate, and there is no sustained use of original field data. Frank maintains that through narratives, the dislocations between past and present – consequent on the interruption occasioned by disease – can be rectified: "Out of narrative truths a sense of coherence can be restored" (p. 61). In telling the illness story and the self-story, therefore, the sick person creates memory and recreates self-identity.

In the course of such narrative reconstruction, the teller emerges from the narrative wreckage, and Frank (1995) celebrates her or him as a kind of narrative hero: "One rises to the occasion by telling not just any story, but a good story. This good story is the measure of an ill person's success" (p. 62). All the examples that Frank cites seem to represent versions of such success. His own metanarrative is one of narrative triumph. Those successful narratives are grounded in what Frank also describes as acts of "witness," in which the sick person constructs a story that is true to lived experience.

If the sick person is a narrative hero, then the physician is portrayed as a narrative villain. Frank (1995), like the other authors I have discussed above, draws on the notion of interruption to characterize the work of the doctor. Equally, he equates contemporary medicine with the project of modernity and a colonializing tendency in which the sick person's story is appropriated by the medical practitioner. Taking, for instance, Parsons's (1951) ideal type of the sick role as a paradigm of modern medicine, Frank highlights the obligation of the sick person to seek and follow the advice of a professional:

> I understand this obligation of seeking medical care as a narrative surrender and mark it as the central moment in modernist illness experience. The ill person not only agrees to follow physical regimens that are prescribed; she also agrees, tacitly but with no less implication, to tell her story in medical terms. "How are you?" now requires that personal feeling be contextualized within a secondhand medical report. The physician becomes the spokesperson for the disease, and the ill person's stories come to depend heavily on repetition of what the physician has said. (p. 6)

Although Frank (1995) illustrates his argument with numerous brief quotations from published accounts, he does not base his analysis on the detailed examination of extensive first-person illness narratives. Consequently, the structure of such narratives remains virtually unexamined. He does, however, undertake analysis of a rather different sort: He deals with them in terms of genre. He emphasizes that any given illness will be told in terms of all three of the types he identifies, and that through those narrative types, cultural forms and personal experiences are brought together.

Restitution narratives tell of the body restored – or at least restorable – to health, through compliance with medical regimes. Frank (1995) suggests that such stories depend on a mechanistic view of the body and on a model of illness as a temporary breakdown that can be repaired. The ill person can only be a hero in such narratives by virtue of the superior heroism of the medical practitioner. By contrast, *chaos narratives* are antinarratives, without the resolution proffered by the restitution type. Indeed, Frank suggests, chaos escapes narrative closure, whereas narrative cannot encompass the disordered, temporally fragmented experience in which control is lost:

> The teller of chaos stories is, pre-eminently, the wounded storyteller, but those who are truly *living* the chaos cannot tell in words. To turn the chaos into a verbal story is to have some reflective grasp of it. The chaos that can be told in story is already taking place at a distance and is being reflected on retrospectively. For a person to gain such a reflective grasp of her own life, distance is a prerequisite. In telling the events of one's life, events are mediated by the telling. But in the lived chaos there is no mediation, only immediacy. The body is imprisoned in the frustrated needs of the moment. The person living the chaos story has no distance from her life and no reflective grasp on it. Lived chaos makes reflection, and consequently story-telling, impossible. (p. 98)

Third, the *quest narrative* constructs illness as a kind of journey. Here, the teller is a hero in his or her own story. There are three subtypes: the memoir, the manifesto, and the automythology. The first type is more or less self-explanatory, recounting an illness story together with other life events. The second combines personal narrative of illness with a prophetic call for social action. The third transforms the story of illness into a "paradigm of universal conflicts and concerns" (p. 126), transmuting the personal into more general metaphors and archetypes.

Whereas Frank (1995) takes his discussion of illness narratives into an exploration of genre and culturally shared resources, his analysis remains stunted. His standpoint is inspired more by ethical than methodological preoccupations. As I have indicated already, he shows little interest in the formal analysis of actual narratives, spoken or written, and is far more committed to the construction of a narrative morality. Like Kleinman (1988), he commends serious attention to illness narratives as the basis for clinical understanding and as the foundation for practical ethics.

Narrators and their narratives are far from equal in Frank's (1995) account. Narratives are celebrated insofar as they construct the active heroism of the ill person. Again, Frank is preoccupied with the authenticity of narratives, with the testimony that they inscribe and the self-identities that they enact. This is grounded in a particular version of postmodernist thought.

Frank (1995) equates contemporary medical practice and medical discourse with modernity and seeks a postmodern position. Drawing on authors such as Giddens and Bauman, Frank identifies personal responsibility as a key issue in postmodernity. Following Giddens, he proposes that the postmodern self is a reflexive project for which the individual is responsible. Such responsibility is enacted through narrative:

> Ill people's storytelling is informed by a sense of responsibility to the com-
> monsense world and represents one way of living *for* the other. People
> tell stories not just to work out their own changing identities, but also to
> guide others who will follow them. They seek not to provide a map that
> can guide others – each must create his own – but rather to witness the
> experience of reconstructing one's own map. Witnessing is one duty to
> the commonsensical and to others. (p. 17)

Like other authors in this vein, however, Frank (1995) seems repeatedly guilty of self-contradiction. Despite his repeated contrasts between the modernism of medicine and the possibilities of a postmodern ethic, he – like Mishler (1984, 1986) and Kleinman (1988) – wants to privilege certain kinds and occasions of narrative performance. He does so to celebrate particular modes of self-expression, in the interest of establishing the authenticity of specific kinds of experience. In the absence of detailed analysis – or even exemplification – of narrative data, it is often difficult to engage systematically with Frank's arguments. Much of his book consists of unsubstantiated assertions, derived from a collection of personal convictions rather than grounded in systematic analysis. So far as one can identify a coherent argument, however, it seems to rest on a similar set of oppositions that can be identified in the work of Kleinman and Mishler. The narratives of medical work are given minimal attention and are dismissed as interruptions. They hold, apparently, no interest and have no features worth documenting. By contrast, the narratives of everyday personal experience (especially quest narratives) are valorized – the more so as they remain innocent of medically derived discourse. The everyday domain of commonsense understanding, like Mishler's lifeworld, is celebrated. Implicitly, different domains of meaning and discourse are evaluated quite differently. Frank eschews any methodological principle of symmetry in his treatment of narratives, while reversing the polarity of credibility that normally distinguishes lay from professional knowledge.

In celebrating the voices that are enacted through narrative, Frank (1995) is as guilty as Kleinman (1988) of treating narrators and narratives in a vacuum. This omission is ironic: The discourse of medicine is held up for criticism because it allegedly decontextualizes illness. Yet, these celebrations of the voice of everyday, lay experience are equally divorced from their contexts. The narratives seem to float in a social vacuum. The voices echo in an otherwise empty world. There is an extraordinary absence of social context, social action, and social interaction. We get, for instance, remarkably little sense of how narratives are forged in face-to-face interaction or how they are elicited in given social contexts. There is little sensitivity to the temporal and spatial distribution of illness stories or how they are embedded in a social division of labor. Frank is, as we have seen, more committed to dismissing the work of others than to incorporating it into a principled sociological or anthropological analysis.

What we are invited to endorse, therefore, is a celebration of some – but by no means all – narratives. These are stripped of social context and social consequences. They are understood in terms of an individualized view of the self. Narratives are the means whereby the narrating subject, autonomous and independent of the medical profession, can achieve authenticity. Narratives are the means whereby illness may be transcended and turned into an apotheosis through self-mythologizing. This represents an almost total failure to use narrative to achieve serious social analysis. Discussions like Frank's (1995) fall between two stools. They are devoid of social context, and no attention is devoted to their formal structures: Both are necessary for an adequate analysis.

The Place of Narrative

So far, I have suggested a small number of simple things. First, that there is a contemporary emphasis on narrative modes in social analysis; second, that medicine may readily be demonstrated to have major narrative occasions and functions; and third, that some applications of narrative understanding – including analyses of medical narrative – are misplaced and misrepresent the fundamental nature of narrative. Finally, I want to consider how narrative approaches might appropriately be located within the formal analysis of social encounters and social order.

Before I do so, let me recapitulate what I take to be the elementary message of this discussion. The narrative organization of health and illness, and of medical work, is unquestionable. The temporal trajectory of illness careers is organized through the narrative unfolding of events and evaluations; the illness trajectory is a situated production, enacted through the occasioned tellings of illness experience. The meaning of illness is projected retrospectively and prospectively through oral and written language acts. Likewise, the attributions of disease and the accounting of medical treatment, the medical history, and the prognosis may also be enacted through narrative performances. As I have suggested, the modern clinic is a densely narrated environment.

There is an economy in which narratives are exchanged and modified over time through repeated transactions, ranging from the most formal to the more informal and fleeting. The oral traditions of medicine are reproduced through such tellings. The formal analyses of health and illness, and the formal analyses of medical settings, are impoverished without due attention to narrative formats and their place in more general organizational work.

Likewise, the biographical work that is embedded in health and medicine is also a narrative accomplishment. In the repeated telling of health and illness, the person of the patient is constituted. Moral work is accomplished through the accounts of health activity. This is true of patients and of health professionals. Through their tellings of cases, physicians, nurses, and others render themselves and their routine work accountable. As Pithouse and I argued in another context, focusing on social work as an occupation, the narrative construction of a case renders the otherwise invisible craft work of the trade visible to colleagues and superiors. The narrative ordering of the case is the object of professional scrutiny and supervision (Pithouse & Atkinson, 1988; see also Atkinson, 1994).

By the same token, there is absolutely no doubt that illness is, in part, a narrative accomplishment. Accounts of symptoms, biographical disruption, the search for causes, lay referral, impairment, healing, and so on are ubiquitous. Narrative formats – like those identified by Frank (1995) – are among the cultural resources that are available for the social construction of health and illness. The data presented or alluded to by authors such as Kleinman (1988), Mishler (1984, 1986), and Frank are ample testimony to the distribution of narratives in such constructions.

But, as I have emphasized throughout this discussion, the ubiquity of the narrative and its centrality to everyday work are not license simply to privilege those forms. It is the work of anthropologists and sociologists to examine those narratives and to subject them to the same analysis as any other forms. We need to pay due attention to their construction in use: how actors improvise their personal narrative or their narratives of work accomplished. We need to attend to how socially shared resources of rhetoric and narrative are deployed to generate recognizable, plausible, and culturally well-formed accounts. We need, in other words, to treat them as "social facts," like any other that is equally conventional, and apply the same canons of methodological skepticism as we would apply to any other acts and social forms. What we cannot afford to do is to be seduced by the cultural conventions we seek to study. We should not endorse those cultural conventions that seek to privilege the account as a special kind of representation.

We are, for instance, surrounded by a culture that stresses and rewards self-revelation and autobiographical work. It is right, therefore, that sociologists and anthropologists should in recent years have paid explicit attention to the autobiographical. What would not be right would be to assume that auto-biographical accounts thereby become privileged kinds of data, with greater or different claims for authenticity. Autobiographical accounts and self-revelations are as conventional and as artful as any other mode of representation. We sell short ourselves and the possibility of systematic social analysis if we implicitly assume that autobiographical accounts or narratives of personal experience grant us untrammeled access to a realm of hyperauthenticity. The collection and reproduction of narratives and the celebration of voices through that work are not guarantees of anything. The assumption of authenticity uncritically reflects dominant beliefs about the self and its revelation. It endorses the romantic image of the interior self – a self that is also anterior to the realm of social action. It takes insufficient account of the traditions of interpretative social science that – as in the classic contribution of George Herbert Mead (1934), for instance – stress the social origins of the gesture and the discursive production of the social self. It is in danger of substituting a psychotherapeutic for a sociological view of the person.

This view surely does not mean that there is no place for narrative analysis. On the contrary, a social analysis without an adequate treatment of narrative, rhetoric, and other features of discourse would be unthinkable. As I have hinted earlier, a sociology or anthropology of the domain of medical and health work that paid no attention to such phenomena would be jejune indeed. What is to be avoided, however, is a reductionist argument that promotes just one form of culture, just one mode of performance, just one kind of text and treats it as the paramount mode of reality. We need, it seems to me, a genuinely *thick description* of medical and other organizational settings.

By thick description, I do not mean simply detailed – any more than did Geertz (1973). Too often, especially in secondary sites of knowledge reproduction, the term thick description is used quite erroneously and in incorrect ways analogous to the violence done to terms like *grounded theory*. Whereas the terms' originators meant to convey something rather complex about the social world and its exploration, in the hands of semischolars they become debased: Grounded theory becomes an apology for qualitative empiricism and thick description becomes a pretentious synonym for rich data. Now I recognize that there is more than one way to interpret the notion of thick description. What I want to emphasize here is that our descriptions of social settings need to do justice to the complex variety of forms through which they are enacted. We do not need a reductionist emphasis on narrative to the exclusion of all else, any more than we need an emphasis on conversational turn taking, or on proxemics and kinesics, or on dramaturgy and self-presentation. Nor, by the same token, do I mean that every analysis must try to analyze out all those issues simultaneously. One can identify and analyze an interaction order that is relatively autonomous and can be studied in its own right, just as one can study the economic order in its own terms; but this is not a single indivisible entity, nor will one analytic strategy exhaustively account for that interaction order.

We need, therefore, to put narrative in its place. The narrative mode of representation is important in everyday life and in professional work. But it is one mode of representation among many. Neither it nor any others can be granted priority. I repeat, narrative does not provide a hyperauthentic version of actors' experiences or selves. A backdoor smuggling in of romantic constructions of the self will not do. We will not produce good research on the social world by stripping out the social, replacing it with solitary voices or individualized versions of experience. We need to put narrative in its place, therefore, by approaching it in the context of the multiple modes of performance, of ordering, of remembering, of interacting. Narrative is but one form of social action. It should not be singled out to the detriment of qualitative health research that is firmly grounded in the multiple forms of action and interaction.

Author's Note

This article is a revised version of an address delivered to the International Qualitative Health Research Conference, Bournemouth, UK, November 1996.

References

Atkinson, P. (1994). Rhetoric as skill. In M. Bloor & P. Taraborrelli (Eds.), *Qualitative research in health and medicine* (pp. 110–130). Aldershot, England: Avebury.

Atkinson, P. A. (1995). *Medical talk and medical work.* London: Sage.

Bosk, C. (1979). *Forgive and remember.* Chicago: University of Chicago Press.

Cappetti, C. (1993). *Writing Chicago: Modernism, ethnography and the novel.* New York: Columbia University Press.

Farrell, J. T. (1988). *Studs Lonigan.* London: Picador.

Foucault, M. (1973). *The birth of the clinic.* London: Tavistock.

Fox, N. J. (1992). *The social meaning of surgery.* Buckingham, England: Open University Press.

Fox, N. J. (1993). *Postmodernism, sociology and health.* Buckingham, England: Open University Press.

Frank, A. W. (1995). *The wounded storyteller.* Chicago: University of Chicago Press.

Geertz, C. (1973). *The interpretation of cultures.* New York: Basic Books.

Holstein, J. A., & Gubrium, J. F. (1995). *The active interview.* Thousand Oaks, CA: Sage.

Hunter, K. M. (1991). *Doctors' stories: The narrative structure of medical knowledge.* Princeton, NJ: Princeton University Press.

Kleinman, A. (1988). *The illness narratives: Suffering, healing and the human condition.* New York: Basic Books.

Maupin, A. (1989). *Tales of the city.* London: Black Swan.

Mead, G. H. (1934). *Mind, self and society.* Chicago: University of Chicago Press.

Mishler, E. (1984). *The discourse of medicine.* Norwood, NJ: Ablex.

Mishler, E. (1986). *Research interviewing.* Cambridge, MA: Harvard University Press.

Phenomenology

43

Nursing, Morality, and Emotions: Phase I and Phase II Clinical Trials and Patients with Cancer

Meinir Krishnasamy

The following interview arose out of an ongoing debate engendered by reflections on practice in a cancer clinical trials unit (CCTU). A desire to explore the moral agency of their work was expressed by a group of three United Kingdom nurses working with patients receiving phases I and II of cancer clinical trials (1). As such, the findings of the interview are representative of the three nurses' working reality, and this article is presented within that cultural context. However, it is hoped that some of the issues raised will prove to be of interest and relevance to nurses working in similar environments elsewhere.

Moral agency has been defined by Raines (1) as actions undertaken in an ethos of care committed to the centrality of the patient. Phases I and II trials are undertaken to determine the efficacy of new drugs and to identify responding tumor types, maximum tolerated dose, and toxicity levels (2). Phase I trials are concerned with finding the best way to administer a new treatment and with identifying its maximum tolerated dose. They involve small numbers of patients whose cancers are known to be unresponsive to other treatments. Although the new treatment will have been well tested in laboratory and animal studies with promising results, its side effects in patients remain unknown until trials have been undertaken.

Phase I drugs may or may not produce anticancer effects, but when drugs demonstrate promising results, they are studied further in phase II trials

Source: *Cancer Nursing*, 22(4) (1999): 251–259.

designed to determine the efficacy of a new drug alongside ongoing monitoring of its toxicity profile. For drugs whose anticancer properties are established, a phase III study comparing standard treatment against the new drug is then undertaken (2,3).

A detailed explanation of the purpose and phases of clinical trials is not provided here, nor a discussion of issues associated with informed consent in relation to cancer clinical trials because these previously were discussed comprehensively (2,3,8). This article focuses on the experiences of three cancer and palliative care nurses, citing their views on the moral dimensions of their work through their own words. It considers their discussion alongside previous work undertaken to explore the moral work of nursing and a consideration of the significance that emotions have to ethical decision making. Reference is made to the competing paradigms of care and cure, and consideration is given to the impact of these on professional cohesion in the clinical trials unit.

Cancer Clinical Trials: Context and Emotion

Cancer research and cancer therapy are often presented as complementary domains (4), activities undertaken by those committed to finding a cure for cancers, alongside the work of those committed to the care of individuals for whom cure may no longer reflect a realistic outcome. Yet, if there is indeed a complementarity, it exists largely as a consequence of the commitment of all involved to sustain a tentative balance between a plethora of emotions:

The doctor : *We will conquer this thing, … perhaps not in your lifetime, but surely not too long from now* (5).

The patient : *I sometimes wonder if the people who are recommending this drug or that drug would subject themselves to the therapy they are recommending* (6).

The patient : *Just before assaults on fortified positions, U.S. Civil War soldiers would pin their names and addresses onto their uniforms to make it easier for the body sorters to do their work. Patients going into these modified protocols could likewise place their names on specific protocol adjustments. Survivors could then proclaim: "This is how I wanted to die-not a suicide and not passively accepting, but eagerly in the struggle* (7).

The nurse (Nurse 2 in the interview):

Patients are so hopeful …. You don't want to dash their hopes, but you just sort of think …, "Are you really that informed about things?" … You almost feel as though you are going along with this sort of jolly positive side that maybe you don't actually believe in.

Grady (8) distinguishes between clinical practice as a set of activities designed to enhance the well-being of the individual patient and clinical research defined as a set of activities intended to test a hypothesis and therefore contribute to or develop knowledge. Many patients, doctors, and nurses express concerns about the efficacy compared with the distressing side effects of clinical trials in treating patients with cancer (e.g., septicemia, oral infections, alopecia, constipation, nausea and vomiting, or isolation from family and friends) who experience repeated hospital admissions necessitated by the trial protocol. Sometimes, these concerns are compounded by emotional claims about experimenting on the dying (9). Along with conflicting perspectives, these concerns can place medical and nursing staff under considerable stress as they work together to balance the objectivity of clinical research with the humanity of clinical practice (2,10).

This article draws in part on literature that compares ethical decision-making models between doctors and nurses. The intention of this article, however, is not to dichotomize the medical and nursing views as either-or models of moral agency belonging solely to care or cure paradigms. The heterogeneity of moral thinking and professional knowledge is undisputed. An acknowledgment that doctors and nurses have personal knowledge of patients that may compete with the depersonalized knowledge of clinical trial statistics also is asserted.

Nursing and Medicine

Medicine has dominated the Western paradigm of professional health care for more than 200 years (11), but the health care system within which it is framed increasingly is recognized as being in a "crisis of transition" (12,13). Political crises, forcing radical changes in the ways by which health care is delivered dominate discussions of health care provision, while at a more fundamental level, a philosophical or intellectual crisis appears to be occurring. According to Kuhn (12), when something happens that forces scientists to question the basic principles and assumptions of their knowledge base, a philosophic crises ensues, caused by the necessity of working with intellectual uncertainty and professional vulnerability.

Nursing, grounded in a knowledge based on caring relationships with people (14), is inextricably caught up in the current uncertainty and vulnerability of medicine, in which an acknowledgment of the significance of personhood and sociocultural facets of health care intervention rest tentatively alongside the dominance of clinical medicine. Increasingly, medicine is being challenged to embrace patients' cultural and contextual reality (15) in a system being driven to manage chronic health care needs.

Furthermore, it can be said that nursing is emerging from its own crisis of transition, in which nurses contribution to the humanness of health care is being recognized through innovative, dynamic ways of working with individuals in the totality of their ill-health experience (16–19).

Somewhere in this complexity, the interplay between nursing and medicine has begun to change (20). The doctor-nurse game (21), characterized by a medical omnipotence covertly challenged by a nursing manipulation is still much in evidence. Yet there is an increasing tendency toward a negotiated-order approach (22). Such an approach emphasizes that a principal way by which things get accomplished in organizations is through people negotiating with each other.

The negotiating capacity of nursing undoubtedly is stronger than it was a decade ago. Also, a consensus exists among the nursing profession that a mutual relationship between medicine and nursing not only is possible, but also is an ethical requirement (23,24). In this shifting dynamic, nurses unquestionably have gained more responsibility for patients and their families (22). However, there still is a corresponding lack of authority for effecting patient centered health care decisions. These decisions still are jealously guarded by many doctors (22,25). Increasingly, nurses are finding themselves in an exposed position between the doctor and the patient (22), a situation potentially heightened when an ethos of cure comes face to face with an ethos of care.

Gilligan (26) and Benner and Wrubel (27) proposed that caring can be at the center of a personal belief system, and that because caring is central to nursing, it is possible to have an ethic based on caring, an assertion vociferously challenged for its obscurity (10). An ethic of caring based on the premise that "to care" is morally good is rejected out of hand. Allmark (10) concluded that "what we care about is morally important; the fact that we care per se is not" (p. 23). Allmark gave no indication as to whether he believes that distinguishing between acknowledged competing value systems in the health care system (i.e., care versus cure) is necessary so that the contribution of each professional group can be recognized and conveyed in a manner that ultimately best supports patients and their families and fosters a respect toward divergent moral reasoning. He asserted that for someone to be caring, the right set of values must be apparent, and that care must be conveyed in the right way.

The preceding view seems to reflect an Aristotelian view of ethics, which is concerned with the process of moral decision making, and not solely with its outcome. In other words, if an endeavor is to be considered ethical, the thoughts, feelings, and desires behind the action must be morally irreprehensible. This clearly involves a requirement that a person be able to explore the feelings, thoughts, and desires accompanying the provision of care before claiming ability to decide whether he or she can act ethically in a given situation.

Emotions and Ethical Decision Making

Oakley (28) defined emotion as a complex of interrelated affects, desires, and cognitions in relation to a given situation and asserted that they are pivotal to moral decision making. He argued that rather than being vilified as unscientific, emotions should be embraced and understood as a powerful means of fostering and understanding ethical interactions. Affects may be bodily feelings (e.g., shivering or dizziness) or psychic feelings (e.g., hope, despair, sadness) that may or may not have physical manifestations). Desires or wishes may be unconscious and not necessarily expressed in behavior, whereas cognitions are defined as incorporating a variety of elements that may effect the way in which a person views a situation as a consequence of his or her beliefs, thoughts, values, socialization, professional or political affiliations, and the like. (28). Professional socialization clearly is appropriate here, and its significance in establishing a moral code of conduct in a clinical trials unit is discussed further in the following discussion.

Nursing and Moral Agency

Traditionally, it has been assumed that the predominant ethical framework within which nursing has functioned has been a principle-orientated ethic (29). Principle-oriented ethics are reliant on rules. Moral decision making involves a consideration of these differing rules and culminates with an objective process of choosing between possible actions (11). Objectivity, impartiality and acting in accordance with preset principles govern the moral process. An ethic of care, whether accepted as viable or not, is presented as being concerned primarily with responsibility in a relationship and is characterized by interdependence and reciprocity (29).

Melia (30), critical of the idealized notions of an ethic of care, proposed that if nursing is to make a contribution to health care ethics, then it should turn to explore the issues as they relate to patients in a very practical manner. In three independent studies of ethical decision making by nurses, a picture of moral reasoning emerged, which represented a process far more complex than one bound solely by a justice or principle-oriented ethic (31–33). Although grounded in a global context of ethics, nursing, if it is to make a unique contribution to health care ethics, must find a way of encompassing the norms, values, and principles that guide the profession within ethical debate (34).

The Interview

The group interview provided an opportunity to explore the views of three nurses on the moral dimensions of their work in caring for patients receiving phases I and II of cancer clinical trials in an attempt to further an understanding of the complexity of this work. Group membership was self-selected after unit nurses were openly invited to participate. Although not employed as research nurses, the unit nurses routinely administered chemotherapy as part of their day to day caregiving.

Three qualified nurses with varying amounts of experience of working in a CCTU took part in the interview. The semistructured, tape-recorded interview lasting 2 hours was led by the author, who has experience working in a trials unit. The nurses met in a chemotherapy day-care ward at the hospital on an afternoon when no chemotherapy day-care patients were present. A group interview was undertaken with the intention of providing the nurses an opportunity to discuss complex issues together away from the unit setting with an impartial but knowledgeable listener. The acceptability of a group discussion was checked with the nurses before the interview was undertaken.

The directness and versatility offered by an interview frequently allows for disclosure of information across contexts (e.g., information about feelings, values, opinions, and motives) (35). Therefore, the interview was highly appropriate to the aim of the study. Participants were invited to talk about any aspect of their work with patients receiving phases I and II clinical trials that they felt demonstrated its ethical or moral dimensions:

> *Please describe in your own words what you consider to be ethical or moral dimensions of your work. Are there any aspects of these dimensions that you find ethically or morally demanding, and why is that?*

The clinical trial experience of the group ranged from 15 months to 4 years. At the time they undertook the interview, two of the nurses were in the process of pursuing diplomas in palliative care. None had been educated to degree level. No signed consent was obtained, but verbal agreement to take part was recorded at the beginning of the interview, as were assurances of anonymity and confidentiality. After verbatim transcriptio n from the tape-recordings, the interview was subjected to a process of thematic content analysis (36), in which the interview was read and reread to elicit and refine emergent themes.

Transcribed data initially was coded into the following 15 microcategories:

1. Perceptions of the value of clinical trials
2. Examples of moral or ethical challenges experienced in relation to named patients or critical incidents
3. What do I think about my work?
4. Communication within the professional team
5. Patient and family expectations of a trial
6. Personal and professional valuing within the health care team
7. Personal and professional contribution within the health care team
8. Acute versus palliative care
9. Setting care boundaries within the unit's remit

10. The need for information and inclusion in decision making
11. Conflict and professional ethos
12. Trust and mistrust
13. The cost of caring
14. The cost of not caring
15. Education and autonomy.

As the interview was read and reread, and the microcategories were re-explored in relation to the context of the whole, the three key categories listed in the next section were developed. Negotiation for the provision of an interview transcript to each participant and an opportunity to proofread this paper provided the participants with a chance to validate the themes presented.

Results

Analysis of the data resulted in the emergence of three key themes:

1. Being valued and moral distress
2. Caring in a climate of scientific research
3. Care, cure, and consequences for moral reasoning.

The themes, discussed in the following section, are not presented in any order of importance. Although presented here as discrete entities, they should be understood as interconnected facets of the nurses' dialogue.

Discussion

Being Valued and Moral Distress

A pervasive element throughout the interview was the conflict caused by a dichotomy between nursing's increased responsibility for and contribution to the care of patients and their families (22) and a recognized continued lack of authority with which to influence patient care decisions (22,25). Working in an environment suffused with moral conflicts appeared to heighten the nurses' awareness of a lack of perceived moral or respectful behavior among medical colleagues. It also increased feelings of having to betray personal values of caring in response to a lack of authority. This led to feelings of being devalued within the health care team and resulted in insecurity and low self-worth, which at times influenced the nurse's ability to act in the best interests of his or her patient:

> *The link person for that trial went to the consultant and still her views were ignored, and coming back to how that makes you feel about your job, I think,*

it's almost you accept it as part of your working in that environment.... You haven't got enough knowledge to make the decision ... to speak up any further than you do. (Nurse 2)

You tend to lose your confidence or I do anyway, and I think, I shouldn't have asked that,... and you just leave it and let it go,... so it would be really helpful just to have a meeting where you could say anything, not feel stupid for it. (Nurse 1)

The feelings expressed by the nurses also appeared to suggest a degree of passivity, which resulted in profound feelings of personal and professional disillusionment and distress:

As nurses, particularly ward nurses, we haven't got a lot of say about choice of treatment or anything like that.... We are just from an outsider almost point of view.... Our opinions aren't that valid.... (Nurse 2) And I think then we can get negative,... and we don't quite understand what hopes ... the medical staff have. (Nurse 3)

You know that their life span is most likely to be very limited,... and they're so hopeful, you're almost, you don't want to dash their hopes, but you just sort of think, "Do you really know, are you really that informed about things?" And ... you almost sort of feel as though you are going along with its sort of jolly positive side that maybe you don't actually believe in. (Nurse 2)

The nurses described a desire to shift their work from within an organizational structure traditionally reliant on the doctor-nurse game (21) perceived to be a significant cause of their distress to one that embraces a negotiated order approach (22) reflecting a desire to have nursing's contribution recognized and incorporated into the unit's dominant decision-making structure. The passivity expressed undoubtedly is a reflection of the cultural context within which these United Kingdom nurses work. However, they spoke little of their responsibility to contribute to the organizational shift they clearly desire. A mistrust and misunderstanding of medical colleagues' intentions and objectives is articulated, resulting in an inherent passivity and devaluation of the nurses, which seemingly discourages them from engaging in the pursuit of a shift in organizational culture.

In those meetings where there's a medical student, they always have time for teaching,... (but) they can't find time to maybe explain data and criteria to us. (Nurse 3)

I think they very much see that everything we would say would be threatening to the decision that they'd made. It's almost as if it's them and us, and we're sort of the ones in the background going, but why? (Nurse 2)

I think we all have our own agendas. I think as nurses ... our priority is patient care, in whatever setting.... I think a lot of the doctors' agenda ... they've got their statistics ... doing work for their research fellowships. (Nurse 3)

The consequences of these feelings of mistrust and misunderstanding for the medical staff is not apparent here, and this must be acknowledged as significant omission in the perspectives offered. Furthermore, a lack in understanding how able doctors are to convey feelings of distress within their cultural and social parameters would add considerably to this discussion.

A communication gap described by Grundstein-Amado (24) and Svensson (22) is evident, resulting from feelings of frustration and exasperation at having nursing's contribution to the care of patients in the unit poorly understood and undervalued:

> *I think that deep down the decision is still made by the doctor, and if they are not aware of the ethical issues of situations that everyone becomes involved with, then they still make a cut and dry medical decision. (Nurse 2)*

> *Everything seems to be very segregated.... You have a doctor's meeting with the presence of one nurse or whatever, or you have a multidisciplinary meeting, but without the doctor. (Nurse 3)*

The consequence for nurses, attempting to support patients and their families when difficult decisions have to be made and they feel unsupported and undervalued themselves, are considerable:

> *How our contribution as nursing is valued, and I would say it's very low, very small, that yes, we do a good job ... for what they see nursing to be, but I don't really think that ... umm ... the medical team have any concept really of our involvement or the contribution we make to the patients. (Nurse 2)*

Erosion of personal integrity and betrayal of personal values are central causes of nursing disillusionment (39). For these nurses, it appeared that working in a system that seems to place greater value on the outcome than on the process of scientific endeavor, and that espouses an unspoken ethical view based on theoretical ethical principles and rules, diminishes the place given to supportive care while also minimizing its therapeutic significance (40–41).

> *We've had patients that have become ... terminal, and almost you feel as though they are being pressurized to get out of the ward because they are taking up a clinical trial beds. (Nurse 2) ... But the doctor would argue very much and would turn round and say, "But this is a clinical trials unit." (Nurse 1) ... But I find that very difficult when you're offering clinical trials for palliative care when just because the clinical trial stops, then your palliative care stops ... you just can't say that. (Nurse 2)*

The confusion of nursing over its negotiating capacity and power status (23,24) is much in evidence here as the nurses describe their affects, desires, and cognitions in relating to the patients under their care. It has been shown that feelings of powerlessness lead to frustration, anger, and personal conflict, with a nurse questioning what she is doing and what she feels she should be doing (39,42). Such emotions result in what has been referred to as emotional inertia. The extracts from the interview are suffused with feelings of uncertainty, of being in an unsafe position, of mediating between patients and doctors, and of yet feeling powerless to effect ethical decisions regarding patient care (25):

> We get so tied up with the work on the ward,... and I don't think at the end of the day any of us have got any energy left to fight, continuously fight, for ethical discussions, or to have the time to be able to go to research lectures, etc., etc. (Nurse 1)

The nurses identified one cause of their powerlessness as their inability to articulate ethical dilemmas in a language that they believed would be acces-sible to medical colleagues. Consequently, they concluded that their opinions would be ignored or dismissed as being "emotionally" driven. Oakley (28) asserted that a person's thoughts, desires, and cognitions, influenced by personal value systems and professional socialization, are central to that person's evaluation of a given situation and its ethical dimension. Emotions, so prevalent in these nurses' discussions of their work and its moral dimension, instead of being denigrated as muddying the waters of principle-oriented ethics, need to be explored and understood in relation to their contribution to nursing and its moral agency (28). It is within this complex and stressful environment that these nurses and doctors work and grapple with the moral dimensions of their roles, which are complicated by an ontologic and epistemologic spilt between the objectivity of scientific research and a determination to care for individuals.

Caring in a Climate of Scientific Research

Swanz (43) argued that a research endeavor should be judged at one level, not in relation to the potential for patient involvement or clinical outcome, but according to whether the patient benefited therapeutically through association with the undertaking. This may be especially significant in a CCTU where the majority of patients have a poor prognosis. Nevertheless, palliative care research, representative of the realistic context wherein many cancer clinical trials are undertaken, exists predominantly within the paradigm of biomedical science (44). Yet, much of the care provided in CCTUs is concerned with establishing close relationships with patients, rejecting an approach based on objective science, and striving instead to establish a personal relationship that promotes integrity, trust, and respect for all involved (45). This relationship is fundamentally associated with the concept of containment (46), in which the health care professional consciously sets out to safe-guard the personal integrity of the patient. Reason (45) asserted that a patient-as-object approach to care delivery is destructive, reducing persons to objects of research endeavor. This dichotomy is not explicitly articulated anywhere in the interview reported here, and yet it would appear to be a fundamental cause of moral distress and emotional inertia for the nurses:

> *You can't isolate it can you … not when there's people involved.… You can't have one [a clinical trial] without the other [people]; you can't separate the issue of holistic care. (Nurse 3)*

Emotional inertia refers to feelings of powerlessness and inner conflict, when people question their professed beliefs or judgments in response to their seemingly contradictory actions (28). The current interview was embued with a language of emotional inertia, with the nurses expressing contradictory emotions and professional beliefs in an attempt to explain the moral agency of their work:

> *You feel as though you're sort of waving them [the patients] goodbye [at the end of a trial].… You want the contact to continue. You want to carry on supporting these people who you've actually come to know very well, but the environment where we work doesn't allow that. (Nurse 2)*

The distress caused by this inertia, manifest throughout the discussion, is reflected by a personal and professional cost akin to that reported by Morrison (47) and Oberle and Davies (37). Where an individual works in a system that espouses values that differ from his or her own, the cost to that person may be high, resulting in an incongruency between what the person believes should be done and what he or she is able to do (48). There also may be far-reaching consequences for the quality of care delivered at the end of the day (42).

Erosion of personal integrity and betrayal of personal values in the context of professional practice have been cited as central causes of nursing disillusionment (39). Nurses whose personal ethic is rooted in caring may feel undervalued when working in a system that places greater value on technical skill, adopting an ethical view based on the application of abstract principles and rules that allows no place for relationships and caring (39). Further evidence of this dissonance and its costs, manifesting as confusion, anger, and hurt, has been reported by Parker (48).

In the study by Erlen and Frost (25), physician control, a lack of knowledge concerning alternative courses of action, and ineffectiveness in exerting any influence on the outcome of a dilemma were the predominant causes for feelings of powerlessness. One nurse stated: "You feel that no one wants to listen to you, or what you have to say is not important" (p. 403). When the nurses made efforts to exercise expert power, they met medical resistance. Similar experiences were reported by the nurses interviewed for the current study:

> *There is an awareness that we are not talking about ethical decisions. We've had a visiting ethicist round to just have a debate.… It was attended by the nurses.… (Nurse 1) It wasn't attended doctor-wise. (Nurse 2)*

Care, Cure and Consequences for Moral Reasoning

Confining an understanding of the ethical decision making patterns of the nurses who participated in this interview to a rigid principle-orientated ethic limits our ability to understand the moral dimensions of their work. At the outset of a nurse-patient relationship, as Cooper (29) reported, a principle-orientated ethic focusing on traditional moral principles of beneficence, autonomy, and respect is foremost. As the relationship between the nurse and the patient develops, however, the nurse increasingly finds herself drawn into an emotionally laden, complex, and unpredictable situation characterized by a moral response guided by an awareness of the patients' experiences. In keeping with an Aristotelian view of ethics, the nurses interviewed during the current study, reflect a concern with the processes involved in moral reasoning:

> *The patients are constantly looking for a cure.... They'll accept ... without really looking at, you know, what it's going to do to my quality of life, how much time am I going to spend in the unit rather than at home. (Nurse 1)*

However, the nurses do not suggest that their medical colleagues are unconcerned with the costs for patients, but instead convey misgivings about the primacy given by doctors to the outcome issues. Evidence cited earlier asserts that doctors and nurses have been shown to demonstrate differences in ethical decision-making patterns. For the nurses interviewed in this study, this dichotomy appears to stem from an ambiguity surrounding the doctors "agendas":

> *I think we all have our own agendas. I think as nurses ... our priority is patient care, in whatever setting.... I think a lot of the doctors' agenda ... they've got their statistics ... doing work for their research fellowships. (Nurse 3)*

For the nurses who were interviewed, a tension existed between an individual's therapeutic potential for involvement in a clinical trial and the utilitarian concept of advancement of scientific knowledge, the very raison d'être of the unit. It appears that it is the omnipotence of a utilitarian outcome that causes them moral disquiet. Committed to the unit and their medical colleagues, the nurses find themselves in "no man's land" caught between a desire to act in the best interests of the patients with whom they enter into intense relationships and wanting to be understood, valued, and respected by medical colleagues as partners and representatives of patients' voices when ethical decisions have to be made. This isolation results in the communication gaps, frustrations, anger, and personal and professional distress highlighted earlier. The degree to which this dichotomy influenced the doctors working in the unit was not explored, but one of the nurses commented as follows:

The doctors haven't got time to even acknowledge that they're concerned,... and almost wouldn't be supported even if they did say ... If a junior doctor raised a concern, it wouldn't be seen as a positive thing really. (Nurse 3)

The ways in which the nurses discussed complex care decisions mirror decision-making patterns described previously, in which a picture of moral reasoning represented a process far more complex than one bound solely by a justice or principle-oriented ethic (29,31–33). A principle-oriented ethic, focusing on tenets of beneficence, autonomy, and respect, adequate to inform decision making at the outset of a nurse-patient relationship becomes inadequate as relationships between a nurse and patient develop. The nurse increasingly finds herself drawn into a complex and emotionally laden interaction:

They come in with all these hopes, and you, you know, you would never ever take those away from them because it's their right to have those hopes, but then ... it's very difficult sometimes. (Nurse 3)

You don't know whether to be, to try to be very realistic with them, or, and to increase their hopes, or whether to say, "Well look, you know, don't get too, too enthused,"... and I almost want to say sometimes, "Oh please, don't put them on that trial," ... but who are we to say that? (N1)

These quotes illustrate that for the interviewed nurses, the decision-making framework within which they function belongs to the practical world of the patient and his family (30). These nurses work at the interface between the quest for a cure and nature's determination to prevail. It is here that nursing rests, exposed and vulnerable, at considerable risk of moral distress and emotional inertia (28).

Conclusion

Issues raised in this interview mirror evidence of the ethical components that comprise nurses' work in various care settings (25,29,32–34,39,47,48). The aim of this undertaking was to further an understanding of the moral agency of nurses working with patients receiving phases I and II of cancer clinical trials undertaken to determine the effectiveness of new drugs and to identify responding tumor types as well as maximum tolerated dose and toxicity levels. These compounds administered to vulnerable individuals, for whom no known effective treatment is available, are at once a consequence of scientific activity (i.e., the quest for cure and the cause of moral debate). However, at whose cost is the quest, and for whose benefit?

It would appear that if nurses are to function effectively and with regard to their emotional well-being in this complex arena of health care provision, we need to be proactive in promoting an exploration of the role that emotions play in moral decision making, examining its contribution to what we care about and why. Also needed is a commitment to a shared understanding and valuing of divergent ethical reasoning within and across professional cultures of care and research paradigms. Future research directed at exploring ways of fostering collaborative, interdisciplinary discussions about these issues and consequent ethical decision making, the outcomes of which are observed and evaluated, may provide one means of moving this difficult area of practice forward.

The complexity of caring for patients being offered phase I and II of cancer clinical trials transcends professional boundaries, and yet, until divergent perspectives brought to ethically laden contexts of care can be shared and understood by all involved, the consequences may be considerable. Seminars or discussion groups set up in practice settings, which are externally facilitated to support all involved, offer another possible avenue for growth and development. The three nurses who took part in this interview have contributed to an appreciation of the potentially painful and damaging consequences for the professionals working in an environment suffused with moral conflicts. The consequences for patients remain unknown because they are, as yet, inadequately researched.

References

1. Raines DA. Moral agency in nursing. *Nurs Forum* 1994;29(1):5–11.
2. Cox K, Avis M. Ethical and practical problems of early anti-cancer drug trials: a review of the literature. *Eur J Cancer Care* 1996;5:90–5.
3. http://cancer.med.upenn.edu/pdq_html/2/engl/203900.htlm NCI/PDQ *Patient statement*. Updated 5/95.
4. Lowy I. *Between bench and bedside: science healing and interleukin-2 in a cancer ward.* Cambridge, MA: Harvard University Press, 1996.
5. Lerner G. A *death of one's own.* New York: Simon & Schuster, 1978:168.
6. Shapiro K. *Dying and living: one man's life with cancer.* Austin, TX: University of Texas Press, 1985:9.
7. Zimmer G. An idea for modifying phase 1 clinical trials: a patient's view, cited in: Daugherty CK, Siegler M, Ratain M, Zimmer G, eds. Learning from our patients: one participant's impact on clinical trial research and informed consent. *Ann Intern Med* 1997;126(11):892–7.
8. Grady C. Ethical issues in clinical trials. *Semin Oncol Nurs* 1991;7(4):288–96.
9. Doyle D, Hanks GWC, McDonald N. *Oxford textbook of palliative medicine.* Oxford, England: Oxford University Press, 1993.
10. Allmark P. Can there be an ethics of care? *J Med Ethics* 1995;21:19–24.
11. Seedhouse D. *Ethics: the heart of health care.* Chichester, U.K.: Wiley, 1988.
12. Kuhn TS. *The structure of scientific revolutions.* Chicago: University of Chicago, 1970.
13. Pope C, Mays N. Researching the parts other methods cannot reach: an introduction to qualitative methods in health and health services research. *BMJ* 1995;311:42–5.
14. Hagell El. Nursing knowledge: women's knowledge: a sociological perspective. *J Adv Nurs* 1989;14:226–33.

15. Silverman D. Communication and medical practice. *Social relations in the clinic.* London: Sage, 1987.
16. Corner J, Plant H, Warner L. Developing a nursing approach to managing dyspnoea in lung cancer. *Int J Palliat Nurs* 1995;1(1):5–11.
17. Faithful S. "Just grin and bear it and hope that it will go away": coping with urinary symptoms from pelvic radiotherapy. *Eur J Cancer Care* 1995;4(4):158–65.
18. Preston N. New strategies for the management of malignant ascites. *Eur J Cancer Care* 1995;4(4):173–83.
19. Lanceley A. Wider issues in pain management. *Eur J Cancer Care* 1996;4(4):153–7.
20. Walby S, Greenwell J. *Medicine and nursing: professions in a changing health service.* London: Sage, 1994.
21. Stein L. The doctor-nurse game. *Arch Gen Psychol* 1967;16:699–703.
22. Svensson R. The interplay between doctors and nurses: a negotiated order perspective. *Soc Health Illness* 1996;18(3):379–98.
23. Dingwall R, McIntosh J (eds.). *Readings in the sociology of nursing.* Edinburgh: Churchill-Livingstone, 1978.
24. Grundstein-Amado R. Differences in ethical decision-making processes among nurses and doctors. *J Adv Nurs* 1992;17:129–37.
25. Erlen JA, Frost B. Nurses' perceptions of powerlessness in influencing ethical decisions making. *West J Nurs Res* 1991;13(3):397–407.
26. Gilligan C. *In a different voice: psychological theory and women's development.* Cambridge, MA: Harvard University Press, 1982.
27. Benner P, Wrubel J. *The primacy of caring: stress and coping in health and illness.* Menlo-Park: Addison-Wesley, 1988.
28. Oakley J. *Morality and the emotions.* London: Routledge, 1992.
29. Cooper MC. Principle-oriented ethics and the ethics of care: a creative tension. *Adv Nurs Sci* 1991;14(2):22–31.
30. Melia K. The task of nursing ethics. *J Med Ethics* 1994;20:7–11.
31. DeWolf M. Ethical decision making. *Sem Nurs Oncol* 1989;5:77–81.
32. Holly CM. The ethical quandaries of acute care nursing practice. *J Prof Nurs* 1993; 9:110–15.
33. Smith KV. Ethical decision making by staff nurses. *Nurs Ethics* 1996;3(1):17–25.
34. Scanlon C. Nursing ethics: Understanding the moral life. *J New York State Nurs Assoc* 1995;26(1):16–17.
35. Morse J. Qualitative nursing research: a free for all? In: Morse J, ed. *Qualitative nursing research: a contemporary dialogue.* London: Sage, 1991:14–22.
36. Glaser BG, Strauss AL. *The discovery of grounded theory.* Chicago: Aldine, 1967.
37. Jameton A. *Nursing practice: the ethical issues.* London: Prentice-Hall, 1984.
38. Jack R, Jack DC. *Moral vision and professional decisions: the changing values of women and men lawyers.* Cambridge: Cambridge University Press, 1989.
39. Oberle K, Davies B. An exploration of nursing disillusionment. *Can J Nurs Res* 1993;25(1):67–76.
40. Dunkel-Schetter C. Social support and cancer: findings based on patient interviews and their implications. *J Soc Issues* 1984;40(4):77–98.
41. Nichols K. *Psychological care in physical illness.* London: Chapman Hall, 1993.
42. Cameron M. The moral and ethical component of nurse burnout. *Nurs Manage* 1986;17(4):42b, 42d-e.
43. Swantz ML. *Milk, blood and death: transformative symbols of the Zamaro of Tanzania.* London: Bergin & Garvey, 1995.
44. Corner J. Is there a research paradigm for palliative care? *Palliat Med* 1996;10(3):201–8.

45. Reason P. Reflections on the purposes of human inquiry. *Qual Inquiry* 1996;2(1):15–28.
46. Judd D. Life-threatening illness as psychic trauma: psychotherapy with adolescent patients. In: Erskine A, Judd D, eds. *The imaginative body.* London: Whurr Publishers, 1993.
47. Morrison P. Nursing and caring: a personal construct theory study of some nurses' self-perceptions. *J Adv Nurs* 1989;14:421–6.
48. Parker RS. Nurses' stories: the search for a relational ethic of care. *Adv Nurs Sci* 1990;13(1):31–40.

44

Quality of Life: A Phenomenological Perspective on Explanation, Prediction, and Understanding in Nursing Science

Patricia Benner

Nursing is concerned with health promotion and the treatment of illness and disease. Health and illness are lived experiences and are accessed through perceptions, beliefs, skills, practices, and expectations. Illness is the human experience of dysfunction whereas disease is concerned with biochemical and neurophysiological functioning at the cell, tissue, and organ system levels.[1] The problem with being concerned with both the phenomenal world – health and illness, and the biophysiological world – disease, is that these two levels of discourse call for different kinds of explanation and prediction in the western tradition. Here the author departs from strict naturalists who hold that the ultimate level of explanation and prediction lies at the biophysiological level and that the phenomenal level is superfluous, an unnecessary trapping of human culture and language. The problem of two levels of discourse, the phenomenological level and the biophysiological level, is made more interesting by the empirical evidence that the phenomenal realms, the experiences of health and illness, are causally related to the disease and recovery processes at the cellular and tissue levels.[2]

Merleau-Ponty[3] states that no strictly bottom-up explanation – that is, explanation from the cellular level up to the lived experience of health and illness – can adequately explain or accurately predict the particular course of an illness, nor can it explain the maintenance of health. We know that laboratory data frequently do not match the illness experience. People do not die or survive strictly according to our best biochemical and physiological accounts.

Source: *Advances in Nursing Science*, 8(1) (1985): 1–14.

Furthermore, the person's understanding of his or her body and illness and experience must be taken into consideration to account for alterations in the disease process at the tissue level. These puzzles leave those who are concerned with both the phenomenal realms of health and illness and the physiological manifestations of disease dissatisfied with the Platonic and Cartesian legacy of a split between the mind and body. Cassell has alluded to the problem succinctly:

> If the mind-body dichotomy results in assigning the body to medicine, and the person is not in that category, then the only remaining place for the person is in the category of the mind. Where the mind is problematic (not identifiable in objective terms), its very reality diminishes for science, and so, too, does that of the person. Therefore, so long as the mind-body dichotomy is accepted, suffering is either subjective and not truly "real" – not within medicine's domain – or identified exclusively with bodily pain. Not only is such an identification misleading and distorting, for it depersonalizes the sick patient, but it is itself a source of suffering.[4(p640)]

The paradox of the subject/object split of Cartesian dualism is that it is either extremely subjectivizing or extremely objectifying. The self is viewed as a possession and attributes are given objectively as possessions by the subject in a purely intentional way. This view cannot take account of the historical, cultural, embodied, situated person. The self of possession[5-7] is a collection of attributes and objective traits that the self freely chooses and has ultimate control over as an autonomous subject. This view of the self overlooks the participative and constitutive side of the person's participation in a social world. The person is involved in a shared history, tradition, and social network that he or she both constitutes and is constituted by. Health and illness cannot be understood by studying a mind that possesses a list of talents, traits, and attributes, nor can they be understood by strictly studying biophysiological states. Health and illness of the person can only be understood by studying the person in context. This becomes painfully clear, for example, when patients refuse blood transfusions because they would cut patients off from God and their communities.

Dreyfus explains that the traditional problem of mind-body split comes from the Cartesian tradition of:

1. taking the self as an isolable present at hand (an objectively, self-possessed, uninvolved) entity rather than a public activity; and
2. trying to generalize a problem that arises in special cases into a problem about every case. This second move only seems possible if one forgets the shared practices, ie, passes over the phenomenon of world.[8(p11)]

In the human sciences this means that we take examples of breakdown and assume that what shows up can also account for normal functioning.

The particular problems of explanation and prediction in the phenomenal realms (health and illness) must be solved before adequate holistic explanations and predictions of prevention and recovery from disease (the biophysiological) can be developed. Covering laws or other strictly naturalistic explanatory and predictive formulas will not work for health and illness because human experience is based on participating in linguistic and cultural practices that are not reducible to context-free elements capable of being related by the kind of covering laws described by Hempel.[9] The closest approximation to similar covering laws in human behavior is rule-governed behavior (although the author argues with Dreyfus,[8] human beings are capable of orderly behavior without recourse to following formal rules). For the sake of argument, Toulmin's[10] claim that positivistic scientists have glossed over the difference between *rule-governed behavior and law-governed action* may be taken seriously.

Action and Behavior

The first mistake is to overlook the distinction between action and behavior. Behavior is purposive where the action of physical objects just describes motion trajectories. Taylor[11] points out the difference between action and behavior by noting the differences between the mere action of "raising the arm" and voting behavior. What counts as an adequate explanation of the motion or action of an arm-raising trajectory is not a satisfactory account of voting behavior. Toulmin points out:

> The essential mark of rule-conforming behavior lies in the normative force of relevant rules. An agent who recognizes that he is deviating from a rule acknowledges a claim on him to correct his behavior. By contrast if we consider natural phenomena of a purely law-governed kind, no such distinction makes sense.... Psychologists ... have played down the differences between rule-conforming and law-governed phenomena of physics and physiology.[10]

According to Taylor[11,12] and Dreyfus,[13] the rules we can expect to find in understanding health and illness are of the *ceteris paribus* kind. They will focus on sufficient conditions and make statements such as, all other things being equal, one can expect such and such to occur. Such a statement leaves room for transformations in meanings and changes in human concerns.

The analysis of variance model of interaction will not be sufficient to capture the relational quality of the person in the situation. That is, separating person variables and situational variables and then calculating their independent contribution to a singular main effect does not capture the configurational relationships inherent in the situation.[14,15] At issue is the understanding that the existence of or freedom from disease may be a necessary condition for certain behavior, but a sufficient condition would be the presence of disease together with the person's experience of the disease and the environment, which constitute together a teleological antecedent. A purely deterministic, tissue-level explanation or a purely psychological description will not suffice. The existence of the diseased organ is not the cause of the state (its sufficient condition) and therefore not the cause (the necessary condition) of the behavior either. As Taylor points out, "The widespread assumption that, because certain physiological states are *necessary* conditions of behavior, behavior must be accounted for by nonteleological physiological laws involves an illegitimate inference."[12(p25)]

Thus, any rules of behavior in explaining health and illness will be teleological or goal oriented in their nature. We cannot expect the same kind of deterministic laws found in nonteleological explanations and predictions of natural science. According to Taylor, such teleological laws will not be able to meet the assumptions of atomism that demand that the two terms, linked in a law, be identifiable separately from each other. Atomism is based on the

> notion that the ultimate evidence for any laws we frame about the world is in the form of discrete units of information, each of which could be as it is even if all others were different, i.e., each of which is separably identifiable from its connections with any of the others.[12(p11)]

Teleological laws are going to be transactional because the self both constitutes and is constituted by situation, language, culture, and history. Taylor says:

> In this way, teleological explanation is, as has often been remarked, connected with some form of holism, or anti-atomistic doctrine.... Whether the stringent atomist requirement can be met by all valid laws, then, is itself an empirical question, which hinges partly on the question whether all teleological explanation – or any other type of explanation which involves holist assumptions – can be done away with. It cannot be decided by epistemological fiat, by a rule to the effect that the evidence for teleological laws must be such that it can be stated by means of nonteleological laws.[12(pp11–15)]

Such an epistemological fiat amounts to "methodolatry." Teleological explanations require the systematic inclusion of meanings and self-interpretations in the study of health, illness, and suffering. Meanings are not relegated to philosophical inquiry[16] but become legitimate aspects for empirical study. As Wolf has observed in medicine:

> The plain fact is that many of the manifestations of the integrative processes in the brain that govern visceral and general behavior of human beings cannot be reduced to numbers: faith and optimism, on the one hand, or surrender and depression on the other, are such processes. Moreover, neither measurements nor numbers will help one to understand the tangible effects of placebos or of confidence in a doctor. Thus, the intensity of

crucially important attitudes, values, and expectations cannot be gauged by the quantity of even the character of a stimulus, but depend on who is involved and in what context.

The recent neglect of descriptive behavioral studies of individual human beings may have resulted in part from an understandable preoccupation with and fascination by increasingly sophisticated technology, but perhaps more important have been an unwarrantedly exclusive concern with quantitation and an unnecessary diffidence in approaching problems of replication, verification, and observer bias.... In medicine, we are just beginning to learn to relegate our preoccupation with quantitation to its proper place and to also ask configurational questions in more than one dimension.[14(pp5,7–8)]

Phenomenology

Pragmatic activity, human concerns, and meanings call for investigative strategies that do not require the kind of decontextualization of strict operationalism. Systematic strategies of study that can be verified or falsified by others and that capture relational and configurational patterns are required. Hermeneutics is one such strategy.[17–21]

Hermeneutics, which allows for the study of the person in the situation, offers a way of studying the phenomenal realms of health and illness, and overcomes the problems of extreme subjectivity or objectivity. Hermeneutics has been used to understand everyday practices, meanings, and knowledge embedded in skills, stress, and coping.[19,20] Hermeneutics assumes that the study of pragmatic activity, that is, everyday understanding and practices, and the study of relational issues are distinctly different from the study of objects or even biophysiological events on the tissue and cellular level.

Hermeneutics stems from the systematic study of texts and was originally developed as a tool of biblical exegesis, jurisprudence, and more recently, historical research and literary criticism. The particular kind of hermeneutics the author has used is congruent with a particular theoretical stance (Heideggerian phenomenology) taken toward human beings and human experience.[8,18] Three essential tenets of this phenomenology are: (1) human beings are self-interpreting. Their interpretations are not just possessions of the self; they are constitutive of the self; (2) furthermore, to be a human being means that the kind of being is an issue, that is, the person takes a stand on the kind of being he or she is. Finally, (3) the self is not a radically free arbiter of meaning. Though the meanings available to the individual can undergo transformations, they are limited by a particular language, culture, and history. No higher court for the individual exists than meanings or self-interpretations embedded in language, skills, and practices. No laws, structures, or mechanisms offer higher explanatory principles or greater predictive power than self-interpretations in the form of common meanings, personal concerns, and cultural practices shaped by a particular history. The goal is to understand everyday practices and the experiences of health and illness.[19-21]

Heideggerian phenomenology offers a critique and an alternative to a strictly cost-benefit approach to the study of quality of life wherein benefit is defined primarily in economic or mastery terms. Quality of life can be approached from the perspective of quality of being, and does not need to be approached merely from the perspective of doing and achieving. Such a perspective is highly relational and requires research strategies that uncover meaning and relational qualities.

The kind of hermeneutics described here has its roots in Division I of Heidegger's work.[17] Others who use this kind of hermeneutics are Taylor,[11] Kuhn,[22] Geertz,[23] and Garfinkel.[24] The goal is to find exemplars or paradigm cases that embody the meanings of everyday practices. The data are participant observations, field notes, interviews, and unobtrusive samples of behavior and interaction in natural settings. Human behavior is treated as a text analogue and the task is to uncover the meanings in everyday practice in such a way that they are not destroyed, distorted, decontextualized, trivialized, or sentimentalized.[25] When the interpreter has done a good job, participants can recognize and validate the interpretation. Participants will be somewhat annoyed or pleased that the interpreter has given a meaningful account of their experience. This is not a hermeneutics of suspicion, used by Marx or Freud or the mid-career-Heidegger, where the goal is to discover some latent causal explanation in theoretical or power terms, such as class struggle, Oedipal complex, dependency needs, or anxiety over ungroundedness, but to accurately portray lived meanings in their own terms.[26]

This method is particularly useful for understanding the phenomenal world of health and illness. It provides an appropriate access to increasing the understanding of disease as it is shaped by experiences of health and illness. It is not a mentalistic view of disease; therefore it is not a subjectivistic or completely relativistic view.[27,28] For example, this view holds that the pathology of diabetes exists irrespective of self-understanding and even before the scientific discovery of the dysfunction. But once the scientific explanation exists and is transmitted culturally, the illness experience is transformed and impacts the disease itself. It is known that psychological stress, even in the form of "fear of diabetic coma," can increase the need for insulin. The person's illness experience both constitutes and is constituted by disease. To try to determine the relative contribution of "uninterpreted disease" and "the cultural interpretation of the disease" to the illness experience is to ignore the constitutive relationship.

Hermeneutic phenomenology is holistic in that it seeks to study the person in the situation, rather than isolating person variables and situation variables and then trying to put them back together.[15] The explanations are teleological and include intentional causality but are not limited to a mentalistic view of pure intentionality. This view allows the explanation of disease through practice and history without having to embrace a purely intentionalistic explanation that would, for example, allocate unconscious responsibility for choosing the site of one's cancer through internal and unconscious conflicts ("unconscious intent").

Underlying all interpretation-laden practices and self-understanding that are handed down through language and culture is the notion of "the background." The full-blown notion of background preunderstanding is one of the major distinctions between Heideggerian phenomenology and Husserlian transcendental phenomenology. It is this background that individuals cannot make fully explicit and cannot get completely clear about or clear of; it gives individuals the conditions of their possibility and the conditions for their perceptions, for their actions, and so forth. It is this background that makes human beings different from the artificial intelligence of the computer that always has to build its story up element by element, whereas human beings always come to a situation with a story, a preunderstanding. This position assumes that background meanings, skills, and practices are not completely rationalizable (cannot be made completely explicit), that this background forms the conditions of possibility, and that the background is handed down and not individually derived. Therefore, this position breaks with the tradition of methodological individualism. In fact, the meaning-giving subject is no longer the unit of analysis. Meaning resides not solely within the individual nor solely within the situation but is a transaction between the two so that the individual both constitutes and is constituted by the situation. Therefore, the unit of analysis is the transaction. This position, however, expects not only the unique or idiosyncratic but commonalities and recurring similarities and differences as well. However, unlike rational empiricism, hermeneutics does not look for these recurring similarities and differences in laws, mechanisms, structures, and processes or even in values that are unrelated to meaning. In this view, meaning is expressive and constitutive as well as designative and denotative.[29]

To review, methodological individualism is avoided by finding commonality and therefore teleological explanation and prediction based on background skills, meanings, and practices shared in a people with a common history and common situations.[8] This position abandons two assumptions of naturalism pointed out by Taylor.[29] The first position is that meaning can be seen in terms of representation of an independent reality (based on the 17th century philosophers, Hobbes and Locke). This is particularly a problem in studying highly skilled performance, pragmatic activities, and human concerns because all of these human activities and capacities are highly relational. The differential attention paid to aspects of the situation varies with the situation in ways that cannot be quantified. Moreover, many of the aspects that are recognized cannot be reduced to mental representations. They are based on perceptual recognitional abilities that Polanyi calls connoisseurship and the author terms graded qualitative distinctions.[19] One strategy for attending to meaningful distinctions in a situation is to reduce the distinctions to an array of patterns, with each pattern signifying a different meaning. This is a decided advance over identifying one variable at a time but cannot cope with the variability and nuances in shifting importance and rapidly changing relevance that can be recognized by human beings in a situation. The mental representation theory is analogous to matching templates on situations, but such an approach is slow and not as skilled as the experienced person who, without knowing the particulars or the reasons, attends to subtle differences in patterns and subtle shifts in relative importance of presenting issues.

The second assumption of naturalism (rational empiricism) that hermeneutic phenomenology questions is that theory can be generated from the standpoint of a monological observer who stands outside the situation and has private meanings that are then tested or matched with public activities.[19] The model of the person (both researcher and participant) in hermeneutic phenomenology does not expect that the person can ever gain a privileged transcendental position. Dreyfus made the point that "There can be no stable science of an entity which as meaning giver is the condition of its own objectification. No science can objectify the skills which make it possible. But this only shows we should abandon the Kantian definition of man."[13(p15)] Dreyfus goes on to note:

> According to Foucault the human sciences involve a unique human self-interpretation, which reaches its fullest expression in Kant. They interpret their domain of investigation, man, as a transcendental/empirical double – a meaning giver who constitutes the world and determines what counts as objects, and yet is an object in the world like any other. This conception of man makes human self-interpretation essential to an understanding of human beings while at the same time stipulating that human beings are meaningless objects amenable to the sort of theory characteristic of the natural sciences.[13(p4)]

Dreyfus[13] points out that this "double aspect theory," ie, the attempt to explain human activity from a totally physicalistic language and the attempt to provide a totally intentionalistic account, ensures that the sciences of man would always be "abnormal" (Kuhn's[30] term for science with competing paradigms). Two schools of thought – one interpretive and one materialistic – would perpetually compete with each other, each with an exclusive and conflicting vocabulary that could not accommodate the explanatory vocabulary of the other.

Heideggerian phenomenology overcomes the problems inherent in the Cartesian "transcendental/empirical double," or subject-object split, by starting with a different notion of the person. The person is studied in the situation and pragmatic involved activity is considered as a way of knowing and being. Dreyfus has called this "embodied intelligence."[31] Self-interpretations based on skills and practices and preunderstanding govern health and illness experiences and influence physiological functioning.

Dreyfus argues, and the author's observation of expert nurses illustrates,[19] that in studying pragmatic activities and human concerns, an approach to theorizing that is dependent on identifying decontextualized features *by definition* leaves out the meaning of the situation or situational understanding. As Dreyfus states: "The meaning of the situation plays an essential role in determining what counts as an event, and it is precisely this contextualized meaning that theory must ignore."[13(p11)] People have direct access to meaningful situations by virtue of education and experience. For example, nurses are trained to approach and interpret situations differently from physicians. Nurses approach clinical situations with a working knowledge of physiology and medicine but also with a knowledge about particular physicians' clinical skills, how available they typically are, and what their typical responses are likely to be. This situational understanding about the physician is augmented by an understanding of the particular patient and his or her typical response patterns in one situation, and even the clinical skill likely to be available on the next shift. Once situational contextual knowledge is spelled out, it becomes clearer why a purely structural account is unsatisfactory. This problem of describing human pragmatic activity with structuralism is illustrated in Bourdieu's criticism of Levi-Strauss's formal structural theoretical account of gift giving:

> It is all a question of style, which means in this case timing and choice of occasion, for the same act – giving, giving in return, offering one's services, paying a visit, etc. – can have completely different meanings at different times.[32(pp5–6)]

It is possible to make a similar comparison about the meaning of a bed bath.[33] The list of decontextualized functions and features of a bed bath could be endless. However, with understanding of the situation, one can judge whether the bed bath is an unnecessary fostering of dependence, an essential tool for making a thorough yet unobtrusive assessment, a means of communicating with a withdrawn patient, or something else. In this case, theoretical access is not more elegant or more efficient than practical expert understanding of the situation. Clinical know-how has been trivialized by the thought that it could completely be captured by formal statements just as the experiences of health, illness, and suffering have been trivialized by analytically separating the mind and body.

Interpretive Research Strategies

Hermeneutics is a systematic approach to interpreting a text. Interview material and observations are turned into text through transcription. The interpretation entails a systematic analysis of the whole text, a systematic analysis of parts of the text, and a comparison of the two interpretations for conflicts and for understanding the whole in relation to the parts, and vice versa. Whole cases can be compared to other whole cases. Usually, this shifting back and forth between the parts and the whole reveals new themes, new issues, and new questions that are generated in the process of understanding the text itself.

The participant offers a depiction of the lived experience and the interpreter seeks commonalities in meanings, situations, practices, and bodily experiences. Interpreters use their distance and perspectives to understand the immediacy of the lived situation but these experience-distant perspectives must take into account the person *in* the situation. The interpreter enters into a dialogue with the text. For example, in proposing a clinical ethnography of an illness trajectory, the author has recommended that the interpreter consider the following experience-distant perspectives as possible starting points for interpretation: (1) the changing experience of the body; (2) changing social relationships as a result of the illness; (3) changing demands and tasks of different stages in the disease process and illness trajectory; (4) predictable responses and effective coping strategies for treatment side effects and sequelae; and (5) the particular – what the illness interrupts, threatens, and means to the individual.[21] Such predictable sources of commonality provide a starting point for the interpretation, but they do not set limits on what can be discovered in the process of allowing the test itself to make claims and raise issues with the interpreter. Three strategies – paradigm cases, exemplars, and thematic analysis – are useful for allowing the particular claims of the text to stand out and for presenting configurational and transactional relationships.

Paradigm Cases

A whole case may stand out as a paradigm case, a strong instance of a particular pattern of meanings. Such a case is a "marker" so that once a paradigm case is recognized because of its particular clarity or vividness, other more subtle cases with similar global characteristics can be recognized.

Paradigm cases are useful as a recognitional strategy because early in the interpretive effort the interpreter may recognize only that this case is a strong instance of a particular relationship or meaning but may not be able to articulate *why* the case stands out or *what it depicts.* Through asking questions such as: Similar in what respect or different in what respect? How does this case stand out in relation to other cases?, the interpreter is able to put into words what this case is depicting. Paradigm cases are also useful as presentation strategies because the pattern of meanings and concerns depicted by the case often cannot be broken down into small units without losing important aspects of the patterns.

Exemplars

Exemplars are also useful as recognitional tools *and* presentation strategies. An exemplar is smaller than a paradigm case, but like a paradigm case is a strong instance of a particularly meaningful transaction, intention, or capacity. An exemplar is a vignette or story of the particular transaction that captures the meaning in the situation so that the reader is able to recognize the same meaningful transaction in another situation where the objective characteristics might be quite different. Both exemplars and paradigm cases are presentation strategies that allow the depiction of the person *in* the situation. They present the context, the intentions of the actors, and the meanings in the situation.

Thematic Analysis

A third interpretive strategy is that of thematic analysis. The interpreter identifies common themes in the interviews and extracts sufficient interview excerpts to present evidence to the reader of the theme. A thematic analysis is useful for presenting common meanings. In all three presentation strategies, sufficient interview documentation is provided to allow the reader to participate in the validation of the findings.

All three interpretive strategies (paradigm cases, exemplars, and thematic analysis) work both as discovery and presentation strategies. They all allow for the presentation of context and meanings. In interpretive research, unlike grounded theory,[34,35] the goal is not to extract theoretical terms or concepts at a higher level of abstraction. The goal is to discover meaning terms and to achieve understanding. If attempts are made to decontextualize the meaning, then the phenomenon is changed or rendered meaningless. This is the same point that Kuhn makes about the practical knowledge of the natural scientist that resides in shared exemplars and not strictly in rules and procedures. He writes:

> When I speak of knowledge embedded in shared exemplars, I am not referring to a model of knowing that is less systematic or less analyzable than knowledge embedded in rules, laws, or criteria of identification. Instead, I have in mind a manner of knowing which is misconstrued if reconstructed in terms of rules that are first abstracted from exemplars and thereafter function in their stead.[30(p192)]

The discovery of paradigm cases, exemplars, and recurring themes can be systematically and rigorously validated by experts and by those who are living out the practical knowledge and meanings presented in these interpretive strategies. However, if the method of validation requires decontextualization, as in operationalism, then the relational issues, that is, the concerns, meanings, and practical knowledge conveyed by presenting the person in context, will be lost. The experiences of health, illness, and suffering are trivialized by analytically separating the mind and body, and by using research strategies that systematically exclude the lived meanings of these experiences.

Bias Control Strategies

Multiple stages of interpretation allow for bias control by exposing contradictions, conflicts, or surprises that cannot be accounted for by an earlier or later interpretation. Actions and practices may not necessarily be rational, but it is assumed that they will have understandable, meaningful patterns. Multiple interviews with the same participants also provide a bias contol strategy inasmuch as they allow patterns to emerge and prevent the interpreter from emphasizing a nonrecurring, idiosyncratic episode, statement, or behavior. Redundancy provides confidence in the interpretation. The interpreter attempts to be "true" to the text and not read in meanings that are not supported by textual evidence. Expert consensual validation is sought for at least a subset of the data to guard against the importation of meanings not actually supported by the text. The assumption is that the interpretations offered are based on shared cultural meanings and are therefore recognizable by other readers who share the same culture. This is congruent with the Heideggerian assumption that the meaning and organization of a culture precedes individual meaning-giving activity.[17]

The goal of this kind of commentary is to make the commonplace visible and understood. In achieving this goal, the interpreter has the same problem as the anthropologist who returns home. The anthropologist at home runs the risk of overlooking key meanings, not because they are so esoteric or uncommon, but rather because they are so pervasive.[17] The reader of the interpretation actively participates in the validation process. The reader should approach interpretive works with the following five criteria of internal validity outlined by Cherniss:

> First, they should help us to understand the lives of the subjects; we should better comprehend the complex pattern of human experience as a result of these. Second, the themes should maintain the integrity of the original "data." Third, the interpretations should be internally consistent. Fourth, data that support the findings should be presented. Usually, these data will take the form of excerpts from interviews. Finally, the reported conclusions should be consistent with the reader's own experience. In qualitative research, the readers must critically scrutinize the results of the thematic analysis, playing a more active role in the process of "validation" than they normally would.[36(pp278-279)]

Cherniss's third point on internal consistency should not be misconstrued to mean that the interpretation should reveal only internally consistent practices and commitments by participants. Conflicting, inconsistent practices and commitments are common and are often what is uncovered in doing the interpretation. Interpretations are considered internally consistent if the textual data presented match the interpretations offered.

The author is enough of a pragmatist to believe that the final proof of the hermeneutic phenomenology position lies in the knowledge it uncovers. We have to ask what our theory and method screens allow us to see. Do theories lend themselves best to a chart audit to determine the completeness of records, or do they tell the clinician how to promote healing and wellness and understand illness and suffering to promote comfort and cure? Do theories allow for mere categorization of information or do they provide guidelines for interpreting the information? Are predictions so deterministic that they overlook human possibilities, change, and growth?

Science at this point needs to return individuals to the things themselves, the experience of health, illness, suffering, and the wisdom and ignorance embedded in practice. There must be a return to the systematic study of practice and of health, illness, and suffering.[21] The study of practice should offer more than a sociological description of role relationships. The goal should be to find out the wisdom, frustration, puzzles, dilemmas, and knowledge embedded in practice. The study of health and illness should offer a new understanding of the lived body in health and illness. The hermeneutics of early Heidegger offers a promising methodological approach.[17]

The author is not a single paradigm expectant scientist,[26,37] because a single paradigm in the human sciences claims that one single perspective provides the *one* explanatory vantage point and that all other paradigms are inferior or subordinate. One paradigm would provide a totalitarian explanatory system for all human behavior and would assume one privileged position exists from which to view situations, capacities, and problems of human beings. Such a singular paradigm works in the natural sciences because the background practices, skills, and assumptions of the scientists are not issues for them. Decontextualizing practices can be ignored after standardization because the natural scientist searches for objectified and decontextualized elements that can be related by strict laws.[13] But as Dreyfus and Rabinow point out:

> If the human sciences claim to study human activities, then the human sciences, unlike the natural sciences, must take account of those human activities which make possible their own disciplines.
>
> Thus, while in the natural sciences it is always possible and generally desirable that an unchallenged normal science which defines and resolves problems concerning the structure of the physical universe establish itself, in the social sciences such an unchallenged normal science would only indicate that an orthodoxy had established itself, not through scientific achievement, but by ignoring the background and eliminating all competitors.[26(pp163–164)]

Such a totalitarian stance is not only unattractive; it simply does not offer much in the way of explanation, prediction, and understanding because the theories in human sciences must always presuppose common background meanings and practices. For example, Taylor[11] points out that objective political science is dependent on cultural practices that are not immutable but subject to change in a constitutive way. Political theory in an individual-based contract society such as the United States will not work on a background of different cultural interpretations such as the Japanese cultural background of consensus and group orientation. The scientist is always in a culture and cannot completely step outside the particular historical understanding available during his or her period. There can be no value-free or interpretation-free data language. Consequently, deterministic monological theoretical schemes will necessarily be time bound and limited in their predictive and explanatory power. Such deterministic theoretical schemes are a part of the cultural press for extreme rationalization and objectification. Weber,[38] Adorno,[39] Foucault,[40] and Dreyfus and Rabinow[26] have been concerned with this pervasive press for rationalization in the western tradition.

Certainly the strain of objectification is felt in the study of health, illness, suffering, and disease. The very labeling and technologizing of symptoms add to the stress of the "target population" at "high risk."[41] Discovering that one is in a high-risk group increases the risk. But coming to view oneself as a collection of needs, wants, and health risks that must be scientifically met creates a stressful, effortful life style based on the premises of control and balance.[20] Such a formula works well until the limits of control are confronted, which for the person experiencing illness or suffering is frequent.[20] As a nurse scientist, the author does not want to increase the rationalization and objectification of the notion of health and the experience of illness and suffering by the formal models and methods used to study individuals.

Extreme objectification and subjectification cannot capture the lived experiences of health and illness because human beings are never fully object or fully subject; they exist in a network of concerns and relations. If the way of doing science objectifies or oversubjectifies (in the sense of making the health-illness experience an extremely private, idiosyncratic one), then those individuals using these approaches will unwittingly contribute to the stress-related diseases so prevalent in today's society, do little to treat illness and disease, and finally blunt the ability to alleviate suffering. Heideggerian phenomenology generates forms of explanation and prediction that offer understanding and choice, rather than manipulation and control. Nursing requires access to concrete problems and dilemmas associated with health, illness, suffering, and disease and an understanding of the power of human practices, skills, and relationships that engender hope and promote healing.

References

1. Kleinman A, Eisenberg L, Good B: Culture, illness, and care: Clinical lessons from anthropologic and cross-cultural research. *Ann Intern Med* 1978;88:251–258.
2. West JW, Stein MS (eds): *Critical Issues in Behavioral Medicine.* Philadelphia, Lippincott, 1982.
3. Merleau-Ponty M: *Phenomenology of Perception.* London, Routledge and Kegan Paul, 1962.
4. Cassell EJ: The nature of suffering and the goals of medicine. *N Engl J Med* 1982;30: 639–645.
5. Sandel M: *Liberalism and the Limits of Justice.* London, Cambridge Univ. Press, 1982.
6. Gilligan C: *In a Different Voice.* Cambridge, Mass, Harvard Univ. Press, 1982.

7. Yankelovich D: *New Rules in American Life: Searching for Self-Fulfillment in a World Turned Upside Down.* New York, Random House, 1981.

8. Dreyfus HL: *Being-in-the-World: A Commentary on Division I of Being and Time.* Cambridge, Mass, MIT Press, to be published.

9. Hempel C: *Aspects of Scientific Explanation.* New York, The Free Press, 1965.

10. Toulmin S: Concepts and the explanation of human behavior, in Mischel S (ed): *Human Action.* New York, Academic Press, 1969, pp 87–88.

11. Taylor C: Interpretation and the sciences of man, in Rabinow P, Sullivan M (eds): *Interpretive Social Science.* Berkeley, University of California Press, 1979.

12. Taylor C: *Explanation of Behavior.* New York, Humanities Press, 1964.

13. Dreyfus HL: Why the study of human capacities can never be scientific. *Berkeley Cognitive Science Report*, no. 11. Berkeley, University of California, Cognitive Science Program, Institute of Human Learning, 1984.

14. Wolf S: Introduction: The role of the brain in bodily disease, in Werner H, Hoger MA, Strunkard AJ (eds): *Brain, Behavior, and Bodily Disease.* New York, Raven Press, 1981, pp 1–9.

15. Lazarus RS, Launier R: Stress-related transactions between person and environment, in Pervin L, Lewis M (eds): *Perspectives in Interactional Psychology.* New York, Plenum Press, 1978, pp 287–327.

16. Weisman A: *Coping with Cancer.* New York, McGraw-Hill, 1979.

17. Heidegger M: *Being and Time*, Macquarrie J, Robinson E (trans). New York, Harper & Row, 1962.

18. Heidegger M: *The Basic Problems of Phenomenology*, Hofstadter A (trans). Bloomington, Ind, Indiana Univ. Press, 1982.

19. Benner P: *From Novice to Expert: Excellence and Power in Clinical Nursing Practice.* Menlo Park, Calif, Addison-Wesley, 1984.

20. Benner, P: *Stress and Satisfaction on the Job: Work Meanings and Coping of Mid-Career Men.* New York, Praeger Scientific Press, 1984.

21. Benner P: The oncology clinical nurse specialist as expert coach. *Oncology Nurse Forum* 1985;12(2):40–44.

22. Kuhn TS: *The Essential Tension.* Chicago, University of Chicago Press, 1977.

23. Geertz C: *The Interpretation of Cultures.* New York, Harper & Row, 1973.

24. Garfinkel H: *Studies in Ethnomethodology.* Englewood Cliffs, NJ, Prentice-Hall, 1967.

25. Lazarus RS: The trivialization of distress, in Rosen JC, Solomon LJ (eds): *Vermont Conference on the Primary Prevention of Psychopathology*, vol. 8. Hanover, NH, University Press of New England, to be published.

26. Dreyfus HL, Rabinow P: *Michel Foucault Beyond Structuralism and Hermeneutics.* Chicago, The University of Chicago Press, 1982.

27. Bernstein R: *Beyond Objectivism and Relativism: Science, Hermeneutics, and Praxis.* Philadelphia, University of Pennsylvania Press, 1983.

28. Palmer RE: *Hermeneutics.* Evanston, Northwestern Univ. Press, 1969.

29. Taylor C: *Dawes Hicks Lecture, Theories of Meaning, Proceedings of the British Academy*, London, British Academy, 1982, pp 283–327.

30. Kuhn TS: *The Structure of Scientific Revolutions*, ed 2, enlarged. Chicago, The University of Chicago Press, 1970.

31. Dreyfus HL: *What Computers Can't Do.* New York, Harper & Row, 1979.

32. Bourdieu P: *Outline of a Theory of Practice.* Cambridge, Cambridge Univ. Press, 1977.

33. Benner P: Issues in competence based testing. *Nurs Outlook* 1982;30:303–309.

34. Glaser BG, Strauss AL: *The Discovery of Grounded Theory.* Chicago, Atherton Press, 1967.

35. Glaser BG: *Theoretical Sensitivity.* Mill Valley, Calif, The Sociology Press, 1978.

36. Cherniss C: *Professional Burnout in Human Services Organizations.* New York, Praeger, 1980.

37. Rabinow P, Sullivan WM (eds): Introduction, The interpretive turn: Emergence of an approach, in *Interpretive Social Science*. Berkeley, University of California Press, 1979.

38. Weber M: *The Protestant Ethic and the Spirit of Capitalism*. New York, Scribner, 1958.

39. Adorno T: *Against Epistemology*, Domingo W (trans). Cambridge, Mass, MIT Press, 1983.

40. Foucault M: *Madness and Civilization: A History of Insanity in the Age of Reason*. Howard R (trans). New York, Random House, 1973.

41. Horowitz MJ, Dimon N, Holden M, et al: Stressful impact of news of risk for premature heart disease. *Psychosom Med* 1983;45(1):31–40.

45

Phenomenologies as Research Methodologies for Nursing: From Philosophy to Researching Practice

Jocalyn Lawler

Introduction

The purpose of this paper is to examine ways in which phenomenologies have been used as means of conducting research in nursing. The term 'phenomenologies' is used in the lower case form and in the plural sense because I am not concerned here with singling out any particular variation of phenomenology. The discussion is aimed at a more general critique of the issues that concern nursing's understanding of human being, human existence and the life world as it pertains to human(e) encounters in practice. The points of anchorage for this paper are: my readings of the different literatures; teaching research to graduate nursing students and examining and supervising higher degree work; and my own struggles to come to terms with difficult material, both in nursing and phenomenologies.

By drawing on my own direct experiences and my being, including my being-a-nurse, and my being-a-researcher, I want to position myself and my thoughts more directly with other scholars and with the materials that are available to me as a researcher and a person who thinks about nursing. I do not want to rely solely on the works and words of others but also to acknowledge my own direct experience as having a bearing on how we can work as researchers. In doing so, however, I am conscious that this is both risky and potentially problematic. I am reminded, for example, of the experience of Mykhalovskiy,[1] who in

Source: *Nursing Inquiry*, 5(2) (1998): 104–111.

writing about his attempts to understand the nature of masculinity, being a man and growing up male, was judged unsuitable as a candidate for a graduate programme in sociology on the grounds that, in writing about himself – and writing in the first person – he was guilty of intellectual self-indulgence. I am not attempting therefore to be self-indulgent; rather, my intention is to raise questions about issues of central importance to nursing's use of phenomenologies for research purposes.

Nursing and Its Research Project

I would like to begin with a 'true' story – in so far as such things exist. I once worked with a surgeon who believed, on the basis of his long experience, that while it was possible to make things waterproof, foolproof, and idiotproof, there was nothing that could be made nurseproof. For this man, nurses had an amazing and, at times, bewildering and frustrating capacity to re-invent, subvert, and investigate almost anything, particularly if it was a dressing or an elaborate and imaginative way of treating and covering a wound. In his view, the more he tried to keep nurses out of things, the more determined they were to keep under the dressing and inspect, at first hand, that which he sought to keep covered.

In many respects, nurses have undertaken similar things in their approach to research, particularly with phenomenologies and other interpretive approaches, which draw from existential philosophies, and in which the design characteristics are not so tightly prescribed or predetermined by hypotheses, sample size and the need to establish control. Just as they have sought to have direct first hand contact with the things they seek to understand in their practice, so too nurses as researchers have not always paid due regard to what might be considered sacrosanct or methodologically pure.

In their research, particularly in clinical settings, nurses are sometimes required to invent methodology and design in order to manage unexpected events or issues on which the textbooks are silent or unhelpful and this has created a number of difficulties. Some of these nurse researchers have shown considerable insight into what they are doing and the discipline is richer for it;[2,3] however, such reporting is not the norm and if many others have had such insights they have remained silent on how (or if) they chose to deal with these issues. Because they have not reported the means by which the gap between philosophically related theory and research practice is resolved, we fail to add to our understanding of the methodological imperatives of investigating nursing – as a distinct research field of inquiry.

There has been relatively more research literature in which the outcomes of phenomenological projects are reported than discussions of the methodological appropriateness – as distinct from the philosophical appropriateness – of such approaches for nursing research. This represents a significant gap in our understanding of how to inquire into nursing and what the methodological demands of nursing are or may be.

Nurse researchers have taken on phenomenologies and other interpretive and interactive research approaches with great enthusiasm; and that enthusiasm has contributed to a number of problems. In a recent article, Thorne has raised concerns about the extent to which there has been a 'slippage from the original objectives of the qualitative research enterprise' such that they are re-casting their studies in some form of pseudo-objective version of reality.[4] She makes a distinction between the need for the researcher to adopt a phenomenological attitude toward the other, and the simultaneous purpose of deriving phenomenological knowledge. Another, more serious, issue that inheres in the fashionableness of phenomenologies is that enthusiasm can overshadow the need for a more circumspect and judicious approach to choosing the most appropriate method for particular questions.

Curiously, there has been very little discussion among nurses about why interpretive/qualitative approaches have been embraced so enthusiastically and on such a large scale. Rather, debates have focused attention on the perceived relative merits, and differences between, quantitative and qualitative research. The more fundamental question that has not been addressed is the appropriateness, *with direct reference to nursing's knowledge base(s) and in the interests of nursing scholarship*, of choosing one particular methodology over another. This is a debate that goes to the heart of what kind of discipline we want nursing to be and to become and what assumptions we make about foundations of nursing knowledge and practice.

One of the more enduring misconceptions about nursing's research endeavours, which results from the choice of qualitative, interpretive, non-numerical work, is the view that, as a group, we are not up to the 'real' thing, that is, experimental, positivist research, or that we are not seriously committed to the academic enterprise. What is not widely understood among nurses and non-nurses alike, is why we should embrace these approaches. This argument gets more complicated in cases where nurses' research focuses on issues that are taboo or which people do not want investigated for socially sensitive reasons.[5]

What is still not well understood is that those who are working in more interactive research modes are not necessarily seeking definitive answers to questions, such as the cause(s) of disease; nor are they seeking to reduce levels of uncertainty and unpredictability about arriving at a diagnosis; nor are they concerned about producing more cost-effective and quantifiable indicators of health care, although such questions need to be pursued. Researchers working with interpretive methodologies are asking different questions and seeking to know the world differently. At its most simplistic level, it is not always understood that nursing, as a discipline concerned with health, illness and medicine, differs from other health groups in relation to the kinds of knowledges on which it relies and which both inform and are drawn from practice; and nursing differs in many respects in relation to its philosophical roots and disciplinary interests. Nursing research reflects these different concerns and points of emphasis. Consequently, a nursing research project will differ in important respects from other health disciplines and it will differ in relation to its cultural context.[6]

Nurse researchers, among other things, seek to understand the experience of uncertainty for its own sake – not to control uncertainty, but to find ways to live (be-as-a-person) with it. Nor are nurse researchers necessarily seeking definitive outcomes, but a kind of shared and deep understanding of what being human and being ill is like for people. And unless nurses know what meanings people attach to the events that disrupt their lives, nurses – as practitioners and people – have a restricted capacity to help their patients or find ways to deal with their own experiences as practitioners.

It is both logical and understandable therefore that nurses turn to methodologies that help to focus on what it is to be human. One of the ironies is that in making this particular choice of methodology, nursing research can be seen as a 'soft' option; but even a half-serious attempt to come to grips with Heidegger's *Being and Time*,[7] for example, would disabuse one of the view that interpretive approaches to understanding the world are easy. Moreover, making sense of a data set that consists of thousands of words of relatively unstructured text is complex, difficult, and often uncharted. In attempting to understand phenomenologies, and indeed nursing, researchers are attempting to understand life as humans live it, find meaning in it, and as we struggle to understand things that can seem to be beyond human comprehension.

When I search for a way to understand why nurses have chosen particular methodologies and approaches to research, there are three issues that stand out. The first is that nursing knowledges, practice and research encompass a very wide range of subject matter; the second – and it is a direct consequence of the first – is that there is no single research paradigm that suits all of the things which are of concern to nursing. Perhaps this is because:

> In practice [nurses] have to span a staggering array of things – the physical and existential concerns of the people around us (patients/clients, relatives, other professionals, nursing colleagues); the unpredicted and the unpredictable; the bodies of people and the problems of living in bodies which do not work properly – much of which is done under less than ideal conditions.
>
> At the academic level, where the discipline is supposed to be articulated and extended for posterity, we face a similarly staggering array of concerns – straddling multiple paradigms and methodologies; diverse and rapidly expanding knowledge bases; and research questions which may have no established trails to guide us (p. 18).[8]

The third issue is that the methodologies nursing has adopted were not necessarily designed to deal with people who are ill and outside their normal contexts and surroundings. A compounding problematic for nursing research is that most of nursing's research and educational literature is biased in favour of works that originate in the USA or that are controlled by publishing interests based there.[6] Such literature has a unique kind of intellectual and scholarly tradition that differs in important respects from what is emerging elsewhere around the globe and this is important for emergent patterns of nursing scholarship and research internationally.

This bias towards the USA creates three major problems for nursing research. First, what is typical of the USA is seen to be typical of nursing generally – an issue which is clear in Crotty's recent text, *Phenomenology and Nursing Research*.[9] Second, works sourced in the USA generally reflect the ethnocentricity of their culture and scholarship as well as the economic imperatives facing their health-care systems.[6] The third point is that other views and voices are marginalised or not heard because they are swamped by the weight of works that reflect American interests.

The intellectual climate of the USA, which typifies their cultural and social mores and history, is also said to have produced a different kind of phenomenology. This is the centrepiece of Crotty's critique of nurses' use of phenomenology in which he argues that nurses have constructed a rather restricted and misguided form of phenomenology.[9] However, because of their capacity to saturate the literature worldwide, the American style of phenomenological research can be (mis)taken as the norm in nursing; and Crotty's critique fails to take account of this.[9] There also is a kind of methodological fundamentalism in much of this interpretive research, including that which is based on phenomenologies, that gives the impression that it is more important to follow the 'right' steps than it is to grasp the theoretical importance and insights that inhere in a particular data set or data gathering experience.

This fundamentalist approach to methodology leads to an emphasis on process rather than the exciting possibilities that can flow from the data. This is an important issue if one takes the view that projects based on the gathering of (relatively) unstructured data or that concern the uncertainties of other people's lives can demand less formal(ised) approaches to the way in which they are reported. Yet there exists a tendency for nursing works (and other works dealing with human experience) to be 'forced' into ill-fitting models, particularly in relation to the language and discourses that are used,[10] or to be passed off as a pseudo-positivist construction of reality.[4]

Phenomenological Philosophies, Culture and Nursing Research

Philosophy, like many human activities, is affected by culture and language. We think of German philosophy as dense and difficult but often brilliant; of English philosophy as more cognitive-rational and intellectual (in its disembodied sense); and of the French as having a more accessible and radical/political and popularised form of philosophy. Matthews put it well when he said:

> French philosophy remains French, however, in that it has assimilated such external influences and given them a particularly Gallic gloss. Again, to write philosophy primarily in France and in French is necessarily to place oneself within a particular cultural tradition, whatever the writer's own original nationality may be (p. 4).[11]

In our thinking about phenomenologies, that is, in our thinking about what it is to be, we also cannot escape culture nor individual circumstances, such as gender, colour, height and shape. One cannot 'be' in a culture-free way. One does not have culture without humans to embody and experience it in a lived and expressed (or expressive) way and to pass it on to successive generations who themselves embody a culturally mediated way to be-in-the-world, to think about that world, reflect on it, or describe it in language.

There are at least three culturally affected and recognizable forms of phenomenology: German, French and American varieties. Within the latter, there is perhaps a doubtful sub-category that Crotty calls nursing phenomenology.[9] Crotty argues that:

> … in being transplanted to the North American continent, phenomenology experienced significant mutations. Transplantation may not be the analogy to use. For the most part, rather than being permitted to set down its own roots west of the Atlantic, phenomenology was grafted onto local stock. The fruit it has produced reflects the American intellectual tradition far more than any features of its parent plant (p. 2).[9]

In Crotty's view, what the North Americans have done is to focus rather more attention on subjectivity and individual meaning than on being itself or the thing(s) that beings are making sense of. He further argues that this emphasis on the subjective, is typical, and consistent with, the strong sense of individualism that characterizes American culture. For example, a strict reading of phenomenology as a philosophical system, particularly in its German(ic) form, is about the nature of being and being conscious of phenomena; that is, it is a predominantly intellectual notion and activity, albeit an embodied one. In its French form, a little more latitude is required to make way for a subtle shift towards embodied, incarnate existence. In many respects, it is the more carnate (or carnal) and sensual qualities of the French philosophical works that sets them apart, particularly those influenced by Merleau-Ponty.[12] And, French philosophy is more overtly gendered and linked to embodiment, particularly in relation to the works of de Beauvoir.[13,14] and many current French feminists, for example, Kristeva.[15]

However, Lyotard's work on the history of phenomenology had this to say:

> ... there are presently *many* phenomenologists, and since its meaning is still 'in process', unfinished precisely because it is historical. There are, in effect, different 'accents' ... yet there remains a common phenomenological 'style' ... and not being able here, except on occasion, to localize the finer or coarser divergences which separate ... philosophers, it is this common style above all which we will seek to outline, **after having rendered unto Husserl that which is Husserl's** (p. 34).[16] (emphasis added)

What then, is the 'accent' that nursing gives phenomenology? If it is the case that different cultures shape the grain and texture of phenomenology, then it may be reasonable to expect that different disciplines will have a characteristic way in which they operationalise philosophies to investigate their particular concerns. What is more, the nature of the material that one investigates and the way in which research participants interact with the project add other qualities that the researcher has to accommodate.

Phenomenologies and the Sub-Culture of Nursing: Pushing the Boundaries Too Far?

Nurses bring to their research their experiences from how they have come to know the world from their practice, as well as from their own lives. The sense of practicality that their clinical practice demands of them inevitably has an influence on what topics they investigate and how they wish to investigate them. Often these topics lurk on the edges of acceptable social boundaries, which are both personal and intimate. That is, nurses bring a kind of professional culture to bear on their constructs of being and their understandings of the being-of-the-other. In their attempts to understand the project of nursing, nurse researchers have sometimes pushed methodologies and methods beyond the purpose for which they were originally intended; and some nurses have used creative combinations of components of different research traditions. At its best, this inventiveness has resulted in works of great imagination, creativity and insight, and at worst the result has sometimes been a mish-mash of unconnected and mis-connected bits.

One major issue that confronts us internationally is the popularity of phenomenologies such that this research approach has become a kind of boutique methodology. Among the choices of qualitative research methodologies that are currently used, phenomenologies are the most common in the reported literature; the only serious rival is grounded theory, which many regard not as a methodology but as a method. Among researchers whose intellectual traditions are more European, however, other interpretive and critical paradigms are more apparent, including those drawn from sociological, political, and anthropological traditions and from cultural studies.

However, in nursing works from the USA, phenomenology is almost universal as the qualitative research design of choice (if one excludes grounded theory) and one sees relatively little work based in symbolic interaction, ethnomethodology and ethnography. With a few notable exceptions, such as Benner's and others' works,[17,18] there is a strong preference for Husserlian phenomenology, particularly as it is reflected in the analysis techniques that are based on it, for example Giorgi.[19] Furthermore, there are few works that draw explicitly on the more critical and politically oriented approaches other than feminism. There also has been a tendency in the literature from the USA to use grounded theory as a singular, unitary and self-contained method(ology) that conveys a kind of fundamentalist approach to methodology.

In other contexts, nurse researchers are more inclined to 'blend' grounded theory with other ways of knowing or to borrow some of its more appealing tools, particularly concepts such as 'saturation', 'theoretical sampling', 'coding' and keeping memos. However, in the recent special issue of *Qualitative Health Research*,[20] there is a sense in which grounded theorists are strengthening the linkages between grounded theory and symbolic interaction with which it shares epistemological roots and a common history. Such links generally are not yet reflected in the analyses that appear in published works. One could conclude therefore that such links are more historical than apparent. The editorial in this same volume suggests strongly that poorly executed grounded theory studies are the result of researchers' deficit that could be attributed to inadequate learning and/or mentoring about the method.[21] This type of commentary resonates with that sense of *déjà vu* reminiscent of the debates about nurses' reluctant to embrace the nursing process – their reluctance was said to inhere in the nurses rather than the nursing process itself because the nurses were not using it 'properly'.

In the hands of nurses, phenomenologies have been expected to be both robust and versatile. Crotty has gone so far as to claim that there is a kind of orthodoxy about phenomenology as it is used by nurses in the USA and that nurses have re-created it to suit circumstances for which it was not intended.[9] In so doing, nurses have drifted so far from the original ideas that they no longer undertake phenomenology, but something quite different; and that *difference* has become well established. He argues that nurses' attempts to find meanings in people's experiences indicate that they are not being true to phenomenology. Another reading of Crotty's text could have him asserting that they are not 'real' phenomenologists – a position which is certainly contestable. Another reading still, could suggest that, in seeking meanings from their phenomenological inquiries, nurses are drifting much closer to the French position – and perhaps this is what concerns Crotty, that (American) nurses have strayed from the German(ic) traditions.

Lyotard has argued, however, that the assumption of meaning is implicit in but omitted from descriptions of methodology, particularly in phenomenologically informed types of sociology – another discipline that has been inventive in its use of phenomenology. Lyotard goes further to state that:

... all human science posits the existence of meaning in what it studies. This meaning is not simply a function of utility: it cannot be correctly identified without referring to the person or persons studied. Thus in every human science there is an implicit 'postulate' of the comprehensibility of humans to humans; and consequently the relation of the observer to the observed in the human sciences is a case of the relation of person to person, of Me to You (p. 100).[16]

Crotty's case, although it is justified and valid in part, is based on works that typify phenomenology as it is conceptualised, taught and conducted in the USA and by nurses in particular.[9] His argument does not necessarily apply outside that country; his text therefore could be more accurately titled *Phenomenology and American Nursing Research*. Phenomenologically inspired nursing research conducted with a more European and particularly French 'accent' (after Lyotard[16]), has a greater emphasis on the body, embodiment and embodied being. In the published nursing research that originates in the USA, the body and embodiment – as mainstream nursing concerns – have a rather more peripheral and sanitised presence than is the case elsewhere. The body of the patient is conspicuously absent in nursing literature from the USA. Likewise, their phenomenological studies, with the exception of Benner's works, are reported in rather more cerebral and cognitive terms (that is with a German 'accent') than they are existential and embodied (that is with a French 'accent').

The influence of Benner's and others' works has been more prominent than that of her American-based colleagues in that she has been influenced by French philosophers, in particular Merleau-Ponty.[17,18] And there is a strong theme of embodiment that runs through her works. However, the embodiment-of-the-patient in Benner's work is positioned in relation to a more central (intellectual and epistemological) concern both with knowing (and knowledge) and caring for the other who is embodied than with the body-of-the-other. Crotty's critique draws extensively on Benner's work, yet curiously, he focuses most of his attention of her treatment of Heidegger's work, making only passing reference (p. 125) about the extent to which the work of Merleau-Ponty is influential in her oeuvre;[9] this is a very selective analysis and one that does not do justice to Benner's published works.

Crotty has been roundly criticised, however, for his analysis of the phenomenological works of Benner who has criticised him for his pejorative tone, his 'wholesale rejection' of what he has described as nursing phenomenology, for confusing issues and, importantly, for his not taking an impartial view.[22] It is difficult to see therefore what Crotty's work adds to the emergent patterns of knowing the lived world in the practice of nursing. What Crotty offers nursing, however, is the impetus to more reflectively and overtly articulate the philosophical and epistemological attractions of interpretive traditions for nursing.

While Crotty's critique of nurses' use of phenomenology (or nursing phenomenology) turns on its philosophical points, it does not go to the heart of the matter in nursing research and methodology.[9] The points for nursing are these: that nursing is in search of methodologies for its project in which the life and times of the other can be given voice; that nursing has turned to phenomenological philosophy because the nature of the subject matter to be investigated invites a human(e) approach that does not reduce the person to a set of physiological or pathological descriptors or probability statements; and if phenomenologies have been found to be wanting as methodologies in nursing research it may be a reflection of the complexity of nursing's project as much as it is a comment on the way in which nursing practice and research are culture-sensitive.

However, in examining the philosophical bases on which nursing's phenomenological research is based there is room for some reflection, particularly in light of Holmes' recent analysis of the relationship between Heidegger's politics and his philosophy.[23] Indeed, Holmes believes that Heideggerian philosophy may ultimately be ruled out as an appropriate basis on which to conduct nursing inquiry because it is fundamentally and essentially incompatible with the values of nursing.

Phenomenological Philosophy and Nursing Research Methodologies

In order to examine how well phenomenologies stand up to the demands of a 'live' research project, it is well to reflect on what students can do with the ideas and systems of thought in what are called phenomenologies. Even the most gifted students struggle with these approaches; it is almost a right of passage to arrive at a glimmer of understanding about philosophers' thinking, and to have achieved a working understanding of differences between transcendental and existential phenomenologies, the cultural and historical influences on the various authors and difficult concepts such as ontology, epistemology, and their relations to methodology in interpretive paradigms. And this is exacerbated both by an increasing uncertainty about what we take to be knowledge in the postmodern period and a view that there is 'a right way' to do these things – a taken-for-granted way of understanding that has a long history in nursing.

One of the great dramas that is lived out by people working in these areas is making the transition from philosophy to methodology to design and the selection of data collection methods. This problem is less prevalent in projects that draw more directly from ethnographic traditions because the gaps between the philosophy, theory, methodology and method are not as large and there has been a sort of simultaneous and parallel development of philosophy, theory, epistemology and method. In the case of phenomenologies, the philosophy seems to overpower methodology; and the methods of data collection are appropriated from ethnography, anthropology and sociology. In these socially oriented disciplines, the intent and orientation of the data collector – in relation to what information is to be collected – can differ. And it is on this issue that phenomenologies are most vulnerable and researchers most troubled because phenomenologies – at least in its post-Husserlian form – were not intended for field work or for empirical inquiry, which is where they are now being employed for nursing research.

In its Husserlian form, phenomenology remains fixed in the modern period and does not allow for the influences of multiple subjectivities, multiple realities or the problematics of discourses. And this can create tension between the research question(s), the philosophical space in which the researcher wants to be positioned, and the means by which the project can be conducted successfully. What may have worked for Husserlian phenomenology as an intellectual exercise in which thought and words were central (but understood unproblematicly), is not necessarily appropriate for a project constructed and conducted in the postmodern period; nor are they necessarily appropriate for a practice discipline.

These are matters that Borbasi,[2] and others[3,24] have highlighted and which go to the nub of our troubles in translocating or transforming philosophical systems into empirical ones for a practice discipline, Borbasi did not immediately know what to *be;* that is, she was unclear how she should position herself as a nurse researching in an environment in which she was familiar.[2] Just as we have many possible selves, and possible positions as researchers, we also have different ways to *be.* Each one of these ways to be has social, personal and contextually defined facets; being is not a unitary notion – and this can be felt acutely in the field.

In response to Borbasi,[2] Rudge,[3] whose research was more overtly ethnographic than Borbasi's phenomenological project, nevertheless identified with Borbasi's troubles. Rudge offered the following comments: 'as with other natives who have come to observe their own cultures, the nurse research destabilizes this dichotomy. We are both; we are neither – we are something else altogether'. In response to Borbasi,[2] I also argued that:

> There are methodological, ethical, ontological, clinical, and pragmatic issues that nurses have to negotiate when they take borrowed methodologies out of what could be called their epistemological ambience-of-origin and into a clinical context. Furthermore, these methodologies are being relocated from a predominantly academic context to the world of practice; nursing is yet to systematically explore the consequences of that relocation both on researchers (as individuals) and methodology (p. 57).[24]

Conclusion

In summary, the popularity of interpretive approaches to research into nursing, particularly phenomenologies, has taken place quickly opening new areas of documenting nursing knowledge and practice. This evolution has taken place without a simultaneous exploration or explication of the issues that inhere in appropriating fundamentally philosophical approaches for investigating questions in a practice discipline. Furthermore, there are areas of confusion about some key concepts in phenomenologies and issues to be explored in the transposition of philosophical systems of thought into methodologies for the field(s) of nursing inquiry.

References

1. Mykhalovskiy E. Reconsidering table talk: Critical thoughts on the relationship between sociology, autobiography and self-indulgence. *Qualitative Sociology* 1996; **19** (1): 131–152.
2. Borbasi S. To be or not to be? Nurse? Researcher? Or both? *Nursing Inquiry* 1995; **1**: 57.
3. Rudge T. Response: insider ethnography: researching nursing from within. *Nursing Inquiry* 1995; **1**: 58.
4. Thorne S. Phenomenological positivism and other problematic trends in health science research. *Qualitative Health Research* 1997; **7**: 287–293.
5. Lawler J. *Behind the Screens: Nursing, Somology and the Problem of the Body.* Melbourne: Churchill Livingstone, 1991.
6. Lawler J. In search of an Australian identity. In: Gray G & Pratt R (eds). *Towards a Discipline of Nursing.* Melbourne: Churchill Livingstone, 1991; 211–227.
7. Heidegger M. *Being and Time* (trans. Macquarrie J & Robinson E). Oxford: Basil Blackwell, 1962.
8. Lawler J. What you see is not always what you get: Seeing, feeling and researching nursing. In: *Nursing Research: Reactive vs. Proactive.* Proceedings of the First International Nursing Research Conference of the Centre for Nursing Research and the Royal College of Nursing, Adelaide, Australia, 1991: 13–21.
9. Crotty M. *Phenomenology and Nursing Research.* Melbourne: Churchill Livingstone, 1996.
10. Lawler J. Knowing the body and embodiment: methodologies, discourses and nursing. In: Lawler J (ed.). *The Body in Nursing: A Collection of Views.* Melbourne: Churchill Livingstone, 1997.
11. Matthews E. *Twentieth-Century French Philosophy.* Oxford: Oxford University Press, 1996.
12. Crossley N. Merleau-Ponty, the elusive body and carnal sociology. *Body and Society* 1995; **1**: 43–63.
13. de Beauvoir S. *The Second Sex.* Harmondsworth: Penguin, 1972.
14. Hughes A & Witz A. Feminism and the matter of bodies: from de Beauvoir to Butler. *Body and Society* 1997; **3**: 47–60.
15. Kristeva J. *Powers of Horror: An Essay on Abjection.* New York: Columbia University Press, 1982.
16. Lyotard J-F. *Phenomenology* (B Beakley, trans.). Albany: State University of New York, 1991.
17. Benner P & Wrubel J. *The Primacy of Caring.* Menlo Park: Addison-Wesley, 1988.
18. Benner P (ed.). *Interpretive Phenomenology: Embodiment, Caring, and Ethics in Health and Illness.* Thousand Oaks: Sage, 1994.
19. Giorgi A. *Psychology as a Human Science.* New York: Harper & Row, 1975.
20. Special issue: Advances in grounded theory. *Qualitative Health Research* 1996; **6** (3).

21. May K. Editorial: Diffusion, dilution, or distillation? The case of grounded theory method. *Qualitative Health Research* 1996; **6**: 309–311.

22. Benner P. Book review: *Phenomenology and Nursing Research* by M. Crotty (1996) in *Nursing Inquiry* 1996; **3**: 257–258.

23. Holmes CA. The politics of phenomenological concepts in nursing. *Journal of Advanced Nursing* 1996; **24**: 579–587.

24. Lawler J. Response to Borbasi: To be or not to be? Nurse? Researcher? Or both? *Nursing Inquiry* 1995; **2**: 57.

Action Research

46

Older People in Accident and Emergency: The Use of Action Research to Explore the Interface between Services in an Acute Hospital

Jackie Bridges and Julienne Meyer

This article presents a case study of the role of an action researcher in a study that aims to evaluate and improve the organisation of care for older people in the accident and emergency (A&E) department of a large United Kingdom NHS Trust. The change project is still underway at the time of writing and the final data analysis has therefore yet to be completed. The work presented here represents a description of the study and the role of the action researcher to date, with findings based on a preliminary analysis of the action research cycles and a set of intermediate interviews carried out with key participants in the study. This article aims to explore the value of action research, with a focus on one interpretation of the role of action researcher, in addressing a complex, large-scale problem in health care with significant implications for patients and staff.

National Background

Growing pressures on acute in-patient beds in the NHS have prompted the development of a variety of strategies designed to keep in-patient stays as short and effective as possible for individual patients of all ages. The management

Source: *Educational Action Research*, 8(2) (2000): 277–289.

of emergency admissions is a current focus of attention (NHS Confederation and Royal College of Physicians, 1997; NHS Executive, 1997b). In recent years, an ongoing rise in emergency admissions coupled with the effect of a number of factors, including some specifically associated with the winter season (NHS Executive, 1997b), have led to problems in the management of emergency admissions. When problems occur, the number of patients requiring acute admission can occasionally exceed the availability of in-patient beds. The growth of 'winter pressures' has led to a recognition of the need for more systematic, longer term planning for the winter months. Recent publications reflect attempts to draw a national picture of the problems and to pool expertise and experience to devise solutions (NHS Executive, 1997a, b). Solutions introduced in some hospitals include primary care services based in A&E, assessment and admissions units, and telephone triage.

Older people are forming an increasingly large proportion of the demands on the acute sector. The increasing demand is due to growing numbers of older people in the general population and the increasing likelihood of multiple health and social care needs with older age (Audit Commission, 1997). American research highlights the special needs of older people at the point of presentation to A&E (Baum & Rubenstein, 1987; Sanders & Morley, 1993) and how the practice of A&E staff needs to develop to meet these needs (Jones et al, 1988; Rahman et al, 1989; Vreeken & Hall, 1990). Very little equivalent research has been done in the UK, and UK policy documents recently produced do not advocate separate or specialist arrangements for the emergency admission of older people (whether admitted through A&E or directly into in-patient beds). There appears to be an implicit assumption that the solutions advocated in the emergency admissions literature, including the A&E literature, will adequately meet the needs of all age groups. Although the A&E literature includes the description of some initiatives specifically designed to meet the needs of older people, for example supporting A&E discharge work through nurse specialist and post-discharge follow-up support (Rajacich & Cameron, 1995; Allen, 1997), only a small number of articles in the literature advocate the fundamental review of A&E services as a whole to meet the needs of older people (Andreoli & Musser, 1985; Sanders, 1992; British Geriatrics Society, 1997).

Local Background

The service for elderly people (SEP) at a large United Kingdom NHS Trust funds my post as Research Fellow in Adult Nursing at City University. I have a background as a clinical nurse specialist in acute-care gerontology and a range of experiences as a change agent in health care. The post was funded by the service to provide a lead in R&D and nursing development activities, and also to use an action research approach to undertake projects in line with service priorities. My work was supervised by Dr Julienne Meyer, Chair in Adult Nursing at

City University. The service director's idea of funding an externally-based post to undertake projects using an action research approach was based on three main beliefs. First, that the post holder could negotiate different relationships with individuals and groups within the trust given the post-holder's lack of position within the trust's hierarchy and politics. Secondly, that action research provides a methodology that would allow a different approach to solving difficult problems. Thirdly, the academic credibility of a university based post and the status of the project as a research study may help garner support for any changes that need to happen. The experience of implementing the post appears to have supported these beliefs, as will be demonstrated below.

The study reported here was commissioned by the SEP service director following a winter period where the acute sector had been under intense pressure. Within SEP, there were concerns about the quality of care of older people during the process of admission to acute care (in the light of long waits for in-patient beds) and the recognition by SEP's service director that there may be scope for greater collaboration between A&E and SEP. This prompted the service director to commission the action research study, although once the work began, I was given a free hand to explore and determine the issues from all perspectives, not just SEP's. The 10-month action research study began in July 1997.

The research questions that this study aims to address are:

What is the nature of the current organisation of care for older people in A&E?

How do older users and carers perceive the care in A&E?

How can improvements in received care be achieved?

What can be learned from attempts to change the organisation of care in A&E?

Approach and Methods Used

My role in the study is as lead researcher and facilitator of change. I began with a period of fieldwork in A&E to gain an understanding of A&E processes. The fieldwork included non-participant observational work and informal interviews with key people (e.g. patients, A&E nursing and medical staff, A&E service director) to encourage them to identify areas for improvement and difficulties in their own work. This period was important in enabling me to understand the processes that patients and staff move through in A&E (I had very little experience of A&E) and to gain an understanding of the reality of the situation from both the patient and staff point of view. The work also aimed to engage A&E staff in the study and enable them to contribute at an early stage to building up a picture of any issues from their point of view and possible solutions.

The main participants in the action research study were recruited through informal recommendation from managers and staff in the two services (A&E and SEP) as the issues to be addressed emerged. All potential participants were invited to take part on a voluntary basis and no one refused. The main participants at the outset of the study are shown in Figure 1.

SEP Research Fellow
A&E service director*
A&E clinical director/consultant*
A&E sister*
A&E primary care consultant
SEP service director*
SEP acute service manager*
SEP consultant*
2 SEP ward managers
Hospital at Home co-ordinator
A&E OT
Trust-wide emergency admissions project (EAP) co-ordinator
Trust board director/EAP leader*
Public health consultant

Figure 1: Main participants in study

* Denotes individual who acted as 'key participant'
A clinical audit facilitator, two health visitors for older people and social services representatives also became involved later as the work developed.

Following the fieldwork and identification of the main participants. I facilitated a multidisciplinary workshop with most of the main participants to share the findings from the preliminary field work, define problems, decide the scope and areas of focus within the study, and brainstorm possible solutions for problems identified. I also held two focus groups with SEP ward nursing staff for the same purpose. Focus groups with A&E nursing staff were planned, but managers or staff could not find a way for these groups to be convened. This represented the first of a number of unsuccessful attempts to engage the A&E nursing staff group in collaboration in the project and the reasons for this are explored later.

Three projects were identified for action within the main study and each follows the action research cycle of problem definition, solution identification, implementation and evaluation. The three subsequent action research cycles and their relationship to the main study are illustrated in Figure 2. Each action research cycle has been taken forward by a multidisciplinary group made up of a mix of professionals appropriate to the task in hand. In two action research cycles ('Discharge from A&E' and 'Care While in A&E'), I meet with the groups on a regular basis to discuss problems and plan the implementation of solutions. In the other action research cycle, the group does not formally meet together and the participation of individuals in the group's work varies as to the relevance of the work. As is evident from the configuration of the work, my role as lead researcher forms the link between the three action research cycles and the main study. My own systematic reflections of progress through the course of the study also inform the progress of the three action research cycles and the main study.

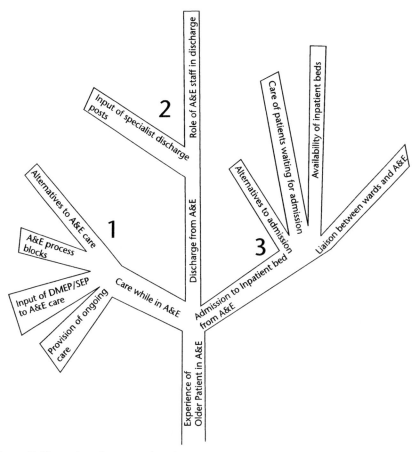

Figure 2: The main action research cycles

A group of key individuals (see Figure 1), who may or may not have been involved in the work of the individual action research cycles, but who has some kind of 'vested interest' in the work in hand, oversee the work, comment on its progress and decide on its focus. I meet with these key 'participants' individually on a regular basis.

The change project has also been informed by information gathered from an extensive literature review of the subject area and by establishing links with other hospitals with experience in tackling similar issues. The university provided library facilities and the help of a research assistant to help with literature collection. The university's positive links with other provider units and my position as a researcher (rather than a representative of a competing Trust) also appears to have helped in gaining open honest accounts of the practical difficulties in improving care in A&E that others were experiencing in different trusts. Other organisations were also approached for help in determining similar work going on elsewhere in the country. These included the Department of Health, the Council of International Hospitals, the Royal College of Nursing and other nurse researchers in A&E. The information gathered from the literature review and contact with other organisations enabled this work and its progress to be viewed in and informed by the national context of work in this area.

During the course of the work, it has become clear that an understanding of the patient's perspective was needed to inform service development. As a consequence, a second researcher has been provided by the university to carry out further observation work and patient interviews of older patients in A&E, for 1 month following their A&E attendance. The data analysis is currently being carried out and it is hoped that this piece of work will also inform understanding of the older patient's experience of A&E.

A number of different data sources have been used to track the progress of the action research study:

> researcher field notes which record meetings, informal conversations, decisions made and events taking place;
> collection of relevant management information, local reports, meeting minutes, correspondence and press cuttings;
> recording of initial workshop and focus groups (see above);
> recorded one-to-one interviews with six of the key participants to review the progress of the study to date, validate some preliminary findings and evaluate the utility of action research in addressing the issues at hand (December 1997/January 1998).

The work of the project is still in progress and, following its completion in April 1998, I aim to conduct a formal analysis of the data collected over the course of the study and validation of the findings with the key participants.

Due to space constraints, it is not possible to present a detailed account of the progress of the whole study. Instead, I will use the working processes and progress within one of the three action research cycles to examine the value of action research in this setting.

Care While in A&E

This action research cycle was set up in response to findings from the initial observation work in A&E. It was observed that nursing systems were set up to assess and initiate treatment for patients as they arrived in A&E. My field notes reflect that nursing systems were not set up to support the delivery of regular planned care over a period of time, the available nurses always needing to attend to the next patient arriving at A&E. In reality, older patients could be in A&E for a number of hours, either because of lengthy A&E processes or because an in-patient bed was not available. Older people are particularly vulnerable to these long waits because of age related changes, and the likelihood their illness is accompanied by other physical and functional disabilities. They need planned and regular pressure area care, nutrition, hydration and help with going to the toilet. The nursing systems allow no more than the *ad hoc* delivery of this type of care. These observations were validated through informal discussions with A&E nurses. The focus group held with ward managers also provided evidence of how the inadequacy of these nursing systems impacted on the outcome of individual patients. Instances were cited of patients arriving on in-patient wards from A&E who had been incontinent of urine, and not been cleaned and changed, and of patients who had not received regular pressure area care.

The action research approach to this issue has allowed a clearer explication of this issue from the perspective of different participants and the subsequent testing of different approaches to improve this part of the care of older people. Three claims about the value of action research will now be illustrated by the project's progress and preliminary findings.

Action Research Enables an Understanding of the Issues from the Perspectives of the Different Participants

It was clear from the initial work (above) that older people had needs for on-going care that were not always met and that the busier A&E became, the less likely these needs were to be met. All participants in the study validated this finding at the initial workshop. However, there was not a shared understanding of primary reason for these needs not being met. Two main perspectives emerged through the initial work on the reasons for the problem and thus the location of the responsibility for change.

The first perspective was shared by participants working outside of the A&E department and this was an assertion that, in their experience. A&E staff did not value older patients and therefore gave older patients' needs lower priority than those of younger patients.

During the focus group for SEP ward managers, one participant highlighted how the problems worsened during the winter:

> When there were problems this winter [1996/97], the elderly very much got the blame for everything and you felt that there was some sort of plague almost down there [A&E] and the attitude was once the decision to admit has been made, then the patient is no longer their responsibility. But then [the elderly patients] fall in this big hole because they are nobodies, they could be there after that time for two or three hours and who is caring for that patient. And at a meeting I went to, the nurses and sisters said 'we came into A&E because we like this nursing, we don't want to do basic nursing care, that's not what we are here for, to feed and wash' which I suppose to some extent is true but if you don't feed [the older patients] and they are there for a long while, they are not going to do well. (WM1)

It is important to note that, while the ward managers had concerns about the quality of care for some patients, they expressed sympathy for the extreme conditions in which A&E staff sometimes worked and a recognition that poor quality of care was not always due to factors within any individual nurse's control. However, there remained an assertion that older people were assigned lower value because of their age and because their needs did not match the expectations of A&E staff of what A&E work should consist of. Data collected through the winter of 1997/98 within the trust's emergency admissions project suggest that people aged 75 and over wait longer for initial A&E medical assessment than younger people. These data do not indicate medical priority, so firm conclusions cannot be drawn that older people are prioritised lower because of their age. However, my field notes reflect informal discussions with some A&E medical staff that indicate the fact that older people were given lower priority not always dependent on their medical needs.

The second main perspective on the reason for older people's ongoing care needs not being met was held mainly by A&E staff. The notes of the discussion from the initial multidisciplinary workshop and subsequent field notes reflect that A&E staff felt that patients did not move out of the department quickly enough because in-patient beds were not always available for the patients to be admitted to. When beds were available, A&E staff felt that ward staff did not always declare them as soon as they became available or, even if a bed was available and 'declared', sometimes the ward would postpone taking a patient if they were busy, short-staffed, or the proposed admission coincided with handover, mealtimes or ward rounds. A&E staff also felt that, apart from the wards' behaviour. Trust-wide issues around bed allocation and bed management also mitigated against optimal bed availability.

The A&E nurses, although recognising the need for ongoing care and feeling frustrated that they are often too busy to provide it properly (particularly when the department becomes overloaded during the winter), felt unfairly blamed for a situation largely outside of their control. They felt that if patients were moved through and out of A&E quicker, older patients would not require this type of attention in A&E. Data collected on 'trolley waits' during 1997 reflect the A&E perspective that, during some periods of time, patients of all age groups waited beyond the national Patient's Charter standard of 2 hours for admission to a bed once the decision to admit had been made. Older patients are perhaps perceived as a greater problem to A&E staff than younger patients during this waiting period because of their greater need for ongoing care.

It is clear from the above that two equally valid perspectives existed on the same issue. The action research approach enabled these perspectives to be explained in a number of ways. A collaborative approach is essential here to ensure that the perspective of each party can be explicated and shared. Good inter-personal skills on the part of the action researcher have also been key in creating opportunities for informal discussion and in encouraging individuals to be open about the problems from their perspective. A number of different data sources were used to explicate and validate the two different perspectives, and a systematic approach was needed to select, gather and analyse this data. The 'multi-methods' feature of action research has enabled the different data to be brought together to form the overall picture.

Action Research Enables Work to Take Place Which Explicitly Takes Account of the Different Perspectives

It is clear from the above perspectives that each party felt the primary responsibility for change lay with the other party. This meant that lone attempts within the study to address, for example, any need for A&E to change their practice, without addressing A&E's perspective on where the change needed to take place, would not have been successful. Because a clearer picture had emerged of the different perspectives through using an action research approach, change in working practice could take place that addressed each aspect of the problem that had been identified.

One piece of work aimed to change the way that nursing care was organised to ensure that ongoing care needs were delivered in a more systematic way. The work included standard setting and piloting new documentation. An A&E sister was actively involved in the work although attempts to engage the wider nursing staff group in the work (through questionnaires and trying to convene group work) were not successful. This appears to be partly due to the relatively low priority of research work in relation to clinical work, but also because the A&E nurses do not feel that altering the nursing care input would solve the fundamental issue from their perspective. Communication in the department seems relatively poor and it could be, that despite my efforts to communicate efforts and progress of the other work of the project through the A&E service director, the majority of A&E staff may not be aware of this work. The work in altering the nursing input to ongoing care needs may thus be seen as the only piece of work aimed at improving care to older patients. Without evidence that their perspective of the problem is being addressed, A&E nurses will probably continue to resist change in their own practice.

The other work that has taken place includes providing information to support re-profiling the grade mix of the nursing staff, advising on the purchase of trolley pads for preventing pressure sores, support to the emergency admissions project to improve bed management and working with ward staff to improve bed availability and explore options for ward nurses helping out in A&E at busy times. It is this kind of work that A&E nurses would see as addressing their perspective. The action research approach has enabled work to take place that supports necessary changes in practice, but has also helped understanding of how a lack of communication may have led to a continuing resistance to changing practice. Other reasons are explored below.

Because my own position lies neither in one 'camp' or the other, I am able to suggest and facilitate changes in a number of different areas. If, for example,

I were a member of A&E staff, my ability to influence the work of ward staff would be limited. Although I have no managerial authority in the organisation, my position as action researcher enables me to legitimately challenge working practices in SEP, A&E and the wider trust. Results of interviews in which key participants were invited to comment on the role of the action researcher reflect the recognition of the value of a multi-factorial approach:

> *I mean I'm sure it's been a power for good, er, not necessarily for just us against A&E but I mean because somebody cares, somebody is trying to sort the issues out on both sides and you're not playing it as if it's one sided, you know you're playing it open minded and talking to people about what they wanted. (SD1, SEP service director)*

The A&E consultant also felt that addressing the problem from different angles had helped:

> *As with any problem, there's always more than one solution, or more than one angle that needs to be looked at. And I think you've handled that wonderfully by bringing forward all the issues with the nurse training, the pressure area care … (CS1)*

The complexity of health care today means that different parts of health services can become isolated from each others and continuing pressures for change within limited resources can lead to further isolation. It appears that the position of the action researcher at the 'interface' between different perspectives can enable an overview of the issues and a legitimacy to tackling these issues from a number of different angles.

Action Research Helps to Explicate the Reasons for Resistance to Change

Throughout the study, daily field notes have been recorded of progress of change, events that have taken place and contextual data. The field notes are used as the basis for ongoing reflection on the progress of the study. These reflections are regularly shared and validated with the key participants, and compared against available literature. These findings enable us to more clearly understand why change is resisted. Two examples are used below to illustrate this.

The first example relates to work that has taken place with ward staff to improve the availability of in-patient beds. This has included putting patients due for discharge that day in the dayroom in the early morning to enable A&E admissions and agreeing spaces where extra beds could be put up on the ward to take patients from A&E when no other options for freeing up in-patient beds remain. This work with the wards, although actively supported by the service manager, has been characterised by reluctance from the ward managers. They have concerns about the quality of care of the patients on their ward, despite the fact that moving more patients on to the ward would probably improve the quality of care for the group of patients waiting for admission as a whole. The ward managers only have responsibility for the care on their ward and not for the care in A&E. They do not, therefore share the problem of the quality of care, of patients waiting for admission. However, following the decision to admit, it is only the physical location of the patient that determines the responsibility to care, not their actual stage in the admission process. Until the ward managers' feeling of responsibility for care extends to any responsibility that SEP as a department may have, 'tussles' over this group of patients will probably continue.

The second example involves the work attempted to change A&E nursing practice in relation to ongoing care needs. One reason for A&E nurses' resistance to change in their practice in this area may be a feeling that the real problem of bed availability is not being addressed and the lack of communication posited above may be a causative factor here. Another reason may be a resistance from A&E nurses to recognising that this aspect of older people's care may be a legitimate part of A&E work, however quickly or slowly patients move out of A&E.

Sociological studies carried out in A&E departments reflect attempts by A&E staff to control the nature of their work by assessing individual patients against implicit criteria (Roth, 1972; Mannon, 1976; Jeffery, 1979; Dingwall & Murray, 1983). Whether or not patients meet these criteria indicates whether or not that patient is a 'deserving' A&E patient, and thus merits the time and input of A&E staff. Reflections on attempts to change practice in this study have indicated that, while acutely ill older people appear to meet the criteria for legitimate A&E attention in terms of their medical needs, other needs such as ongoing nursing care needs are not seen as legitimate work for A&E nurses. The longer the period of time patients need this care, particularly when the length of time is outside A&E control (i.e. waiting for an in-patient bed), the less legitimate those patients' needs are perceived to be by A&E nurses.

Although Sbaih (Sbaih, 1997b) noted the use of terms such as 'inappropriate patient' is now becoming explicitly addressed and disallowed in the A&E world, the actual organisation of work in relation to judgements about legitimacy of presentation has not changed. This assertion is supported by Sbaih's findings from her ethnomethodological work (Sbaih, 1997a,b) and the findings from this action research study also support this conclusion in the care of older adults.

The above examples demonstrate how systematic recording of and reflection on the change process has enabled insights on resistance to change. The formal data analysis and further development of these ideas should hopefully throw further light on real problems for staff and patients in the realities of everyday practice. This knowledge can then be used to inform future efforts at change, in defining what change is seeking to achieve and in planning how change is to be achieved.

Conclusions

An action research approach appears to be playing a valuable role in this study in working at the interface between two acute hospital services. Action research has enabled explication of the differing perspectives of the stakeholders. The independent position of the action researcher has enabled work to take place that addresses these multiple perspectives, and the systematic collection of data on the process and outcomes of change has thrown light on what the reasons for resistance to change may be. In the example used here, the study findings illuminate very real issues in attempting to integrate the approaches to care of two very different acute hospital specialities. The data also suggest that action research may be a key approach in bridging gaps between services and addressing the issues at play.

References

Allen, D. (1997) Telephone Follow up for Older People Discharged from A&E, *Nursing Standard*, 11(46), pp. 34–37.

Andreoli, K. & Musser, L. (1985) Challenges Confronting the Future of Emergency Nursing, *Journal of Emergency Nursing*, 11(1), pp. 16–21.

Audit Commission (1997) *The Coming of Age: improving care services for older people.* London: Audit Commission.

Baum, S. & Rubenstein, L. (1987) Old People in the Emergency Room: age-related differences in emergency department use and care, *Journal of the American Geriatrics Society*-35, pp. 398–404.

British Geriatrics Society (1997) *The Elderly Patient in the Accident and Emergency Department.* London: British Geriatrics Society.

Dingwall, R. & Murray, T. (1983) Categorisation in Accident and Emergency Departments: 'good' patients, 'bad' patients and 'children', *Sociology of Health & Illness*, 5(2), p. 127–148.

Jeffery, R. (1979) Normal Rubbish: deviant patients in casualty departments, *Sociology of Health & Illness*, 1(1), pp. 90–107.

Jones, J., Dougherty, J., Schelble, D. & Cunningham, W. (1988) Emergency Department Protocol for the Diagnosis and Evaluation of Geriatric Abuse, *Annals of Emergency Medicine*, 17(10), pp. 1006–1015.

Mannon, J. (1976) Defining and Treating 'Problem Patients' in a Hospital Emergency Room, *Medical Care*, 14(12), pp. 1004–1013.

NHS Confederation and Royal College of Physicians (1997) *Tackling NHS Emergency Admissions: policy into practice.* London: NHS Confederation.

NHS Executive (1997a) *Developing Emergency Services in the Community.* London NHSE.

NHS Executive (1997b) *Report to the Chief Executive on Winter Pressures.* London: NHSE.

Rahman, A., Salend, E., Liston, M., Lee, G., Dees, G. & Morgan, M. (1989) An Educational Program to Improve Geriatric Emergency Care, *Journal of Emergency Nursing*, 15(4), pp. 313–317.

Rajacich, D. & Cameron, S. (1995) Preventing Admissions of Seniors into the Emergency Department, *Journal of Gerontological Nursing*, 21, pp. 36–40.

Roth, J. (1972) Some Contingencies of the Moral Evaluation and Control of Clientele: the case of the hospital emergency service, *American Journal of Sociology*, 77(5), pp. 839–856.

Sanders, A. (1992) Care of the Elderly in Emergency Departments: conclusions and recommendations, *Annals of Emergency Medicine*, 21, pp. 830–834.

Sanders, A. & Morley, J. (1993) The Older Person and the Emergency Department, *Journal of the American Geriatric Society*, 41, pp. 880–882.

Sbaih, L. (1997a) The Work of Accident and Emergency Nurses: part 1. An Introduction to the Rules, *Accident and Emergency Nursing*, 5, pp. 28–33.

Sbaih, L. (1997b) The Work of Accident and Emergency Nurses: part 2. A&E Maxims: making A&E work unique and special, *Accident and Emergency Nursing*, 5, pp. 1–87.

Vreeken, A. & Hall, B. (1990) Emergency Care and the Geriatric Population, *Emergency Care Quarterly*, 6(1), pp. 27–34.

47

Frontiers in Group Dynamics: *Channels of Group Life; Social Planning and Action Research*

Kurt Lewin

A. Social Channels

1. If one is confronted with producing widespread social changes, perhaps changing food habits of a population through some method of education, certain basic problems of procedure immediately demand attention and require decision.

Should one use radio, posters, lectures, or other means and methods for changing efficiently group ideology and group action? Should one approach the total population of men, women, and children who are to change their food habits? Or would it be sufficient and perhaps even more effective to concentrate on a strategic part of the population? In other words, do all members of the population have equal importance in determining what is eaten? If not, the more important obviously should get special attention. At first glance it would seem that the housewife plays a particular role in determining food habits. To the extent that this proved to be correct, an efficient educational campaign should concentrate upon housewives. Similar problems come up in nearly all problems of social management. As a rule there is not enough time, personnel, and money to approach all members of the population which is to be affected. How can one find which members are the most important?

Source: *Human Relations*, 1 (1947): 143–153.

In answering this question the practitioner customarily looks for persons in "key positions." Thus if an attempt were to be made to reduce racial discrimination in a state, one might think of such key persons as certain types of community workers, industrialists, or politicians and concentrate efforts on these crucial areas in the community. I happened to encounter this problem in change experiments for the first time in regard to family food habits and would like to use this example for analyzing some of the factors involved.

2. Since the percentage of food that is wasted after it has once reached the family table is relatively small, one can state that changing food habits will be accomplished if one can change the character of the food that comes to the family table.

Food comes to the family table through certain "channels." One channel, and by far the most important in modern urban society, is buying at the grocery store. There may be, however, a number of such channels as, for example, growing vegetables in the garden. Within these channels food proceeds in definite steps. Figure 1 (p. 149) distinguishes in the buying channel a number of sections which correspond either to states of affairs or to significant happenings. If we consider the buying channel, the first segment of interest in this analysis is food at the grocery. It then proceeds into the segments, buying, and transportation home. Once the food is home the channel may be divided into at least two parallel arms corresponding to such alternatives as storage in the ice box or storage in the pantry. From here the food may go, with or without being cooked, to preparation for the table. Finally the food reaches the table.

By and large, changing food habits of the family is equivalent to changing the food that moves through this channel. If, therefore, we are to make a realistic analysis of the most efficient methods for bringing about changes in food habits, we have to ask what are the factors which determine the movement of food into and through the channels. To approach an answer to this question, we may ask: (a) What are the patterns of forces in the various sections; (b) What are the main variables which determine the forces?

3. If one follows the pattern of forces which determines the movement of food from one section to another, one finds that the buying situation plays an interesting role. Food does not move by itself but is moved directly or indirectly by an individual. For our purposes, however, it is quite permissible to represent the socio-psychological forces which influence the person who directs the movement of the food by forces acting directly on the food.

The buying situation may be characterized as a conflict situation. Let us assume that food one (Figure 1) is attractive, that the force ($f_{P,EF}^1$) toward eating is large. At the same time, however, the food may be very expensive, yielding an opposite force ($f_{P,SpM}^1$) against spending money which is also large. Since the opposing forces are both large, there will be considerable conflict involved in the purchase of this food. In the figure it is assumed that food number two is both unattractive and cheap. Here, too, there will be conflict, but in this case the conflict will be small. The force toward buying food may

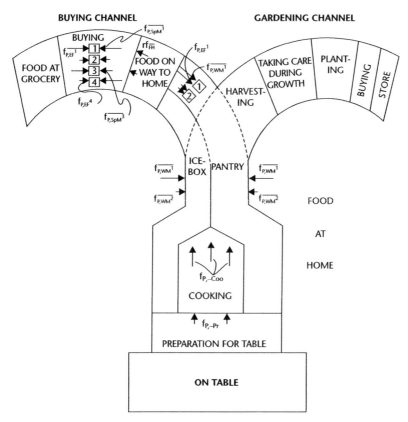

**CHANNELS THROUGH WHICH FOOD REACHES
THE FAMILY TABLE**

Figure 1

be composed of a number of components, such as the buyer's own like of the food, her knowledge of family likes and dislikes, or her ideas about which foods are "essential." The opposing forces may arise from a lack of readiness to spend a certain amount of money, a dislike of lengthy or disagreeable forms of preparation, unattractive taste, lack of fitness for the occasion, etc. Food is bought if the total force toward buying becomes greater than the opposing forces. Food number three in the figure illustrates such a case. Food of the type of number one may be called conflict food.

In a study of food habits conducted during the war in a mid-western community, a conflict rating was prepared for various foods on the basis of interviews with housewives. It is culturally significant that the average conflict rating was considerably higher in the middle economic group that in the high or low group. This conflict seemed to result from the greater discrepancy between the standards which this group wanted to keep up and their ability to do so in a situation of rising prices. If one compares, in this study, the conflict ratings of different foods for the same group of people, one finds that meat stands highest for the low economic group, whereas it is second for the middle, and third for the high economic group. These findings seem to indicate that the conflict between "like" and "expense" in the low economic group is most outspoken for meat. The relatively high conflict rating of vegetables for the high and middle economic groups seem to be due to conflicting forces corresponding to a desire to give healthy food to the family and the fact that vegetables are less well liked, or less easily prepared.

It is of the utmost importance to note that once food has passed through the segment of the channel, "buying," some of the forces change their direction. Let us assume that the housewife has finally decided to buy the high conflict food number one. Now, the situation will be quite different for the housewife. Having invested a substantial sum of money in the food, she will be especially insistent that the food safely reach the table and be eaten. The force against spending money, instead of keeping the food from moving through the channel, will now completely reverse its direction. In other words, the force ($f_{P,WM}{}^1$) against wasting money will have the same direction as the force toward eating this food, or it will have the character of a force against leaving the channel.

This example indicates that a certain area within a channel may function as a "gate"; the constellation of the forces before and after the gate region is decisively different in such a way that the passing or not passing of the unit through the whole channel depends to a high degree upon what happens in the gate region. This holds not only for food channels but also for the travelling of a news item through certain communication channels in a group, for movement of goods, and the social locomotion of individuals in many organizations. A university, for instance, might be quite strict in its admission policy and might set up strong forces against the passing of weak candidates. Once a student is admitted, however, the university frequently tries to do everything in its power to help everyone along. Many business organizations follow a similar policy. Organizations which discriminate against members of a minority group frequently use the argument that they are not ready to accept individuals whom they would be unable to promote sufficiently.

4. Gate sections are governed either by impartial rules or by "gate keepers." In the latter case an individual or group is "in power" for making the decision between "in" or "out." Understanding the functioning of the gate becomes equivalent then to understanding the factors which determine the decisions of the gate keepers and changing the social process means influencing or replacing the gate keeper.

The first diagnostic task in such cases is that of finding the actual gate keepers. In regard to food habits of the family, the answer was rather easily found. First of all, it is interesting to note that the gate keeper in the buying channel and the one in the gardening channel was frequently different. Very often the decision concerning the type of vegetables to be planted in the garden was made by the husband, rather than the wife. Once the decision has been made to grow a certain food, the forces operating on the food to pass through the channel to the table are similar in nature to those found in the buying channel. Efforts to change the family's eating habits, therefore, need to be directed towards the husband insofar as the family eats food grown in the garden. The gate keeper in the buying channel, on the other hand, was found to be most frequently the housewife, though in a small number of families within the highest economic group, it was found that the maids do the buying and thus determine what foods will enter the buying channel.

This is an example of a sociological investigation to determine who the gate keeper is and therefore to determine whose psychology has to be studied, who has to be educated if a change is to be accomplished. We shall not attempt here to give a detailed analysis of the factors determining the forces acting on the gate keeper. It should be realized, however, that the forces in the gate segment of the channel will vary considerably, depending on who the gate keeper is, and upon the total situation within the channel. If the pantry and ice box are getting too full, for example, the forces against buying any food will be increased. The amount of food available in the buying situation also plays a role. The preferences and aversions of the other family members are also important, their ideology about eating, status considerations, difficulties in preparing meals, etc.

It should be realized, however, that "supply and demand" in case of family buying as well as in larger economic settings does not directly affect the constellation at the gate. What counts is the effect which the situation in the various sections of the channel has on the gate keeper. (This is one of the reasons why a combination of economics with other social sciences is necessary for predicting actual group conduct.) Similarly, the effect of husband and children and any change of their desires will affect what comes on the table only to the degree that it affects the housewife.

Similar considerations hold for any social constellation which has the character of a channel, a gate and gate keepers. Discrimination against minorities will not be changed as long as forces are not changed which determine the decisions of the gate keepers. Their decisions depend partly on their ideology, that is their system of values and beliefs which determine what they consider to be "good" or "bad," and partly on the way they perceive the particular situation. Thus if we think of trying to reduce discrimination within a factory, a school system, or any other *organized institution*, we should consider the social life there as something which flows through certain channels. We then see that there are executives or boards who decide who is taken into the organization or who is kept out of it, who is promoted, and so on. The technique of discrimination in these organizations is closely linked with those mechanics which make the life of the members of an organization flow in definite channels. Thus discrimination is basically linked with problems of management, with the actions of gate keepers who determine what is done and what is not done.

5. The relation between social channels, social perception, and decision is methodologically and practically of considerable significance. The theory of channels and gate keepers helps to define more precisely how certain "objective" sociological problems of locomotion of goods and persons intersect with "subjective" psychological and cultural problems. It points to sociologically characterized places, likes gates in social channels, where attitudes count most for certain social processes and where individual or group decisions have a particularly great social affect.

The particularly impressive changes in food habits which were attained by means of group decision emphasizes the relation of channels to the position of the group and to social diagnosis. This relation is twofold: (*a*) Group decisions depend partly on how the group views the situation, and it therefore can be influenced by a change in this perception; (*b*) Group perception of the result of social action is essential to decision about the next step. This latter point we should like to consider somewhat more closely by discussing certain problems of planning.

B. Feedback Problems of Social Diagnosis and Action

1. Many channels of social life have not simply a beginning and an end but are circular in character. The large section of the channel which leads food from the grocery store into the mouths of the family members or into the garbage can is actually a part of another circular process. This process includes dishwashing, receiving money from the husband, and other sections of housekeeping which follow each other in a circular way. Many of the sections are interdependent in that finishing one starts the next.

Organized social life is full of such circular channels. Some of these circular processes correspond to what the physical engineer calls feedback systems, that is, systems which show some kind of self-regulation. One of these systems will be discussed here as an example of problems of social steering or self evaluation.

2. Planned social action usually emerges from a more or less vague "idea." An objective appears in the cloudy form of a dream or a wish, which hardly can be called a goal. To become real, to be able to steer action, something has to be developed which might be called a "plan." The transition from an idea to a plan presupposes that: (i) The objective has to be clarified; (ii) The path to the goal and the available means have to be determined; (iii) A strategy of action has to be developed. These three items together make up the "general plan" which is to precede action.

It should be noted that the development of a general plan presupposes "fact-finding." The original state of the idea of the goal corresponds to an area in the social field or the life space of the individual that is but little structured in itself (Figure 2) and the relation of which to the rest of the field is not clearly determined. Fact-finding is necessary to structure the goal, its relation to the

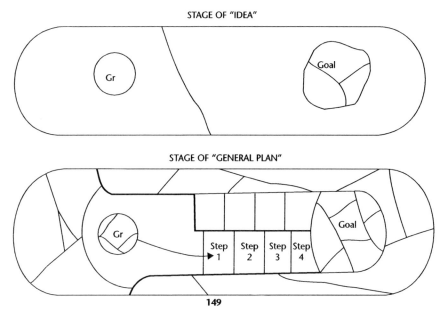

STAGE OF "IDEA"

STAGE OF "GENERAL PLAN"

149

Figure 2

total setting and the path and means which may lead to the goal. On the basis of this fact-finding the goal is usually somewhat altered in light of the findings concerning the means available.

The emerging "general plan" corresponds to a field (lower diagram in Figure 2) which contains the structure of the goal, and the steps to the goal in sufficient detail to serve as a blueprint for action. It is important, however, that such a plan be not too much frozen. To be effective, plans should be "flexible." The flexibility of plans requires the following pattern of procedure: Accepting a plan does not mean that all further steps are fixed by a final decision; only in regard to the first step should the decision be final. After the first action is carried out, the second step should not follow automatically. Instead it should be investigated whether the effect of the first action was actually what was expected.

In military terms, reconnaissance should provide data about where one now stands and whether the field has changed significantly. The result of the reconnaissance after the first step of action should be twofold: (i) It might be necessary to alter the "general plan"; (ii) The basis is given for a final decision on the second step. After the second step again reconnaissance follows, leading again to an alteration of the general plan and the decision on the next step Figure 3 (p. 149).

This pattern of planned group action is probably developed in most detail in the army. It is widespread, however, in many areas of social life, frequently though in a rather rudimentary form. To understand what kind of social organization is required for efficient planned group action one can refer to the pattern of certain goal seeking machines.

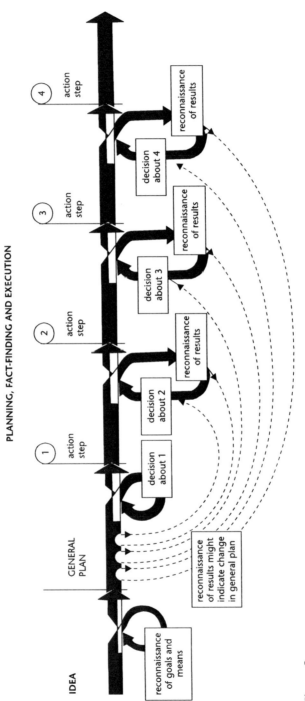

PLANNING, FACT-FINDING AND EXECUTION

Figure 3

3. During the war a multitude of self-steering missiles were developed, goal seeking machines which can reach their target with a remarkable degree of precision. Basically, these goal seeking machines have two components: one is equivalent to a sense organ, perhaps a radar eye; the other is an action organ, for instance, a gun which shoots bullets. If the beam from the target hits the eye of center, a mechanism is set into motion which automatically turns the eye to the center and changes the direction of the action organ toward the target. In other words, the eye functions as a steering mechanism. Technically this is achieved by so-called "feedback" processes which link three entities, namely: (i) the position of the target, (ii) the sense organ, (iii) the action organ. The action organ is continuously steered toward the goal with the help of the sense organ which "seeks" to eliminate divergencies between action and goal.

Some actions of human beings such as driving a car or reaching for a glass of water are steered by a functionally equivalent process. The individual watches the discrepancy between the direction of his action and the direction toward the goal, and this perceived discrepancy more or less automatically steers his action.

Is there anything equivalent in social life to steer social action? What are our social sense organs? How about the steering process?

The engineer knows of steering processes which have no reference to the outside. An example is the system which assures that the rudder of a ship follows every turn of the steering wheel at the captain's bridge. This system lies entirely within the ship and has no relation to points outside. In administration such steering corresponds to a case where a superintendent reports back to the manager of the factory that he has carried out the required action of hiring an expert. That, of course, does not assure that the action has the desired effect of improving the course of the organisation. Of similar nature is the following example: Citizens who feel that certain group relations do not follow an appropriate course get together and try to give the wheel a turn toward the right direction by arranging a brotherhood day. They are elated for having done a good job if the meeting was impressive. Perhaps, however, they should be compared with the captain who hears that his course is too much to the left, rushes to the wheel, turns it to the right and, having done so, goes happily to dinner. In the meantime, his boat goes around in circles.

A good number of our social or administrative actions are of a similar nature. The effort might lead to the satisfaction of the action but actually it does not reach the objective. The reason for the shortcoming, expressed in terms of feedback systems, is that all the inter-dependent parts of the process lie within the moving boat. What is missing is a link which steers the action by its effect on the outside rather than by the effect within the organization.

In many fields of social management as, for instance, in those dealing with minority problems, education, conducting conferences, or committees, we lack signposts of exactly where we are and in what direction we are moving with what velocity. As a result, the actors are uncertain of themselves, they are at the mercy of likes or dislikes of bosses, colleagues, or the public. Perhaps even more important, however, they are unable to "learn." In a field that lacks objective standards of achievement, no learning can take place. If we cannot judge whether an action has led forward or backward, if we have no criteria for evaluating the relation between effort and achievement, there is nothing to prevent us from making the wrong conclusions and to encourage the wrong work habits. Realistic fact-finding and evaluation is a prerequisite for any learning. No wonder that a recent survey of workers in group relations revealed that one of their great difficulties is their feeling of unclearness about what they should do.

An efficient steering of social action presupposes that fact-finding methods have to be developed which permit a sufficiently realistic determination of the nature and position of the social goal and of the direction and the amount of locomotion resulting from a given action. To be effective, this fact-finding has to be linked with the action organization itself: it has to be part of a feedback system which links a reconnaissance branch of the organization with the branches which do the action. The feedback has to be done so that a discrepancy between the desired and the actual direction leads "automatically" to a correction of actions or to a change of planning.

Accounting systems in business are designed to function as reconnaissance parts in the feedback system of a social group. The effectiveness of these and other methods of fact-finding depend upon the frequency with which the reconnaissance is carried out, whether it reaches the really essential data, whether the reconnaissance is transmitted to a sufficiently powerful level in the hierarchy of steering, without channeling so many fact-findings into that steering group that it is overburdened.

4. The research needed for social practice can best be characterized as research for social management or social engineering. It is a type of action-research, a comparative research on the conditions and effects of various forms of social action, and research leading to social action. Research that produces nothing but books will not suffice.

This by no means implies that the research needed is in any respect less scientific or "lower" than what would be required for pure science in the field of social events. I am inclined to hold the opposite to be true. Institutions interested in engineering, such as the Massachusetts Institute of Technology, have turned more and more to what is called basic research. In regard to social engineering, too, progress will depend largely on the rate with which basic research in social sciences can develop deeper insight into the laws which govern social life. This "basic social research" will have to include mathematical and conceptual problems of theoretical analysis. It will have to include the whole range of descriptive fact-finding in regard to small and large social bodies. Above all, it will have to include laboratory and field experiments in social change.

Field experiments are basically not different from laboratory experiments. An experiment as opposed to a mere descriptive analysis tries to study the effect of conditions by some way of measuring or bringing about certain changes under sufficiently controlled conditions. The objective is to understand the laws which govern the nature of the phenomena under study, in our case the nature of group life.

A change (ch) refers to the difference between a preceding situation (S) and a following situation which has emerged out of the first as a result of some inner or outer influences. (Ch $= S_{after} - S_{before}$). A law is found if this change, ch, can be linked to a function, f, of certain factors x and y which are found to be responsible for that change. Not all laws have this form. However, this form represents one of the simplest patterns of a law and characterizes also a certain type of experimental procedure and analysis.

This type of experiment, whether laboratory or field experiment, has as its objective the study of three situations or processes, namely: (*a*) the character of the beginning situation, (*b*) some happenings designed to bring about certain change, (*c*) a study of the end situation to see the actual effect of the happening on the beginning situation. A diagnosis of the before and after situation permits us to define the change or effect; studying the happening should be designed to characterize the factors which brought about this change.

It is obvious that the quality and exactness of the conclusions that might be drawn cannot be larger than the degree to which all three parts of the process can be analyzed. It demands a measurement of the situation before and after but equally a careful description and analysis of those happenings which brought about the change.

In case of a field experiment such as a workshop, this means that an analysis of the situation before and after the workshop is needed to define the change created by the workshop. It means also that the workshop itself would have to be described as carefully and accurately as possible with the objective of finding out as much as possible exactly what type of happening had created this change.

Here, I feel, research faces its most difficult task. To record the content of the lecture or the program would by no means suffice. Description of the form of leadership has to take into account the amount of initiative shown by individuals and subgroups, the division of the trainees into subgroups, the frictions within and between these subgroups, the crises and their outcome, and, above all, the total management pattern as it changes from day to day. These large-scale aspects, more than anything else, seem to determine what a program of action will accomplish. The task which social scientists have to face in objectively recording these data is not too different from that of the historian. We will have to learn to handle these relatively large units of periods and social bodies without lowering the standards of validity and reliability to which we are accustomed in the psychological recording of the more microscopic units of action and periods of minutes or seconds of activity.

One of the difficulties which a description of happenings as extended as the workshop presents to the psychologist is the mere size. Historians have been accustomed to dealing with units of decades and hundreds of years. Psychologists have been more accustomed to minutes and seconds. The particular meaning which the term analysis had to the scientist in the nineteenth century and in the beginning of the twentieth, has identified scientific procedure to many psychologists with procedures which deal with minute time periods. It is only recently that some of us have lost the prejudice according to which the description of a large unit is less scientific than the description of a small unit.

Even those among us who in principle do not like to discriminate against large units have to face a task which is new and a bit frightening even to the brave soul. It raises the question: can we hope to use as objective a description and measurement of large social units as we have been able, at least to the degree we have learned to characterize and measure small units? Is there any way to keep up our standards of reliability and objectivity? At present I feel the social scientist is threatened by the Scylla of losing his "objectivity" by the attempt to deal with sufficiently large and meaningful units on the one hand, and by the Charybdis of losing the "validity" of his study by dealing with inadequate and frequently too small units.

5. Any research program set up within the framework of an organization desiring significant social action must be guided closely by the needs of that organization, and must help define those needs more specifically. Usually there will be three kinds of problems to which the research staff must apply themselves:

Immediate problems. There will be a number of problems requiring some immediate program of action. Experience has shown that the research social scientist can make two contributions here: (*a*) As consultants on methods of action. The accumulation of scientific findings concerning social action techniques is mounting daily and only a technician in this field can be expected to keep up with them. (*b*) As evaluation experts. Major actions should not be launched without proper provisions being made for the evaluation of the success of the action and for the discovery of more effective modifications which may be found. Adequate evaluation is a technical research problem.

Pre-testing. Pre-testing by experimental trying-out of certain potential lines of action with properly selected groups and adequately defined controls is one of the most practical refinements of science, and one of the surest guides to sound administrative policy.

Long-term policies and action programs. As research proceeds, it will become more and more valuable for determining long term policies and action programs. By delegating to the research worker certain responsibilities and freedoms to carry on what is sometimes called "pure research" in a general area of dynamics it is safe to assume that certain basic data for long term planning will gradually emerge. While research of this type sometimes does not look immediately "practical," those in the past who have backed this line of activity have reaped a rich harvest of efficiency, economy and effectiveness.

6. Obviously social management in the various areas of modern society have to face a tremendous task. Its solution presupposes social fact-finding of an unheard of magnitude. It requires basic research about social steering systems. The fear of fascism seems to have driven some people into the greatest kind of misunderstanding which identifies democracy with planlessness. The survival and development of democracy depends not so much on the development of democratic ideals which are wide-spread and strong. Today, more than ever before, democracy depends upon the development of efficient forms of democratic social management and upon the spreading of the skill in such management to the common man.

The social scientists, perhaps more than the natural scientists, have to learn to be unafraid and at the same time fair-minded. To my mind, fair-mindedness is the essence of scientific objectivity. The scientist has to learn to look facts straight in the face, even if they do not agree with his prejudices. He must learn this without giving up his belief in values, that is, without regressing to the pre-war cynicism of the campus. He has to learn to understand how scientific and moral aspects are frequently interlocked in problems, and how the scientific aspects may still be approached. He has to see realistically the problems of power, which are interwoven with many of the questions he is to study, without his becoming a servant to vested interests. His realism should be akin to courage in the sense of Plato, who defines courage as wisdom in the face of danger.

The problem of our own values, objectives, and of objectivity are nowhere more interwoven and more important than in action-research. Fortunately the work of social scientists during the war has created in a good many people just this spirit.

Research in group dynamics is, as a rule, group research. It requires the cooperation of persons who steer group life and who record and measure various aspects of group life. One cannot overemphasize the importance of the spirit of cooperation and of social responsibility for research on group processes. To my mind it is equally important that the same spirit of cooperation dominate the relations between the various institutions which happily have become active in this field.

Editors' Note

When Professor Lewin wrote the article which appeared in the first issue of HUMAN RELATIONS, he planned to follow it with a second. Before his untimely death he was working on the manuscript of this article. Although it was far from finished and in a very preliminary form, what he had written seemed sufficiently complete to warrant publication. The present organization of the material has been made by the editors from the manuscript which Professor Lewin had prepared.

Bibliography

1. Lewin, K. Forces behind food habits and methods of change. *Bulletin of the National Research Council*, 1943, *108*, 35–65.
2. Lewin, K. Action research and minority problems. *J. Soc. Issues*, 1946, *2*, 34–46.
3. Lewin, K. Frontiers in group dynamics. I. Concept, method and reality in social science; social equilibria. *Human Relations*, 1947, *1*, 5–40.

48

An Assessment of the Scientific Merits of Action Research

Gerald I. Susman and Roger D. Evered

Crisis in Organizational Science

There is a crisis in the field of organizational science. The principal symptom of this crisis is that as our research methods and techniques have become more sophisticated, they have also become increasingly less useful for solving the practical problems that members of organizations face.

Many of the findings in our scholarly management journals are only remotely related to the real world of practicing managers and to the actual issues with which members of organizations are concerned, especially when the research has been carried out by the most rigorous methods of the prevailing conception of science. Whatever its shortcomings in method and conception, early research such as that by Fayol, Barnard, Urwick, Roethlisberger, and even Taylor, unlike the more recent organizational research, was at least grounded in the actual problems faced by organizational members and was carried out in close collaboration between researcher and practitioner. Sometimes researcher and practitioner were the same person.

The crisis in organizational science is also reflected in the failure to recognize latent values behind the claim to neutrality about how knowledge is generated. The methods of organizational science have generated knowledge that has led to improvements in the effectiveness and efficiency of organizations, but often at the expense of the quality of working life of their members (Davis and Taylor, 1972).

Source: *Administrative Science Quarterly*, 23(4) (1978): 582–603.

Additionally, the crisis in organizational science is reflected in a conception of research as an accumulation of social facts that can be drawn on by practitioners when they are ready to apply them. This conception encourages a separation of theory from practice because published research is read more by producers of research than by practitioners. As a result, practitioners and their clients complain more and more frequently about the lack of relevance of published research for the problems they face and about the lack of responsiveness of researchers to meeting their needs.

What appears at first to be a crisis of relevancy or usefulness of organizational science is, we feel, really a crisis of epistemology. This crisis has risen, in our judgment, because organizational researchers have taken the positivist model of science which has had great heuristic value for the physical and biological sciences and some fields of the social sciences, and have adopted it as the ultimate model of what is best for organizational science. By limiting its methods to what it claims is value-free, logical, and empirical, the positivist model of science when applied to organizations produces a knowledge that may only inadvertently serve and sometimes undermine the values of organizational members.

This article describes the deficiencies of positivist science for generating knowledge for use in solving problems that members of organizations face. Action research is presented as a method for generating knowledge that corrects these deficiencies. Action research is then tested against the criteria of positivist science and is found not to meet its critical tests. Action research is shown to be able to base its scientific legitimacy in philosophical traditions that are different from those which legitimate positivist science. Criteria and methods of science appropriate to action research are offered.

Deficiencies of Positivist Science

The positivist conception of science has dominated the physical, biological, and social sciences for more than a hundred years. Comte (1864) who is generally credited with the term positivism, used the word "positive" to refer to the actual in contrast to the imaginary, to what can claim certainty in contrast to the undecided, to the exact in contrast to the indefinite. We will use the term positivist science for all approaches to science that consider scientific knowledge to be obtainable only from sense data that can be directly experienced and verified between independent observers. Although commitment to an empirical base for scientific knowledge characterizes what we are calling positivist science, the term subsumes different approaches to generating scientific knowledge. In one approach, which Oquist (1978) labels empiricism, rigorous observation is all that is needed to generate scientific knowledge. Theory is avoided because adherents of this approach believe that theory leads to multiple interpretations and distortions of the observed data. This approach is not widely used in organizational research. Organizational research using behavior modification techniques comes closest to this approach (Luthans and Kreitner, 1975). Radnitsky (1970) labels five "schools" of philosophy which are committed to an empirical base for scientific knowledge as Formalist, Reconstructionist, Pragmatist, Pragmaticist, and Anglo-linguistic. The most representative members of the Formalist school are Russell, members of the Vienna Circle such as Carnap, and, more recently, Hempel. The most well-known member of the Reconstructionist school is Bergmann. The Pragmatist school includes Dewey and James, the Pragmaticist school consists of Peirce, and the Anglo-linguistic school includes Wittgenstein, Austin, and Anscombe.

Radnitsky uses the term "worldpicture" for a conception of the world that Reconstructionists formally acknowledge and Formalists unintentionally encourage. This worldpicture may be characterized by the following four assumptions.

1. The world exists a priori as a unified and causally ordered system.
2. The structure of the world can be inferred from empirical observation.
3. Data about the world can be logically reconstructed into laws which are applicable regardless of the meaning humans may give to the terms of such laws.
4. A morphological correspondence can be established between the structure of logic and the structure of the world Since propositions about the world can be hierarchically organized from the more abstract and general to the more concrete and specific, the world must be so organized. The discovery of a general scientific proposition from which all other scientific propositions can be deduced is considered to be, at least, a realistic possibility.

Since laws are hierarchically organized, according to this worldpicture, knowledge advances either by deduction or by induction. In the first case, new propositions are deduced from previously accepted laws. These new propositions are considered confirmed when their terms can be linked to objects or events, and the relationships between these objects or events can be shown empirically to correspond to relations between the terms of the proposition. In the second case, objective and undistorted observations of associations between discrete objects or events are noted. These associations are scientifically explained only if they can be shown to be particular cases following under more general laws. According to the Formalist and Reconstructionist worldpicture, inductions developed from raw data will meet deductions developed from yet more general propositions creating ultimately a unified hierarchical system of knowledge.

Both Formalists and Reconstructionists have confidence that a universal denotative language such as mathematics or logic can further the growth of scientific knowledge. Mathematics and logic allow a community of scientists to achieve consensus on the validity of scientific propositions. Observational language, another specialized type, reduces sentences used in ordinary speech to sentences that can be verified by direct observation. For example, the sentence "The bear frightens me" can be transformed into "The sight of the bear is associated with the beads of sweat forming on my brow and the trembling of my hands." One of the objectives of Formalists and Reconstructionists is to unite logic and mathematical sentences with observational sentences through "correspondence rules" (see Carnap, 1936, 1937), e.g., if A (bear), then B (beads of sweat), and C (trembling hands).

The Formalist and Reconstructionist worldpicture is an inadequate basis for generating knowledge about organizations and more particularly for developing problem-solving methods if one adapts the following perspective on organizations.

1. Organizations are artifacts created by human beings to serve their ends. Organizations obey laws that are affected by human purposes and actions. In this sense, they do not exist independently of human beings, like the planets, just waiting for an Isaac Newton of organizational theory to discover an equivalent of the laws of planetary motion.
2. Organizations are systems of human action in which the means and ends are guided by values. Consequently, judging the morality of proposed solutions to organizational problems is inescapable.
3. Empirical observation and logical reconstruction of organizational activities are not sufficient for a science of organization because:

    A. Organizations are planned according to their members' conception of the future. But statements about the future have no truth value according to any criterion of confirmation acceptable to positivist science.
    B. Organizations can be understood experientially by organizational researchers so that the truth of many propositions about organizations need not be supported empirically or validated logically.

4. Organizations can be legitimate objects of scientific inquiry only as single cases without considering whether such cases are subsumable under general laws. Knowledge about what actions are appropriate for problem-solving need not be derived by reference to a general category of similar organizations from which we know what the best action to take is on average.

Pragmatists and Pragmaticists differed from Formalists and Reconstructionists in not believing that any worldpicture was a necessary foundation for scientific inquiry. They believed that claims to knowledge were legitimized not by their relationship to an underlying reality but, rather, by the norms and rules of inquiry itself which are themselves open to rational criticism. Peirce (1955) characterized the pragmaticist criterion of truth as the ideal limit of the ultimate opinion of an indefinite community of investigators.

Anglo-linguists did not believe that a universal denotative language such as mathematics or logic could be united with observational language through correspondence rules. Although a Formalist, Hempel (1950) did not believe this either. He and the Anglo-linguists rejected the exclusive use of specialized languages for scientific inquiry. The Anglo-linguists pursued their investigations with language in everyday use.

Although Pragmatists, Pragmaticists, and Anglo-linguists avoid the difficulties that Reconstructionists and Formalists create for organizational research by support of their worldpicture or by the search for correspondence rules between types of language, we find all positivist approaches to science (P.S.) to be deficient in their capacity to generate knowledge for use by members of organizations for solving the problems they face. The following arguments explain this deficiency.

P.S. assumes that its methods are value neutral. As Habermas (1971) points out, knowledge and human interests are interwoven, as reflected in the choice of methods and the ends toward which such methods are put. The primary criteria of confirmation for P.S. are prediction and control of its objects of study, whether they be human or otherwise. When the objects of study are human, methods based on deception and manipulation are not uncommonly used to assure that the experimenter will get the results he or she predicted. It is not too difficult to translate the word "experimenter" into that of "manager" to see the moral implications of extrapolating methods and ends from the "laboratory" to the organization. Habermas pointed out that unless we reflect on the ends to be served by science, we may unwittingly find that prediction and control and its attendant methods will exclude other ends such as improved understanding among persons and the release of human potential. P.S. treats persons as objects of inquiry, even though they are subjects or initiators of action in their own right. Humans differ from objects in their capacity for self-reflection and their ability to collaborate in the diagnosis of their own problems and in the generation of knowledge.

P.S. eliminates the role of history in the generation of knowledge. Individuals and organizations are not born in an instant with their present structures and functions intact. Rather, present patterns of behavior can many times only be understood as the product of shared definitions held by organizational members regarding what their common endeavor is about. These definitions may have evolved from the unique history of a particular organization, its periods of exceptional performance, the psycho-social defenses of its members, its prior leaders, etc.

P.S. assumes that a system is defined only to the extent that a denotative language exists to describe it. However, any representational system is always less than the actual system leaving the practicing manager to rely on intuition, hunch, interpretation, etc. P.S. generally acknowledges that such methods can be precursors to scientific knowledge, but it does not consider them by themselves to be legitimate scientific methods. As Polanyi (1958) has pointed out, such methods generate "tacit knowledge." Rather than poor substitutes for articulation, such methods encourage a deeper understanding of organizational values, encourage consideration of new organizational forms, and facilitate recognition of clues to the new forms the organization might take.

P.S. is itself a product of the human mind, thus knowledge of the inquirer cannot be excluded from an understanding of how knowledge is generated. If a human's consciousness, worldviews, language, etc., are a product of the history of ideas as well as of social and economic development, then a social science model that ignores this product will ratify the past rather than help to create a better future.

Our view is that action research is a mode of inquiry more congenial to the perspective on organizations we characterized above and avoids the deficiencies of positivist science for generating knowledge for application to organizational problems.

Origins of Action Research

The term "action research" was introduced by Kurt Lewin in 1946 to denote a pioneering approach toward social research which combined generation of theory with changing the social system through the researcher acting on or in the social system. The act itself is presented as the means of both changing the system and generating critical knowledge about it.

Lewin gave us a clear picture of what he meant by action research and how it differed from traditional positivist science. His letters between 1944 and 1946 expressed profound concern and urgency for finding methods to deal with critical social problems (fascism, anti-Semitism, poverty, inter-group conflict, minority issues, etc.) (Marrow, 1969). He characterized action research as "a comparative research on the conditions and effects of various forms of social action and research leading to social action (1946: 202–203). The immediacy of critical social issues forms an essential ingredient of action research. Indeed, the first article containing the term action research (Lewin, 1946) was entitled "Action Research and Minority Problems," indicating Lewin's concern that traditional science was not helping in the resolution of critical social problems.

Lewin's laboratory is the change experiment on the social system in which the practitioners and social scientists collaborate to find ways to bring about needed changes. The process is conceived as "a spiral of steps, each of which is composed of a circle of planning, action, and fact-finding about the result of the action" (1946: 206). Workshops conducted jointly by the practitioners and scientists would have the triple function of action, research, and training "as a triangle that should be kept together for the sake of any of the corners" (1946: 211). Training referred to "the training of . . . social scientists who can handle scientific problems but are also equipped for the delicate task of building productive hard-hitting teams of practitioners" (p. 211).

Action research had a parallel but independent development in Britain during the same years that Lewin was formulating his ideas. It began with a World War II group which later formed the Tavistock Institute of Human Relations. This interdisciplinary group drew more on psychoanalysis and social psychiatry than on social and experimental psychology, as did Lewin. But like Lewin, the group was committed to the social engagement of the social sciences, both as a strategy for advancing fundamental knowledge and as a way of enabling the social sciences to contribute solutions to important social problems. One of the group's first projects was the civil repatriation of prisoners of war. Twenty transitional communities were designed partly on data contributed by the repatriated prisoners and partly on the results of the experiments (Wilson, Trist, and Curle, 1952) at Northfield, a military psychiatric hospital with self-governing wards, in which pioneering group therapy techniques were developed by Bion (see Bion, 1946; Bridger, 1946). Subsequently, the Tavistock Institute has broadened its original medical orientation to action research by focusing on engagement with large-scale social systems (see Trist, 1976).

John Collier (1945), who was Commissioner of Indian Affairs from 1933–1945, must also be credited with recognizing the need for developing an approach to generating action-oriented knowledge that requires collaboration between researcher, practitioner, and client.

Definition of Action Research

Rapoport's (1970: 499) definition of action research is, perhaps, the most frequently quoted in contemporary literature on the subject:

> Action research aims to contribute both to the practical concerns of people in an immediate problematic situation and to the goals of social science by joint collaboration within a mutually acceptable ethical framework.

To the aims of contributing to the practical concerns of people and to the goals of social science, we add a third aim, to develop the self-help competencies of people facing problems.

Foster (1972) suggested that the two aims of action research in the Rapoport definition be sought through the process of changing the problem situation itself. The small face-to-face group is the primary medium through which the problem situation may be changed, as well as in which the interests and ethics of the various parties to this process may be developed "within a mutually acceptable ethical framework." An infra-structure of ad hoc and permanent face-to-face groups is generally developed within a client system to conduct action research. A client system is the social system in which the members face problems to be solved by action research. It may be one of the face-to-face groups, an organization, a network of organizations (Trist, 1977), or a community.

While Rapoport's definition of action research focuses on aim, action research can also be viewed as a cyclical process with five phases: diagnosing, action planning, action taking, evaluating, and specifying learning. The infrastructure within the client system and the action researcher maintain and regulate some or all of these five phases jointly (Figure).

We consider all five phases to be necessary for a comprehensive definition of action research. However, action research projects may differ in the number of phases which are carried out in collaboration between action researcher and the client system. Chein, Cook, and Harding (1948) use the term "diagnostic action research" when the researcher is involved only in collecting data for diagnosis and feeding the data back to the client system. Chein, Cook, and Harding use the term "empirical action research" when the researcher only evaluates the actions undertaken by the client system and feeds data back to it. They use the term "participant action research" when diagnosing and action planning are carried out in collaboration between researcher and client system. Finally, they use the term "experimental action research" when researcher and client system collaborate in all or nearly all phases to set up an experiment for taking an action and evaluating its consequences.

In addition to the number of phases that can be carried out in collaboration between action researchers and the client system, contemporary applications of action research can use different techniques for data collection especially in

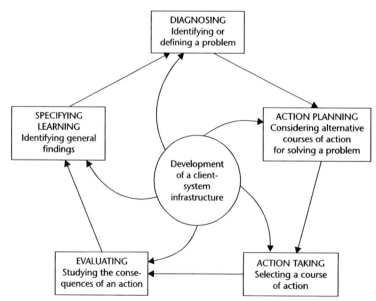

Figure: The cyclical process of action research

the diagnosing and evaluating phases. Action researchers with a background in psychology tend to prefer questionnaires for such purposes, e.g., those affiliated with the Institute for Social Research at the University of Michigan (Mann, 1957; Seashore and Bowers, 1964; Nadler, 1977), while action researchers with a background in applied anthropology, psychoanalysis or sociotechnical systems tend to prefer direct observation and/or in-depth interviewing (Jaques, 1951; Rice, 1958; Whyte and Hamilton, 1964; Duckles, Duckles, and Maccoby, 1977; Trist, Susman, and Brown, 1977) Action researchers with any of these backgrounds may also retrieve data from the records, memos, and reports that the client system routinely produces.

Action Research as a Corrective to the Deficiencies of Positivist Science

Six characteristics of action research provide a corrective to the deficiencies of positivist science we discussed earlier. These characteristics are representative of the methods and objectives of key developers and practitioners of action research (A.R.).

A.R. is future oriented. In dealing with the practical concerns of people, A.R. is oriented toward creating a more desirable future for them. Human beings are therefore recognized as purposeful systems (Ackoff and Emery, 1972) the actions of which are guided by goals, objectives, and ideals. In being future-oriented, A.R. has close affinities to the planning process, so that planning research may be potentially useful in informing A.R. and vice versa.

A.R. is collaborative. Interdependence between researcher and the client system is an essential feature of action research, and the direction of the research process will be partly a function of the needs and competencies of the two. On the one hand, A.R., as Cherns, Clark, and Jenkins (1976: 33) state, "challenges the position of the social scientist as privileged observer, analyst, and critic." On the other hand, it prevents him from taking the role of disinterested observer and obliges him to clarify and represent his own ethics and values so that they, along with those of the client system, can serve as guidelines against which to assess jointly planneed actions.

A.R. implies system development. The action research process encourages the development of the capacity of a system to facilitate, maintain, and regulate the cyclical process of diagnosing, action planning, action taking, evaluating, and specifying learning. The aim in action research is to build appropriate structures, to build the necessary system and competencies, and to modify the relationship of the system to its relevant environment. The focus is on generating the necessary communication and problem-solving procedures. The infrastructure of the system, which the action research generates, is the key instrument for (1) alleviating the immediate problematic situation, and (2) generating new knowledge about system processes.

A.R. generates theory grounded in action. In action research, theory provides a guide for what should be considered in the diagnosis of an organization as well as for generating possible courses of action to deal with the problems of members of the organization. This is the case for psychoanalytic theory, Lewinian field theory, and general systems theory (see Susman, 1976). Furthermore, A.R. contributes to the development of theory by taking actions guided by theory and evaluating their consequences for the problems members of organizations face. Theory may then be supported or revised on the basis of the evaluation.

A.R. is agnostic. The action researcher recognizes that his or her theories and prescriptions for action are themselves the product of previously taken action and, therefore, are subject to reexamination and reformulation upon entering every new research situation. The action researcher also recognizes that the objectives, the problem, and the method of the research must be generated from the process itself, and that the consequences of selected actions cannot be fully known ahead of time.

A.R. is situational. The action researcher knows that many of the relationships between people, events, and things are a function of the situation as relevant actors currently define it. Such relationships are not often invariant (Blumer, 1956) or free of their context, but can change as the definition of the situation changes. Appropriate action is based not on knowledge of the replications of previously observed relationships between actions and outcomes. It is based on knowing how particular actors define their present situations or on achieving consensus on defining situations so that planned actions will produce their intended outcomes.

Is Action Research Scientific?

One criterion of positivist science for judging whether action research is scientific is whether relationships between actions and their consequences can be explained as particular cases falling under more general laws governing types of actions and their consequences. If relationships between actions and consequences can be explained in this way, then the action researcher will know what action to take in future settings by reference to types of actions having lawful relationships to consequences. "Covering law" is the term which Hempel (1965), a leading contemporary philosopher of the Formalist school, applied to a general law which explains a particular case by "covering" or subsuming it. Covering laws are the basis for the only two kinds of explanation that Hempel considered as meriting the label of being scientific; that is, the *deductive-nomological* and the *inductive-statistical* forms. In terms of organizational action, the deductive-nomological type of explanation has the following form: (a) Actions of type A always produce consequences of type C in a given class of situations, (b) Person X takes action A in a particular situation, thus (c) A consequence of type C occurs. In a deductive-nomological explanation, sentence (a) must state a general law about the consequences of human action, while (b) cites a particular fact or event. Sentence (c) (the explicandum) is derived from sentences (a) and (b) (jointly the explicans). Sentence (a) is considered to be a strictly universal form. It asserts that in all cases in which certain specifiable conditions are realized, the action A implies consequence C (that is, the outcome is certain to occur).

The inductive-statistical type of explanation asserts that if certain specifiable conditions are realized, then a particular event will occur with a certain statistical probability. Inductive-statistical explanations have the following form: (a') The likelihood that a consequence of type C will follow action of type A, is some value L, (b') Person X takes action A, thus (c') A consequence of type C will occur with a particular likelihood.

The value of L is not any particular mean of a sampling distribution that represents a long-run frequency with which events of type A are followed by consequences of type C. Rather, it refers to the "degree of rational credibility" (Carnap, 1950) or logical inductive probability which sentence c', the explicandum possesses relative to sentences a' + b', the explicans.

Hempel considered the deductive-nomological model the more desirable, since it provides a higher degree of certainty in the explanation of events. Furthermore, if the explicans precedes the explicandum in time, the model is called a causal model (Evered, 1976). On the other hand, the inductive-statistical model is superior in that any single falsified prediction will not invalidate the explanatory model, as it would for the deductive-nomological model.

Although most contemporary organizational research uses the inductive-statistical model of explanation, Hempel considered it less desirable than the deductive-nomological on these grounds: (1) It cannot predict an outcome with certainty; (2) It cannot explain why any unpredictable outcome has actually occurred, and is therefore, strictly speaking, a noncausal model; (3) Statistical regularity does not allow one to make a specific choice in a concrete situation; and (4) Statistical regularities do not explain why two kinds of events or things are strongly associated.

Although Hempel believed that the logic of all scientific explanations is of the covering-law variety, he did not believe that all empirical phenomena were scientifically explainable or that they are all governed by a system of determinable laws. He acknowledges that there are other ways by which we may explain why some thing or event exists or happens; he just would not call them scientific explanations. On the other hand, he considered it the task of the philosopher to determine together with the scientist whether or not these other forms of explanation could be translated into covering-law terms and be tested. Hempel did not believe we could determine which explanations were scientific a priori.

We will now examine whether actions and their consequences can be subsumed under covering laws, thus permitting them the status of scientific explanation by positivist criteria.

Status of an Action as a Thing or Event

The search for generalizations about the relationship between actions and consequences is ill-conceived if actions are assumed to have a meaning independent of their associations with the outcomes they are intended to produce. Unlike behavior that follows a caused event, i.e., the man trips over a crack in the sidewalk (Anscombe, 1958, confers causal status on events like these), actions are undertaken because of beliefs concerning the ends they are intended to produce, i.e., I am shuffling through the papers on my desk in order to find my glasses. As Hempel pointed out, we cannot explain the actions undertaken without reference to the ends pursued or vice versa, e.g., why is he shuffling through the papers on his desk? He is looking for his glasses. Or the question, Is he looking for his glasses? Well, he is shuffling through papers on his desk. Answers to our questions about ends or actions are provided by considering beliefs about actions and about the ends pursued, in conjunction with an appraisal concerning the rationality of actions undertaken. In Hempel's words, beliefs, ends, and rationality are "epistemically interdependent."

Malcolm (1964) doubts that actions undertaken to pursue intended outcomes can be properly understood in terms of functional laws. He challenges stimulus-response (S-R) laws of association that join actions and consequences based on their prior association. Instead, purposeful actions are connected to their intended outcomes by logic, that is, by their "in order to" quality. For example, "I am rummaging about my desk in order to find my spectacles." The action derives its meaning from the end pursued. Malcolm demonstrates (p. 151) how strange it would sound if a person were to reason in strictly S-R associationist terms:

> Here I am rummaging about my desk. When I have done this in the past my activity has terminated when I have caught hold of my spectacles. Therefore, I am probably looking for my spectacles!

Action Taken in Concrete Setting

Statistical studies that relate two or more organizational variables may increase our understanding of the structure and functioning of organizations if (1) the variables refer to things or events that can be defined independently of the variables to which they are to be related, and (2) the form of the relationship is invariant with respect to the definition of the situation in which the variables are embedded. Studies relating certain aspects of organizational structure to other aspects within the organization or in its environment generally meet such criteria, e.g., size and structure (Blau and Schoenherr, 1971) or technology and structure (Hickson, Pugh, and Pheysey, 1969). These criteria are not met when one of the variables refers to a planned intervention, i.e., human action in a social system.

Furthermore, planned interventions usually take place in only one organization at a time and would not be interpreted within different organizations in the same way. However, suppose such actions could be classified into categories of actions and that the consequences of these actions were observed in 50 different organizations and shown to produce desirable consequences at better than a chance level. The change agent who reads the report of such a study still has to make an intervention in the one organization in which he or she had been invited to intervene. His or her chosen action would be judged good or poor, right or wrong in the singular concrete setting in which it was undertaken. He or she does not intervene in 50 organizations so as to judge whether the chosen action produced the desired outcome at better than the chance level, e.g., in 40 organizations out of 50 rather than in 25 out of 50. Reliance on Bayesian notions of subjective probability of success may have limited value. Any system as complex as a social system has a unique configuration of parameters which was not measured, but which would influence where the organization might fall in the sampling distribution. Thus, the intervener without knowledge of the unique configuration of parameters in the concrete setting in which action is contemplated would not know if an action will produce an outcome at the mean of the sampling distribution or perhaps three standard deviations from it. Without such knowledge, the chosen action may produce an outcome that is less desirable than an outcome chosen on the basis of good judgment of the relevant factors in the concrete setting.

Actions Are Seldom Discrete Events

Some thought should be given as to what kinds of human actions can be considered interventions into an organization. An intervention may be construed as a cause when members of a supra-system or other system take actions to alter the internal or external conditions a targeted organization faces without consultation with members of the targeted organization. The interventions of concern to this discussion are acts of communication between two or more self-reflecting subjects, requiring mutual understanding of the meaning of the acts and common consent as to their presumed consequences. Such interventions have an element of surprise or unexpectedness to them so that they are unlike other actions routinely undertaken within the organization. The meaning of the routine actions is understood because they fit in the context created by a history of previous commitments affecting the goals, structure, and technology of the organization and the language and definitions of situations that led to these commitments.

The element of surprise evoked by an intervention results when the change agent offers members of the target organization a new way to conceptualize an old problem and offers it in a language or framework that differs from that by which members of the organization define their present situation (Susman, 1976).

Interventions may be much less direct. Change agents may serve as catalysts to help organizational members define a problem or reconceptualize an existing one. In these cases, acts of communication take the form of helping organizational members to articulate a desired future against which to compare the present situation (Blake and Mouton, 1974), or pointing out discrepancies between stated intentions and actual behavior (Schon and Argyris, 1974). In areas such as these, successful interventions break patterns of shared expectations and codes of conduct. It must be recognized, however, that the history that produced such expectations and codes, also produced the decisions that limit the possibilities for new action in the immediate future because of previous commitment to physical plant, technology, and current personnel.

Unlike deterministic physical systems, the nonrandomness of the structuredness of a social system results from shared codes of conduct or rules of its members. Even if the intended target of an intervention were changing the physical aspects of a system, e.g., layout, machinery, etc., it still would be mediated by communicating such intentions to members of the social system and gaining the consent of at least its most influential members. Thus, initially, the target of most proposed change efforts concerns the conceptions and ideas of members of the system. If we also consider the personal investments that organizational members have in a particular structure, technology, etc., because of how these arrangements have allowed them to accommodate to conflicts over power, prestige, and attention, we can see that the social system is open ended with respect to the consequences of any proposed change. Acts of communication are unlike actions taken toward physical objects in that acts of communication may simultaneously convey multiple meanings, i.e., manifest and latent content, conscious or unconscious, or they may be subject to different interpretations by sender and receiver. Also, the targets of a proposed change will not know what their reactions will be to a proposed change until they have a chance to contemplate their reactions by mentally rehearsing them or by experiencing the changes first hand.

Positivist Science and Action Research: Contrasting Conceptions of Science

We have shown that actions and their consequences cannot be explained according to the positivist criteria of a scientific explanation. This leaves us with the choice as to whether we ought to declare action research ascientific, or reconsider using positivist criteria to judge the scientific status of action research. We have chosen the second alternative and, on this basis, we propose that action research can be legitimated as science by locating its foundation in philosophical viewpoints which differ from those used to legitimate positivist science. We also propose alternative criteria of science and alternative methods as appropriate for action research. Finally, we consider what action research can contribute to the growth of knowledge.

Philosophical Viewpoints that Legitimate Action Research

While adherents of positivist science can cite several philosophical viewpoints as a foundation for legitimating its methods, action researchers can do the same with different philosophical viewpoints. These viewpoints are as follows:

Praxis. The concept of praxis, originally from Aristotle, refers to the art of acting upon the conditions one faces in order to change them. From Aristotle's writings, Bernstein (1971) interprets praxis to deal with "the disciplines and activities predominant in man's ethical and political life" (p. x). Aristotle contrasted praxis with *theoria*, "those sciences and activities that are concerned with knowing for its own sake" (p. ix), and presented them as two necessary dimensions of a "truly human and free life" (p. x). Aristotle also contrasts praxis with *techne*, which is the "skillful production of artifacts and the expert mastery of objectified tasks" (Habermas, 1973: 42). While *techne* may be improved by training and informed by mathematical calculation, praxis is cultivated and guided by good judgment or "prudence" (p. 42). Marx made praxis the central concept in his theories of alienation, economics, and society. He enlarges upon Aristotle's usage of praxis in that by taking action to change conditions one is personally changed in the process (Marx, 1963).

Hermeneutics. Hermeneutics originally referred to the art of interpreting texts, mainly of biblical, judicial, and, more generally, historical texts (Gadamer, 1975). Contemporary references to hermeneutics focus on its role in the interpretation of languages, culture, and history. It has been a more influential approach to the social sciences on the European continent than positivist approaches have been, with its leading forerunners being Hegel, Dilthey, Weber, and, more recently, members of the Frankfurt school, e.g., Habermas, Horkheimer, Adorno, and Marcuse.

Its most important contribution to action research is its concept of the hermeneutical circle. The idea of the circle is that no knowledge is possible without presuppositions. This idea has been recognized also by philosophers not associated with hermeneutics as, for example, in Popper's (1959) acknowledgement that the framing of any scientific question assumes some foreknowledge of what it is we want to know. In the social sciences, the hermeneutical circle takes the form of attempting an initial holistic understanding of a social system and then using this understanding as a basis for interpreting the parts of the system. Knowledge is gained dialectically by proceeding from the whole to its parts and then back again. Each time an incongruence occurs between part and whole, a reconceptualization takes place. The learning process is not unlike the spiral formulated by Lewin. The frequency of reconceptualization decreases as the match improves between the researcher's conception of the social system and that held by its members. The hermeneutical tradition strengthens the action researcher's methodological position by forewarning him that his interpretation of a social system will never be exactly the same as that held by the members of the social system. This provides the action researcher with a base for understanding his own preconceptions better and by contrast, those held by system members, and also allows him to see possible solutions not seen by system members.

Existentialism. Action research has much in common with existentialism. Both arose out of concern with the limitations of rationalistic science, both assert the importance of human choice and human values, both are keyed to the importance of human action, and both avoid giving traditional causal explanations of human actions.

The existential viewpoint was first articulated by Kierkegaard in the 1840s and Nietzsche in the 1870s, and systematically developed by Heidegger, Sartre, and Jaspers, among others (see Reinhardt, 1952; Barrett, 1958). Central to the existential position is the theme that behind every action, individual choice is based on human interest. The possibility of choice is central to taking action, and the necessity to choose is central to human development.

Pragmaticism and pragmatism. Pragmaticism, as Peirce called it, and Pragmatism, as developed by James and Dewey, belong to the positivist tradition in that they accepted an empirical base as the ultimate source of scientific knowledge. However, their adherents considered the role of scientist as actor within the world rather than a spectator of it. Instead of focusing on formal criteria for establishing the truth of a statement, they shifted the criterion of truth toward what human difference it would make if an action were taken based on a tentative acceptance of the statement; that is, what are the practical consequences for adopting a particular statement. Dewey applied such methods to determine the practical consequences of accepting certain values.

Process philosophies. One of the most salient features of organizations is change. Where Heraclitus observed that "you cannot step into the same river twice," his modern counterpart could comment that you cannot step into the same social system twice. Although action research derives much of its epistemological power from this viewpoint, it is only in the twentieth century that the epistemological implications have been articulated by Bergson (1911), Smuts (1926), Whitehead (1929), Cassirer (1957), and Heidegger (1962)', among others.

Phenomenology. Phenomenology, in its broadest sense, insists on the primacy of immediate subjective experience as the basis for knowledge. As Schacht (1972) pointed out, a person may proceed by minimizing the constraints of preconceptions (Husserl, 1931), or by acknowledging one's preconceptions (Heidegger, 1962) so that, by contrast, one allows another's experience to be communicated in relatively undistorted fashion. Phenomenology has been applied in the social sciences by Lewin (1946, 1951), Rogers (1961), Merleau-Ponty (1963), Perls (1965), and Schutz (1967), each of these researchers has developed psychological theories based on the concept of the phenomenological field of an individual or group. Whether the focus is a person or group, the ends that each pursues to bring about a more desirable future as well as the values and norms that guide the actions undertaken have no objective reality that can be empirically determined as required by positivist science, if such concepts are to enter its domain of inquiry legitimately. However, such ends, values, and norms have a phenomenological reality from the perspective of the person or groups taking action, and knowing them is essential to the action researcher in predicting and understanding the behavior of the person or groups engaged.

Alternative Criteria and Methods of Science

Explanation versus understanding. Human behavior can be explained in other ways than subsuming it under a covering law. Dray (1957) considered the covering law model as "peculiarly inept" for use in explaining human action and urged its replacement in applications to human action by what he called "principles of action." These express a judgment of the form: when in a situation of type S, the action to take is A. Dray called this kind of explanation a "good reason" explanation. Silverman (1971) drawing on Weber and Schutz to describe explanations of this type stated that they were easiest to apply when one could assume that actors were rational and continuously weighed the means, ends, and secondary consequences of their actions. Bateson (1972) had a similar type of explanation in mind with his expression "cybernetic explanation" in which all explanations (save one in the limiting case) were deemed improbable because they were mismatched with what was known of the context within which action was taken.

Reliance on an empirical base alone for explaining behavior can lead an observer to search for a cause of an action taken. When an empirical base is used, changes in behavior are sought through manipulation of the cause of the behavior instead of through the consent and understanding of those whose behavior is to be changed. Trist, Susman, and Brown (1977) have commented that the language and metaphors used by organizational researchers reveal that organizational change is conceptualized as externally caused. Change is often described with energy metaphors, as if it were a force aimed at those parts of an organization the researchers wish to displace while holding other parts of the organization constant.

From a phenomenological perspective, behavior is understood by knowing the ends toward which the action is taken, as well as by sharing the same time frame and universe of moral concerns.

Prediction versus making things happen. Positivist science encourages two conceptions of the researcher's role in prediction in organizational science: (1) the researcher is sole possessor of knowledge from which actions will be drawn and (2) the researcher is sole originator of actions to be taken on an essentially passive world. The degree to which these conceptions are at variance with taking action within a social system is evident from the extraordinary precautions undertaken in many controlled experiments to ensure that human beings will react to the researcher's treatment rather than to the researcher as another human being.

The action researcher, on the other hand, coproduces (Ackoff and Emery, 1972) solutions through collaboration with the client system. Friedmann's (1973) concept of transactive planning provides a basis for synthesizing the contributions that action researcher and clients can bring to solving a problem. The action researcher brings theoretical knowledge as well as breadth of experience to the problem-solving process. The clients bring practical knowledge and experience of the situations in which they are trying to solve problems. Neither client nor researcher has better knowledge; in a sense, they are both experts.

According to positivist conceptions, once the researcher predicts that an outcome will follow taking a particular action, he or she then takes the action and waits to see if the predicted outcome occurs. Any interference by the researcher in the events that intervene between action and outcome nullifies the significance of the prediction. The action researcher collaborates with clients in diagnosis, selection of alternative actions, and evaluation of outcomes. The objective of the collaboration is to bring about a better future, i.e., with a problem solved. The values that guide the client's choice of goals and objectives are ones with which the action researcher becomes "directively correlated" (Sommerhoff, 1969) to increase the relevance of his or her contributions. If the researcher is effective in such circumstances, the hoped for outcome will occur because of the researcher's involvement not from trying to avoid it.

Deduction and induction versus conjectures. Peirce (1955) was one of the earliest to criticize the Formalist and Reconstructionist conception of the manner in which knowledge is advanced. For example, he felt that the deductive mode offered no new knowledge about the world as one uses this mode only to work out the consequences of what one already accepts. Popper (1962) criticized the inductive mode as not having been really the basis for significant advances in knowledge. A Popper-like example of the shortcomings of the inductive mode would be; question: Why does ice float on water? Answer: Because it always does! I've seen it do that a thousand times! Popper claims that significant advances in knowledge occur when the inquirer goes beyond the data; performs a conceptual leap of the imagination to consider analogies, metaphors, models, myths, etc. as a way to explain the data. Popper called such leaps of the imagination conjectures. Leach (1961) has a similar process in mind with his term "inspired guesswork." According to Popper, conjectures are created in the same manner as myths are. He distinguishes conjectures from myths in that tests can be devised for conjectures that could potentially falsify them. They gain in scientific stature the more they survive such tests.

We believe that most of our significant knowledge about social systems has grown by conjecturing, e.g., by conceptualizing the social system as a biological cell (as in general systems theory) or as a machine (scientific management). We make assumptions about organizations by pattern recognition (organizational climate), or by imagining the whole from knowledge of some of its parts. Consistent with an action mode of inquiry, we often test out the consequences of our conjectures by taking actions and either strengthen or weaken our belief in such conjectures as a result.

Detachment versus engagement. The positivist assumption of a detached, neutral, independent, objective researcher is incompatible with the requirements of action research. Once one accepts organizations as artifacts, created by humans for the purpose of serving human needs, then one cannot escape the realization that actions in an organization have moral consequences that must be faced. The success of action research hinges on understanding the values of the relevant actors since such values guide the selection of means and ends for solving problems and develop the commitment of the actors to a particular solution. Empathy, taking the role of the other, participant observation, etc. may be the most effective means for making the theoretical or practical knowledge the researcher possesses really useful and accepted by clients.

Contemplation versus action. If the world were structured logically as Formalists and Reconstructionists assume, then one could work out possible consequences of taking an action without ever having to take the action. Within the context of taking action in an organization, only the most trivial of consequences can be known in this way. By contrast, in action research, not only is knowledge gained by acting in the real situation, but the situation itself is simultaneously a product of the current level of knowledge. Torbert (1972) captures the process with the phrase "Inquiry in action can lead to learning from experience" (p. iv).

Contributions of Action Research to Growth of Knowledge

If action research has its own legitimate epistemological and methodological base, then it can contribute to the growth of knowledge differently from what positivist science can contribute. The focus of organizational knowledge may shift from prescribing rational rules of operation (as with machines) to the emergence of action principles or guides for dealing with different situations. Action research provides a mode of inquiry for evolving criteria by which to articulate and appraise actions taken in organizational contexts. Our relative lack of understanding of action and its effects is further evidence of the epistemological shortcomings of positivist science.

Action research facilitates the development of techniques which we will call "practics" (to distinguish from positivist techniques). Practics would provide the action researcher with know-how such as how to create settings for organizational learning, how to act in unprescribed nonprogrammed situations, how to generate organizational self-help, how to establish action guides where none exist, how to review, revise, redefine the system of which we are part, how to formulate fruitful metaphors, constructs, and images for articulating a more desirable future. Such know-how is difficult to develop or even consider within the positivist framework.

Action research is directed toward the development of action competencies of members of organizations, and can be described as an "enabling" science. Typically, the kinds of skills which action research develops are interpersonal and problem-defining. Competence is developed in interpretation and judgment, in establishing problem-solving procedures, acting in contingent and uncertain situations, learning from one's errors, generating workable new constructs from one's experiences. Such skills are needed by persons in organizations, and positivist science has generally made negligible contributions in providing such skills.

The action researcher establishes conditions for the development of others. He or she acquires increasing skills at developing organizational infrastructures and networks for enabling members of organizations to plan, organize, learn, and help themselves. The action researcher learns how to use earlier infrastructure efforts as models so that persons in other organizations can learn from and improve upon their example. The researcher's own behaviors are even more influential and become a model of how to act in unprescribed nonprogrammed situations.

Collaboration between the researcher and the client system enlarges the domain of inquiry in organizational research from them to us. The knowledge we generate affects us not others; the researcher is necessarily a part of the data he or she helps to generate.

A Contingency View of Science

The Table summarizes the differences between positivist science and action research we have discussed. As we have seen, the differences are extensive. We now consider the question of which approach is better. Our answer is that it all depends on the phenomena one wants to study and the conditions under which they are to be studied. It would be very difficult to state definitively when positivist science is appropriate. However, like Vaill (1976) who questions the use of positivist science ("the expository model of science") for designing organizations, we suggest that the researcher ought to be skeptical of positivist science when the unit of analysis is, like the researcher, a self-reflecting subject, when relationships between subjects (actors) are influenced by definitions of the situation, or when the reason for undertaking the research is to solve a problem which the actors have helped to define.

Table: Comparisons of positivist science and action research

Points of comparison	Positivist science	Action research
Value position	Methods are value neutral	Methods develop social systems and release human potential
Time perspective	Observation of the present	Observation of the present plus interpretation of the present from knowledge of the past, conceptualization of more desirable futures
Relationship with units	Detached spectator, client system members are objects to study	Client system members are self-reflective subjects with whom to collaborate
Treatment of units studied	Cases are of interest only as representatives of populations	Cases can be sufficient sources of knowledge
Language for describing units	Denotative, observational	Connotative, metaphorical
Basis for assuming existence of units	Exist independently of human beings	Human artifacts for human purposes
Epistemological aims	Prediction of events from propositions arranged hierarchically	Development of guides for taking actions that produce desired outcomes
Strategy for growth of knowledge	Induction and deduction	Conjecturing, creating settings for learning and modeling of behavior
Criteria for confirmation	Logical consistency, prediction and control	Evaluating whether actions produce intended consequences
Basis for generalization	Broad, universal, and free of context	Narrow, situational, and bound by context

Summary

We have examined the scientific merits of action research both in the narrow terms of positivist science and more broadly in terms of its capacity to generate knowledge for use in solving problems faced by members of organizations. We find that action research is not compatible with the criteria for scientific explanation as established by positivist science. Hempel's covering-law model of explanation would not grant to action research the status of a valid science. However, in action research, the ultimate sanction is in the perceived functionality of chosen actions to produce desirable consequences for an organization. Action research constitutes a kind of science with a different epistemology that produces a different kind of knowledge, a knowledge which is contingent on the particular situation, and which develops the capacity of members of the organization to solve their own problems.

We hope that this article will enable others to assess the scientific merits of action research. We believe that action research is both ascientific in terms of the criteria of positivist science and relevant in terms of generating good organizational science. As a procedure for generating knowledge, we believe it has far greater potential than positivist science for understanding and managing the affairs of organizations.

Acknowledgement

The authors would like to thank Susan Clark, Max Elden, Eric Trist, and *ASQ* anonymous reviewers who read earlier drafts of this article and offered many valuable suggestions for improving it.

References

Ackoff, Russell, and F. E. Emery 1972 *On Purposeful Systems*. Chicago: Aldine-Atherton.

Anscombe, G. E. M. 1958 *Intention*. Oxford: Blackwell.

Barrett, William 1958 *Irrational Man*. Garden City, NJ: Doubleday.

Bateson, Gregory 1972 *Steps to an Ecology of Mind*. New York: Ballantine.

Bergson, Henri 1911 *Creative Evolution*. New York: MacMillan.

Bernstein, Richard J. 1971 *Praxis and Action*. Philadelphia: University of Pennsylvania.

Bion, W. R. 1946 "The leaderless group project." *Bulletin of the Menninger Clinic*, 10: 77–81.

Blake, R. R., and J. S. Mouton 1964 *The Managerial Grid*, Houston: Gulf.

Blau, P. M., and R. A. Schoenherr 1971 *The Structure of Organizations*. New York: Basic Books.

Blumer, Herbert 1956 "Sociological analysis and the 'variable.'" *American Sociological Review*, 21: 683–690.

Bridger, Harold 1946 "The Northfield experiment." *Bulletin of the Menninger Clinic*, 10: 71–76.

Carnap, Rudolf 1936 "Testability and meaning." *Philosophy of Science*, 3: 419–471.

——— 1937 "Testability and meaning." *Philosophy of Science*, 4: 1–40.

——— 1950 *Logical Foundations of Probability*. Chicago: University of Chicago.

Cassirer, Ernst 1957 The Philosophy of Symbolic Forms, 3: The Phenomenology of Knowledge. Ralph Manheim, trans. New Haven: Yale University Press.

Chein, Isador, Stuart W. Cook, and John Harding 1948 "The field of action research." *American Psychologist*, 3: 43–50.

Cherns, A. B., P. A. Clark, and W. I. Jenkins 1976 "Action research and the development of the social sciences." In Alfred W. Clark (ed.), *Experimenting with Organizational Life: The Action Research Approach*: 33–42. New York: Plenum.

Collier, John 1945 "United States Indian administration as a laboratory of ethnic relations." *Social Research*, 12: 275–276.

Comte, Auguste 1864 *Cours de Philosophie Positive*, 2d ed. Paris: Bailliere.

Davis, Louis E., and J, Taylor (eds.) 1972 *Design of Jobs*. Baltimore: Penguin.

Dray, William 1957 Laws and Explanation in History, chap 5. Oxford: University Press.

Duckles, Margaret M., Robert Duckies, and Michael Maccoby 1977 "The process of change at Bolivar." *The Journal of Applied Behavioral Science*, 13: 387–399.

Evered, Roger D. 1976 "A typology of explicative models." *Technological Forecasting and Social Change*, 9: 259–277.

Foster, Michael 1972 "The theory and practice of action research in work organizations." *Human Relations*, 25: 529–556.

Friedmann, John 1973 *Retracking America: A Theory of Transactive Planning*. Garden City: Doubleday.

Gadamer, Hans-Georg 1975 *Truth and Method*. New York: Seabury.

Habermas, Jurgen 1971 Knowledge and Human Interests. Boston: Beacon.

——— 1973 *Theory and Practice*. Boston: Beacon.

Heidegger, Martin 1962 *Being and Time*. New York: Harper & Row.

Hempel, Carl G. 1950 "Problems and changes in the empiricist criterion of meaning." *Revue Internationale de Philosophie*, 11: 41–63.

Hempel, Carl G. 1965 *Aspects of Scientific Explanation, and Other Essays in the Philosophy of Science*. New York: Free Press.

Hickson, David J., D. S. Pugh, and Diana C. Phesey 1969 "Operations technology and organization structure: an empirical reappraisal." *Administrative Science Quarterly*, 378–397.

Husserl, Edmund 1931 *Ideas: General Introduction to Pure Phenomenology*. London: Allen and Unwin.

Jaques, Elliott 1951 *The Changing Culture of a Factory*. London. Tavistock.

Leach, E. R. 1961 *Rethinking Anthropology*. London: Atholone Press.

Lewin, Kurt 1946 "Action research and minority problems." *Journal of Social Issues*, 2: 34–46.

—— 1951 *Field Theory in Social Sciences*. New York: Harper.

Luthans, Fred, and R. Kreitner 1975 *Organizational Behavior Modification*. Glenview, IL: Scott, Foresman.

Malcolm, Norman 1964 "Behaviorism as a philosophy of psychology." In T. W. Wann (ed.), *Behaviorism and Phenomenology*: 141–155. Chicago: University of Chicago.

Mann, Floyd C. 1957 "Studying and creating change: a means to understanding social organization," In Conrad M. Arensberg (ed.), *Research in Industrial Human Relations: A Critical Appraisal: 146–167*. New York: Harper.

Marrow, Alfred J. 1969 *The Practical Theorist*. New York: Basic Books.

Marx, Karl 1963 Economic and philosophical manuscripts. In T. B. Bottomore (ed.), *Karl Marx: Early Writings*: 61–219. New York: McGraw-Hill. (Originally written in German in 1844.)

Merleau-Ponty, Maurice 1963 *The Structure of Behavior*. Alden L. Fisher, trans. Boston: Beacon. (Originally published in French, by Presses Universitaries de France, 1942.)

Nadler, David A. 1977 *Feedback and Organization Development: Using Data-Based Methods*. Reading, MA: Addison-Wesley.

Oquist, Paul 1978 "The epistemology of action research." *Acta Sociologica*, 21, 143–163.

Peirce, Charles S. 1955 *Philosophical Writings of Peirce*. J. Buckler (ed.). New York: Dover.

Perls, Frederick, Ralph F. Hefferline, and Paul Goodman 1965 *Gestalt Therapy*. New York: Dell. (Originally published 1951.)

Polanyi, Michael 1958 *Personal Knowledge: Towards a Post-Critical Philosophy*. Chicago: University of Chicago Press.

Popper, Karl 1959 *The Logic of Scientific Discovery*. New York: Basic Books.

—— 1968 *Conjectures and Refutations*. New York: Harper. (Originally published 1962.)

Radnitsky, Gerard 1970 *Contemporary Schools of Metascience*. Gateway. (Originally published 1968 by Scandinavian University Books, Göteberg, Sweden.)

Rapoport, Robert N. 1970 "Three dilemmas of action research." *Human Relations*, 23, 499–513.

Reinhardt, Kurt F. 1952 *The Existential Revolt*. New York: Frederick Vugan.

Rice, A. K. 1958 *Productivity and Social Organization: The Ahmedabad Experiment*. London: Tavistock.

Rogers, Carl R. 1961 *On Becoming a Person*. New York: Houghton Mifflin.

Schacht, Richard 1972 "Husserlian and Heideggerian phenomenology." *Philosophical Studies*, 23, 293–314.

Schon, Donald, and C. Argyris 1974 *Theory in Practice: Increasing Professional Effectiveness*. San Francisco: Jossey-Bass.

Schutz, Alfred 1967 *The Phenomenology of the Social World*. George Walsh and Frederick Lehnert, trans. Evanston: Northwestern University. (Originally published in German in 1932.)

Seashore, Stanley, and David G. Bowers 1964 *Changing the Structure and the Functioning of an Organization*. Ann Arbor: Survey Research Center.

Silverman, David 1971 *The Theory of Organizations*. New York: Basic Books.

Smuts, Jan C. 1926 *Holism and Evolution*. New York: Viking.

Sommerhoff, Gert 1969 "The abstract characteristics of living systems." In F. E. Emery (ed.), *Systems Thinking*: 147–202. Baltimore: Penguin.

Susman, Gerald I. 1976 *Autonomy at Work: A Sociotechnical Analysis of Participative Management*. New York: Praeger.

Torbert, William R. 1972 *Learning from Experience*. New York: Columbia University Press

Trist, Eric L. 1976 "Engaging with large-scale systems." In Alfred W. Clark (ed.), *Experimenting with Organizational Life: The Action Research Approach*: 43–57. London: Plenum.

—— 1977 "A concept of organizational ecology" *The Australian Journal of Management*, 2: 171–175

Trist, Eric L., Gerald I. Susman, and Grant R. Brown 1977 "An experiment in autonomous working in an American underground coal mine" *Human Relations*, 30: 201–236.

Whitehead, Alfred N. 1929 *Process and Reality*. Cambridge: University Press.

Whyte, William Foote, and Edith L. Hamilton 1964 *Action Research for Management*. Homewood, IL: Irwin, Dorsey.

Wilson, A. T. M., E. L. Trist, and A. Curle 1952 "Transitional communities and social reconnection: a study of the civil resettlement of British prisoners of war" In G. E. Swanson, T. M. New-comb, and E. L. Hartley (eds.), *Readings in Social Psychology*, 2d ed: 561–579. New York: Holt.

Vaill, Peter B. 1976 "The expository model of science in organization design." In R. H. Kilmann, L. R. Pondy, and D. P. Slevin (eds.), *The Management of Organization Design*, vol. 1: Strategies and Implementation: 73–88. New York: Elsevier North-Holland.

49

Using Qualitative Methods in Health Related Action Research

Julienne Meyer

The barriers to the uptake of the findings of traditional quantitative biomedical research in clinical practice are increasingly being recognised.[1,2] Action research is particularly suited to identifying problems in clinical practice and helping develop potential solutions in order to improve practice.[3] For this reason, action research is increasingly being used in health related settings. Although not synonymous with qualitative research, action research typically draws on qualitative methods such as interviews and observation.

What Is Action Research?

Action research is not easily defined. It is a style of research rather than a specific method. First used in 1946 by Kurt Lewin, a social scientist concerned with intergroup relations and minority problems in the United States, the term is now identified with research in which the researchers work explicitly with and for people rather than undertake research on them.[4] Its strength lies in its focus on generating solutions to practical problems and its ability to empower practitioners – getting them to engage with research and subsequent "development" or implementation activities. Practitioners can choose to research their own practice, or an outside researcher can be engaged to help them identify problems, seek and implement practical solutions, and systematically monitor and reflect, on the process and outcomes of change.

Source: *BMJ*, 320(7228) (2000): 178–181.

Most definitions of action research incorporate three important elements: its participatory character; its democratic impulse; and its simultaneous contribution to social science and social change.[5]

Participation in Action Research

Participation is fundamental to action research: it is an approach which demands that participants perceive the need to change and are willing to play an active part in the research and the change process. All research requires willing subjects, but the level of commitment required in an action research study goes beyond simply agreeing to answer questions or be observed. The clear cut demarcation between "researcher" and "researched" that is found in other types of research may not be so apparent in action research. The research design must be continually negotiated with participants, and researchers need to agree an ethical code of practice with the participants.[6] This is especially important as participation in the research, and in the process of change, can be threatening.[7, 8] Conflicts may arise in the course of the research: outside researchers working with practitioners must obtain their trust and agree rules on the control of data and their use and on how potential conflict will be resolved within the project. The way in which such rules are agreed demonstrates a second important feature of action research – namely, its democratic impulse.

Democracy in Action Research

"Democracy" in action research usually requires participants to be seen as equals. The researcher works as a facilitator of change, consulting with participants not only on the action process but also on how it will be evaluated. One benefit of this is that it can make the research process and outcomes more meaningful to practitioners, by rooting them in the reality of day to day practice.

Throughout the study, findings are fed back to participants for validation and to inform decisions about the next stage of the study. This formative style of research is thus responsive to events as they naturally occur in the field and frequently entails collaborative spirals of planning, acting, observing, reflecting, and replanning. However, care needs to be taken in this process as it can be threatening: democratic practice is not always a feature of health-care settings. An action researcher needs to be able to work across traditional boundaries (for example, between health and social care professionals or between hospital and community care settings) and juggle different, sometimes competing, agendas. This requires excellent interpersonal skills as well as research ability.

Contribution to both Social Science
and Social Change

There is increasing concern about the "theory-practice" gap in clinical practice; practitioners have to rely on their intuition and experience since traditional scientific knowledge – for example, the results of randomised controlled trials – often does not seem to fit the uniqueness of the situation. Action research is seen as one way of dealing with this because, by drawing on practitioners' intuition and experience, it can generate findings that are meaningful and useful to them.

The level of interest in practitioner led research is increasing in Britain, in part as a response to recent proposals to "modernise" the NHS through developing new forms of clinical governance.[9] This and other national initiatives (the NHS Research and Development Strategy, the National Centre for Clinical Audit, the NHS Centre for Reviews and Dissemination, the Cochrane Collaboration, Centres for Evidence Based Practice) emphasise that research and development should be the business of every clinician. Practitioner led research approaches, such as single case experimental designs,[10] reflective case studies,[11] and reflexive action research,[12] are seen as ideal research methods for clinicians concerned with improving the quality of patient care.[13]

In considering the contribution of action research to knowledge, it is important to note that generalisations made from action research studies differ from those made on the basis of more conventional forms of research. To some extent, reports of action research studies rely on readers to underwrite the account of the research by drawing on their own knowledge of human situations. It is therefore important, when reporting action research, to describe the work in its rich contextual detail. The researcher strives to include the participants' perspective on the data by feeding back findings to participants and incorporating their responses as new data in the final report. In addition, the onus is on the researcher to make his or her own values and beliefs explicit in the account of the research so that any biases are evident. This can be facilitated by writing self reflective field notes during the research.

The strength of action research is its ability to influence practice positively while simultaneously gathering data to share with a wider audience. However, change is problematic, and although action research lends itself well to the discovery of solutions, its success should not be judged solely in terms of the size of change achieved or the immediate implementation of solutions. Instead, success can often be viewed in relation to what has been learnt from the experience of undertaking the work. For instance, a study which set out to explore the care of older people in accident and emergency departments did not result in much change in the course of the study.[14] However, the lessons learnt from the research were reviewed in the context of national policy and research and carefully fed back to those working in the trust; as a result, changes have already been made within the organisation to act on the study's recommendations. Some positive changes were achieved in the course of the study (for example, the introduction of specialist discharge posts in accident and emergency departments), but the study also shed light on continuing gaps in care and issues that needed to be improved in future developments. Participants identified that the role of the "action researcher" had enabled greater understanding and communication between two services (the accident and emergency department and the department of medicine for elderly people) and that this had left both better equipped for future joint working. In other words, the solutions emerged from the process of undertaking the research.

Different Types of Action Research

Four basic types of action research have been identified: experimental, organisational, professionalising, and empowering (table).[3] Though this typology is useful in understanding the wide range of action research, its multidimensional nature means that it is not particularly easy to classify individual studies. For instance, a study might be classified as "empowering" because of its "bottom up approach" in relation to the fourth distinguishing criterion of "change intervention," but the other distinguishing criteria may be used to classify the same study as a different action research type (experimental, organisational, or professionalising). This situation is most likely to occur if the researcher and practitioners hold differing views on the nature of society. It may be more fruitful to use this typology as a framework for critiquing individual studies and, in particular for thinking about how concepts are operationalised, the features of particular settings, and the contribution of the people within those settings to solutions.[15]

Action Research in Health Care

At a time when there is increasing concern that research evidence is not sufficiently influencing practice development,[16] action research is gaining credibility in healthcare settings.[17] For example, the Royal College of Physicians in England has become involved in an action research study exploring the roles of clinicians, clinical audit staff, and managers in implementing clinical audit and ways of overcoming organisational barriers to audit.[18] The NHS Research and Development Programme has commissioned a systematic review of the action research. Elsewhere Ong has used "rapid appraisal," a type of action research, to engage users in the development of health care policy and practice.[19]

Action research has also been used in hospital settings to facilitate closer partnerships between staff and users, notably in a study which focused on the introduction of lay participation in care within a general medical ward of a London teaching hospital (box). This study used a range of methods,

Tabel: Action research typology (adapted from Hart and Bond)[3]

Action research type: distinguishing criteria	Consensus model of society — Rational social management		Conflict model of society — Structural change →	
	Experimental	*Organisational*	*Professionalising*	*Empowering*
1 Educative base	Re-education; Enhancing social science or administrative control and social change towards consensus	Re-education or training; Enhancing managerial control and organisational change towards consensus	Reflective practice; Enhancing professional control and individuals' ability to control work situation	Consciousness raising; Enhancing user control and shifting balance of power; structural change towards pluralism
	Inferring relationship between behaviour and output; identifying causal factors in group dynamics	Overcoming resistance to change or restructuring balance of power between managers and workers	Empowering professional groups; advocacy on behalf of patients or clients	Empowering oppressed groups
	Social scientific bias, researcher focused	Managerial bias or client focused	Practitioner focused	User or practitioner focused
2 Individuals in groups	Closed group, controlled, selection made by researcher for purposes of measurement, inferring relationship between cause and effect	Work groups or mixed groups of managers and workers, or both	Professional(s) or (inter-disciplinary) professional group, or negotiated team boundaries	Fluid groupings, self selecting or natural boundary or open/closed by negotiation
	Fixed membership	Selected membership	Shifting membership	Fluid membership
3 Problem focus	Problem emerges from the interaction of social science theory and social problems	Problem defined by most powerful group; some negotiation with users	Problem defined by professional in group; some negotiation with users	Emerging and negotiated definition of problem by less powerful group(s)
	Problems relevant for social science or management interests	Problem relevant for management/social science interests	Problem emerges from professional practice or experience	Problem emerges from members' practice or experience
	Success defined in terms of social sciences	Success defined by sponsors	Contested, professionally determined definitions of success	Competing definitions of success accepted and expected

(Continued)

(Continued)

Action research type: distinguishing criteria	Consensus model of society / Rational social management			Conflict model of society / Structural change
	Experimental	*Organisational*	*Professionalising*	*Empowering*
4 Change of intervention	Social science experimental intervention to test theory or generate theory, or both	Top down, directed change towards predetermined aims	Professionally led, predefined, process led	Bottom up, undetermined, process led
	Problem to be solved in terms of management aims	Problem to be solved in terms of management aims	Problem to be resolved in the interests of resolved in the interests of research based practice and professionalisation	Problem to be explored as part of the process of change, developing an understanding of meaning of issues in terms of problem and solution
5 Improvement	Toward controlled outcome and consensual definition of improvement	Towards tangible outcome and consensus definition of improvement	Towards improvement in practice defined by professionals and on behalf of users	Towards negotiated outcomes and pluralist definitions of improvement: account taken of vested interest
6 Cyclic processes	Research components dominant	Action and research components in tension; action dominated	Research and action components in tension; research dominated	Action components dominant
	Identifies causal processes that can be generalised	Identifies causal processes that are specific to problem context or can be generalised, or both	Identifies causal processes that are specific to problem or can be generalised, or both	Changes course of events; recognition of multiple influences upon change
	Time limited, task focused	Discrete cycle, rationalist, sequential	Spiral of cycles, opportunistic, dynamic	Open ended, process driven
7 Research relationship, degree of collaboration	Experimenter or respondents	Consultant or researcher, respondent or participants	Practitioner, or researcher or collaborators	Practitioner researcher or coresearchers or co-change agents
	Outside researcher as expert or research funding	Client pays an outside consultant – "they who pay the piper call the tune"	Outside resources or internally generated, or both	Outside resources or internally generated, or both
	Differentiated roles	Differential roles	Merged roles	Shared roles

Box: Lay participation in care in a hospital setting: an action research study

---

Participation

- Careful negotiation to recruit willing volunteers to examine practice and initiate lay participation in care
- "Bottom up" approach to change via weekly team meetings
- Researcher as facilitator and multidisciplinary team member

Democracy

- Goal of empowering practitioners and lay people in this setting
- Working collaboratively with multidisciplinary team
- Participants given "ownership" of the data to determine how it might be shared with wider audience

Contribution to social science and social change

- Case study of multidisciplinary team on one general medical ward in London teaching hospital using:
  Qualitative methods to highlight key themes emerging in the project
  Quantitative methods for comparison of subgroups

Main action-reflection spirals

- Reorganising the work of the ward:
  Changes in patient care planning
  New reporting system, including bedside handover with patient
  Introduction of modified form of primary nursing system
- Multidisciplinary communication:
  Weekly team meetings instituted
  Introduction of a handout for new staff and team communication sheet
  Closer liaison with community nurses before discharge
- Lay participation in care:
  Development of resources for patient health education
  Introduction of medicine reminder card system
  Patient information leaflet inviting patients to participate in care

Results

- Insights into health professionals' perceptions of lay participation in care
- Some positive changes achieved (for example, improved attitudes to lay participation in care, patient education, improved ward organisation)
- Identified barriers to changing healthcare practice

---

including depth interviews, questionnaires, documentary analysis, and participant observation to generate data about, health professionals' perceptions of lay participation in care and the difficulties encountered in changing practice.[20, 21] In this study, health professionals expressed extremely positive views about user and carer involvement when completing an attitude scale, confirming the results of previous research on health professionals' attitudes towards user and carer involvement in care.[22] However, the interview data showed that they had some serious doubts and concerns, and observation of practice revealed that these doubts and concerns were inhibiting the implementation of lay participation. This action research was able to explore the relation between attitudes and practices and explain what happened when lay participation was introduced into a practice setting. It showed that although current policy documents advocate lay participation in care (user and carer involvement), some health professionals were merely paying lip service to the concept and were also inadequately prepared to deliver it in practice. By working closely with practitioners to explore issues in a practical context, the researcher gained more insight into how the rhetoric of policy might be better translated into reality.

Conclusions

Action research does not focus exclusively on user and carer involvement, though clearly its participatory principles makes it an obvious choice to explore these issues. It can be used more widely – to foster better practice across interprofessional boundaries and between different healthcare settings, for example.[14, 23] It can also be used by clinicians to research their own practice.[10] It is an eclectic approach to research and draws on a variety of data collection methods. The focus on the process as well as the outcomes of change helps to explain the frequent use of qualitative methods by action researchers.

Competing interests: None declared

Notes

1. Sackett DL, Richardson WS, Rosenberg W, Haynes RB. *Evidence-based medicine: how to practise and teach EBM*. Edinburgh: Churchill Livingstone, 1997.
2. Hicks C, Hennessy D. Mixed messages in nursing research: their contribution to the persisting hiatus between evidence and practice. *J Adv Nurs* 1997; 25:595–601.
3. Hart E, Bond M. *Action research for health and social care: a guide to practice*. Buckingham: Open University Press, 1995.
4. Reason P, Rowan J. *Human inquiry: a sourcebook of new paradigm research* Chichester: Wiley, 1981.
5. Carr W, Kemmis S. *Becoming critical: education, knowledge and action research*. London: Falmer, 1986.
6. Meyer JE, New paradigm research in practice: the trials and tribulations of action research. *J Adv Nurs* 1993;18:1066–72.
7. Webb C, Action research: philosophy, method and personal experiences. *J Adv Nurs* 1989; 14:403–10.
8. Titchen A, Binnie A. Changing power relationships between nurses: a case study of early changes towards patient-centred nursing. *J Clin Nurs* 1993;2:219–29.
9. Secretary of State for Health. *The new NHS*. London: Stationery Office, 1997. (Cm 3807.)
10. Carey LM, Matyas TA, Oke LE. Sensory loss in stroke patients: effective training of tactile and proprioceptive discrimination. *Arch Phys Med Rehab* 1993;74:602–11.

11. Stark S. A nurse tutor's experience of personal and professional growth through action research. *J Adv Nurs* 1994;19:579–84.
12. Titchen A, Binnie A. What am I meant to be doing? Putting practice into theory and back again in new nursing roles. *J Adv Nurs* 1993;18:1054–65.
13. Rolfe G. *Expanding nursing knowledge: understanding and researching your own practice.* Oxford: Butterworth Heineman, 1998.
14. Meyer J, Bridges J. *An action research study into the organisation of care of older people in the accident and emergency department.* London: City University, 1998.
15. Lyon J, Applying Hart and Bond's typology; implementing clinical supervision in an acute setting. *Nurse Researcher* 1999;6:39–53.
16. Walshe K, Ham C, Appleby J. Given in evidence. *Health Serv J* 1995:105:28–9.
17. East L, Robinson J. Change in process: bringing about change in health care through action research. *J Clin Nurs* 1994;3:57–61.
18. Berger A. Why doesn't audit work? *BMJ* 1998; 316:875–6.
19. Ong BN. *Rapid appraisal and health policy.* London: Chapman Hall, 1996.
20. Meyer JE. Lay participation in care: a challenge for multi-disciplinary teamwork. *J Interprofess Care* 1993;7:57–66.
21. Meyer JE. Lay participation in care: threat to the status quo. In: Wilson-Barnett J, Macleod Clark J, eds. *Research in health promotion and nursing.* London: Macmillan, 1993:86–100.
22. Brooking J. Patient and family participation in nursing care: the development of a nursing process measuring scale (PhD dissertation). London: University of London, 1986.
23. Street A, Robinson A. Advanced clinical roles: investigating dilemmas and changing practice through action research. *J Clin Nurs* 1995; 4:343–57.

Quality in Qualitative Research

50

Rationale and Standards for the Systematic Review of Qualitative Literature in Health Services Research

Jennie Popay, Anne Rogers and Gareth Williams

The crossing of boundaries between social sciences and non-social sciences is now a feature of much empirical, methodological, and theoretical work in health services research (HSR), and inter- and multidisciplinary working is rapidly becoming the model for many researchers in the health field. This process of working across disciplines has inevitably led to calls for greater pluralism in attitudes to and use of different methods and, in particular, to increasing recognition of the role that qualitative research can play within HSR (Black, 1994).

This greater openness to different methods has a number of likely determinants, including public skepticism about expertise and a willingness to challenge experts' scientific knowledge (Brown, 1992; Gabe, Kelleher, and Williams, 1994; Rogers & Pilgrim, 1995a; Williams & Popay, 1994); the expectations of purchasers or commissioners in quasi-markets, with regard to the evidence base of health care and, in particular, the role of consumer or user voices (Popay & Williams, 1994); and the extent to which many health problems and processes of care do not fit easily into experimental research designs (Britten & Fischer, 1993; Pope & Mays, 1995; Secker, Wimbush, Watson, & Milburn, 1995). There is also a growing recognition that enlargement of our theoretical understanding of phenomena depends on the collection and interpretation of richer and deeper forms of data (Plummer, 1983).

Source: *Qualitative Health Research*, 8(3) (1998): 341–351.

Alongside these developments, there has been growing enthusiasm for the use of systematic reviews, and the methodology for conducting such reviews has developed considerably (Mulrow, 1994). This has included the development of a framework for establishing a hierarchy of evidence to be used during such reviews (Woolfe, Battista, & Anderson, 1990). The systematic review methodology and the associated framework for assessing the quality of research evidence is concerned in particular with the pursuit of evidence-based practice and therefore with evidence on the effectiveness of health care (Rosenberg & Donald, 1995). Given this context, these reviews, predictably, have been concerned primarily, if not exclusively, with quantitative research (such as those undertaken by the international Cochrane Collaboration), and the evidence framework established is similarly focused on quantitative research, distinguishing between study designs according to their susceptibility to bias, and reinforcing the view that evidence from randomized control trials represents the highest level (Woolfe, Battista & Anderson, 1990).

Despite the growth in qualitative research and the importance attributed to its utility in health services research in particular, little attention has been paid to outlining a rationale or developing standards for the systematic review of qualitative research. Moreover, the debates that have taken place concerning standards in qualitative research have tended to focus almost exclusively on techniques, with little attention being paid to differences in the nature of knowledge that sociologically informed qualitative research entails and the philosophical underpinnings of the methods being deployed (Popay, Rogers, & Williams, 1996).

Why Do We Need Standards for the Evaluation of Qualitative Research?

Few commentators would question the importance of the current and long-overdue emphasis on the need for evidence on effectiveness to play a more prominent role in decision making at all levels of health care. However, although effectiveness is a necessary aspect of clinical and policy decision making, it will never be sufficient. Health economists have argued the case for cost to be a compulsory prefix to effectiveness (Maynard, 1991). Managers and others have highlighted the complex nature of decision making at all levels of health care, with political and other constraints and priorities often displacing cost-effectiveness concerns (Frankford, 1994; Tanenbaum, 1994; Zimmern, 1995). Apart from these issues, there are at least two other critical fields of evidence that should inform policy and practice alongside evidence on effectiveness. These are evidence on appropriateness (i.e., the extent to which care can be said to meet the self-perceived needs of the person to whom it is being offered) and evidence of the factors that affect decision making among policy makers, clinicians, and patients (i.e., why people, both lay and professional, behave as they do when they do). However, in the absence of any attempt to develop standards, there is a danger that qualitative research evidence will be misunderstood and judged inferior by those whose field of vision is firmly fixed on a hierarchy of evidence that makes randomized control trials (RCTs) the gold standard.

There are four further and related reasons why the development of criteria or standards for the evaluation of qualitative research has become more urgent in recent times. First, in addition to the questions of appropriateness and the need to better understand lay and professional decision making already noted, health care procedures and interventions are proposing other questions that cannot be explored or explained by way of the RCT (Fitzpatrick & Boulton, 1994). If health care assessment and evaluation is to extend beyond the preoccupation with effectiveness, valuable as this is, then we need to develop criteria to judge the quality of other forms of research. Second, criteria to be applied in assessing standards in qualitative research during systematic reviews are necessary for rational decision making and the integration of existing information (Mulrow, 1994). In addition, health care providers, researchers, and policy makers are inundated with information and need to be discriminating. In view of the relative unfamiliarity of many health service workers and researchers with qualitative research, some guidelines for how to review and assess such work are needed. Third, many researchers who come to use qualitative methods within health service contexts have little or no familiarity with the disciplines in which the methods were developed and the assumptions underlying them. Although this does not preclude the conduct of good quality research, it limits the capacity of the researcher to maximize the potential contained within the approaches. Finally, from within the qualitative tradition itself, there have been calls for a renewed focus on criteria for assessing interpretive validity (i.e., calls for a focus not just on the technical features of particular methods but on the wider methodological and epistemological context within which the methods are applied) (Altheide & Johnson, 1994). This concern is applicable particularly to social science research in applied fields, such as health services research, in which these wider issues may not be routinely addressed.

What Criteria Should Be Used for Assessing the Validity of Qualitative Research in HSR?

The search for criteria for assessing the validity of qualitative research is not a new preoccupation. Social scientists have identified a number of different ways in which qualitative research can be assessed and good interpretation ensured (Denzin & Lincoln, 1994; Hammersley, 1987). These commentaries on what makes good qualitative research and how it should be judged, broadly speaking, fall into three camps. On one side, there are those who argue that there is nothing unique about qualitative research and that traditional definitions of reliability, validity, objectivity, and generalizability apply across both qualitative and quantitative approaches. On the other side, there are those postmodernists who contend that there can be no criteria for judging qualitative research outcomes (Fuchs, 1993). In this radical relativist position, all criteria are doubtful and none can be privileged. However, both of these positions are unsatisfactory. The second is nihilistic and precludes any distinction based on systematic or other criteria. If the first is adopted, then, at best, qualitative research will always be seen as inferior to quantitative research. At worst, there is a danger that poor-quality qualitative research, which meets criteria inappropriate for the assessment of such evidence, will be privileged.

There are certainly some common problems in evaluating the quality of all research output. For example, reports, articles, and books rarely provide enough detail of the methods used for an adequate judgment to be made about the quality of the study being reported. Moreover, many of the prima facie criteria used to assess the quality of research are similar no matter which method is adopted. These would include sufficient explanation of the background; a succinct statement of objectives or research questions; a full description of the methods used; and a clear presentation and discussion of the main findings, with some statement of their relevance to policy or practice when appropriate. Hammersley (1987) suggests that qualitative research needs to be assessed in terms of its capability to generate theory, be empirically grounded and scientifically credible, produce findings that can be transferable to other settings, and be internally reflexive with regard to the roles played by the researcher and researched. On cursory consideration, only the last of these marks a significant departure from research undertaken from within a quantitative tradition.[1]

However, beyond such minimalist criteria, a judgment about whether what is presented is good or bad requires the invocation of criteria that is more tailored to the particular features of the work in question. For example, qualitative researchers may use conceptions of trustworthiness and authenticity to replace the traditional criteria of validity reliability and objectivity, or the fit of the research with social and political action may be the key criterion (Rogers & Pilgrim, 1995b). Denzin and Lincoln (1994) have argued for efforts to be deployed in the construction of a set of validity criteria that flow from the qualitative project, stressing subjectivity and other antifoundational factors.

The works of Denzin and Lincoln (1994), Hammersley (1987), and others provide the basis for a third approach to the development of standards for assessing evidence from qualitative research. Here, it is accepted that some criteria may be equally applicable to the evaluation of any research product, regardless of the methods. However, this third approach also acknowledges differences. In giving greater recognition to the similarities between research traditions, we must not lose sight of two fundamental differences: the type of knowledge that different methods can generate (i.e., the epistemological difference) and the type of reality or object to which different methods are relevant (i.e., the ontological difference). As we have already noted, we recognize that there is no absolute list of criteria as to what constitutes good qualitative research. However, in the context, in particular, of research questions concerned with the appropriateness of care and with the basis of lay and professional decision making, these differences are fundamental. Therefore, they must inform the development of any framework for establishing hierarchies of evidence relevant to these questions.

The Primary Marker: Lay Accounts and the Privileging of Subjective Meaning

Research concerned with the appropriateness of care and with understanding the basis of lay and professional behavior and action must privilege subjective meaning or lay knowledge if it is to provide good evidence to inform practice and policy. We would term this the primary marker of standards in qualitative research relevant to these questions. In evaluating qualitative research output in terms of this primary marker, the key question to be addressed is, "Does the research, as reported, illuminate the subjective meaning, actions, and context of those being researched?"

This is where the epistemological and ontological differences need to be addressed. First, the most important marker of the caliber of studies seeking to illuminate lay knowledge is the extent to which the research adopts a *verstehen* approach to knowledge, illuminating the meanings people attach to their behaviors and experiences (i.e., it should seek to show how behaviors are viewed from within a culture, society, or group). To make use of Max Weber's (cited in Marsh, 1982) distinction, the point of the explanation is not in the first instance that adequacy is at the level of cause but in the first instance that adequacy is at the level of meaning. An explanation that is meaningful may help us to understand why something has happened or is the way it is.

Related to this is the key ontological reality with which research aimed at providing adequacy at the level of meaning must deal. In contrast to research that examines the lay or patient's view through the prism of professional knowledge or methods, research must attempt to find ways of according lay knowledge equal worth to other forms of knowledge (Stacey, 1994) based on the assumption that lay people and patients are a major source of expertise and skills and are knowledgeable about the management of health and illness. The work of Graham (1987), which explored lay women's accounts of smoking, is an example of an attempt to use verstehen methods and to accord primacy to lay knowledge, rather than professional knowledge, about what lay people think and do.

The case for awarding lay knowledge equal worth to other forms of knowledge rests on the contention that the former has the capacity to address key policy issues that have eluded the efforts of many policy makers. Lay knowledge may also be a prerequisite for more effective and therefore, by definition, more innovative ways of dealing with persistent policy failures or challenges. For example, the management of demand in primary care requires a deeper understanding of the link between health need and use of services than we have at present. A lay perspective on these issues has a vital contribution to make (Williams & Calnan, 1996). Similarly, illuminating the reasons why people act in the way they do at the time they do is central to understanding the perpetuation of variations in health among groups in the population. In studying the way in which actors act and employ their knowledge and experience, we can better understand the interaction between the experience of ill health, health action, and the use of services.

In short, in ensuring that emphasis is given to the interpretations of those being researched, the researcher and the research design will be informed by a position that privileges the lay view rather than resorting to the constructs brought in from professional discourse, such as medicine or psychoanalysis. Of importance, this is equally applicable to research that aims to understand the basis of professional behavior. It is important that the research recognizes and deals with the juxtaposition of professional and lay knowledge – different ways of knowing – among professionals (Edwards & Popay, 1994).

The primacy of the knowledge marker in assessing standards in qualitative research aiming to elucidate lay knowledge and behavior should be reflected in the way other markers for data quality and adequacy are developed. Thus, in the rest of this article, our focus is not on assessing the adequacy of techniques but with identifying criteria that might be used to highlight the ontological differences discussed previously.

Evidence of Responsiveness to Social Context and Flexibility of Design

One key consequence of the ontological and epistemological differences to which we have referred is that qualitative research has a different relationship to the context of the research than is the case with most quantitative research. Whereas the latter seeks to develop methods and produce findings that are independent of the context, qualitative research seeks to maximize the use of context as a means of locating lay knowledge and understanding subjective meaning.

Here, the key question is, "Is there evidence of the adaption and responsiveness of the research design to the circumstances and issues of real-life social settings met during the course of the study?"

One of the most obvious differences between qualitative and quantitative studies is the apparent absence of standardized procedures (or codes) to follow when using particular qualitative methods. For example, judgments about the equation of sample size, statistical significance, and power, which routinely inform our evaluation of quantitative studies, have no equivalent in qualitative studies. In contrast to most quantitative studies, the phases of the research process – sampling, data collection, data analysis, and interpretation – are not separate. Sampling, for example, is interdependent with data collection, data collection overlaps with data analysis, and the movement from analysis to interpretation is not clear-cut. In view of the attention to meaning, qualitative methods need to be able to be responsive to circumstances as they exist, rather than attempt to create a situation in which the variables of interest can be controlled and their relationships examined and compared across all other similarly controlled situations. For this reason, the hallmark of good qualitative methodology is its variability, rather than its standardization. Thus, there should be some evidence of adaption and redesign in the writing up of research.

Evidence of Theoretical or Purposeful Sampling

In view of the very different purpose of qualitative research aiming to illuminate the subjective meanings shaping action and behavior, it should not be surprising that different rules and standards need to be applied than those applied in assessing evidence from experiments or surveys. This is true of sampling, in which randomness and representativeness are of less concern than relevance. Therefore, the key question to be asked in assessing standards of sampling is, "Does the sample produce the type of knowledge necessary to understand the structures and processes within which the individuals or situations are located?"

Particular types of sampling will influence whether the criteria of adequacy at the level of subjective meaning is met. Rather than randomness and calculations based on statistical power, the process by which individuals or cases were theoretically or purposefully sampled needs adequate description. The use of key informants is frequently a preferred way of ensuring the selection of respondents with the appropriate knowledge. As Blumer (1979) has suggested,

> A half dozen individuals with such knowledge constitute a far better "representative sample" than a thousand individuals who may be involved in the action that is being formed but who are not knowledgeable about that formation, (p. 156)

In mixed methods studies, cases for in-depth study can also be sampled from a larger survey population, which may then serve as a context and a basis for empirical generalizations.

Evidence of Adequate Description

One commonly held view is that the hallmark of qualitative research lies in its ability to provide in-depth descriptions. Thus, one marker of adequacy is the richness of the picture that such research produces. However, whereas description may be seen as a resource that is able to provide information about a particular topic, description is also important for analytic inquiry (Stanley, 1990). Therefore, the key question here is not concerned simply with depth but with purpose. Thus, the question should be, "Is the description provided detailed enough to allow the researcher or reader to interpret the meaning and context of what is being researched?"

The process of describing in detail the circumstances surrounding an event or an experience and of exploring people's perceptions of and responses to those circumstances in the situation in which they occur may constitute the grounds for explanation. The distinction between thin and thick description made by Geertz (1973) is useful here. Thin description merely states a set of facts that are independent of intentions or circumstances. In contrast, thick description provides the context of an experience, states the intentions and meanings that feed into that experience, and exposes the experience as a process. The extent to which a text shows evidence of thick description is a part of the claim to authenticity and substantiation because it indicates the depth versus the superficiality of the accounts and observations on which the written research report is based. As Denzin and Lincoln (1994) have noted, thick description makes thick interpretation possible.

Evidence of Data Quality

A number of questions might be asked to assess the quality of data in qualitative research. However, although triangulation might be appropriate, a more broad question should be asked, namely, "How are different sources of knowledge about the same issue compared and contrasted?"

This question is not just to ensure that accounts coincide, as in triangulation, but helps illuminate different facets of the reality being investigated. A second important question directly addresses the ontological issues discussed earlier. "Are subjective perceptions and experiences treated as knowledge in their own right?"

In the context of this marker, it is important to recognize that data are never pure. As Plummer (1983) has noted, there is a continuum of contamination in both the collection and the presentation of the data. In any research report, it is necessary to examine the ways in which the data have been shaped by the researchers' questions or observations and used in the context of a particular set of arguments. Given the involvement of the researcher in the research process, the question is not whether the data are biased, but to what extent has the researcher rendered transparent the processes by which data have been collected, analyzed, and presented. Qualitative research treats all data as the product of interaction. Thus, the time, extent, and nature of the researchers' involvement have to be extensive if the complexities of accounts and social situations are to be adequately revealed.

Evidence of Theoretical and Conceptual Adequacy

Data have no meaning in themselves and validity is a concern common to all research methods. However, in relation to qualitative research, we are principally concerned with interpretive validity, which requires a degree of reflexive accounting on the part of the researcher. Here, the key question is, "How does the research move from a description of the data, through quotation or examples, to an analysis and interpretation of the meaning and significance of it?"

Although in a full report one would expect to find some evidence of the constant comparative method whereby the researcher compares statements and indexes of behavior that occur over time and in a range of periods during the study, a journal article is more limited. However, in an article for review, one should be able (albeit in a limited way) to decipher the views and analysis undertaken by the researcher from the description of the setting and the interactions and accounts given by those who have been studied.

Potential for Assessing Typicality

In undertaking systematic reviews of research evidence, the central question to be asked of the findings of any single study is whether the findings are generalizable. This, of course, is one of the most problematic aspects of qualitative research for many critics. The main point to highlight here is that generalization from a case study or a small theoretical sample is of a different order to the kind of generalization that one can make from an experiment or a survey. The key question to be asked here is, "What claims are being made for the generalizability of the findings to either other bodies of knowledge or to other populations or groups?"

To say that a case is typical is to say that it contains certain features that are found in many other cases. The aim is to make logical generalizations to a theoretical understanding of a similar class of phenomena rather than probabilistic generalizations to a population. Settings or cases do not have to be typical for generalizations to be made. Indeed, the general relevance may derive from their atypicality. This is particularly true of settings and research that are at the forefront of change. Consider the following contemporary United Kingdom example from the British National Health Service: In-depth study of an initial exemplar of total purchasing pilot schemes as an extension of *fundholding* within general practice will allow for the generation of the logical features of a type against which further cases can be examined with gradual evolution of our theoretical understanding of total purchasing. In part, typicality and generalizability can be obtained by relating purposefulness to representativeness. As discussed previously, for example, the characteristics of a sample can be chosen to match the features of particular groups of people associated with certain patterns of health service use, health behavior, or illness.

Because the way in which a case study fits into a body of theory or other findings is important, the reporting of research should provide background information sufficient to make these judgments. Parts of a setting may be studied and then generalized to the whole of a setting, which may in turn be treated as typical of a larger number of settings. Events at one time can sometimes be generalized to events at others if time, place, and setting are made explicit. Confidence in judgments about the typicality of findings can be enhanced by using sources of information such as official and nonofficial statistics, policy documents, and congruent pieces of research.

Conclusion: Relevance of Qualitative Research to Policy

In the context of HSR, qualitative research should have some clear implications for policy and practice. For modern health services, this means indicating the relevance of research to a variety of different stakeholders for whom research of any sort is only one of a number of sources of guidance in decision making. In this context, the development of criteria, markers, or key questions is an important way to aid the reading and assessment of the products of qualitative research by a variety of different audiences with varying agendas. The questions identified previously are just the beginning of formulating standards for the assessment of qualitative research within the context of systematic reviews. The particular focus here is on research evidence that will help to illuminate questions concerning the appropriateness of care and aid understanding of the basis of lay and clinical behavior. To take advantage of the rapidly expanding wealth of qualitative review articles being published in the health field that are relevant to these central questions for contemporary health policy, the preliminary markers presented here will require further development. In addition, attention will have to be given to the adaptation of the methodology for systematic review, including ways of devising appropriate search strategies and of clarifying questions to be asked in relation to specific topic areas. Such developments would, however, make a significant and much needed contribution to systematic review methodology.

Note

1. Even here, quantitative researchers are reflexive, albeit in a limited way, by taking cognizance of sources of contamination; this is similar to the Hawthorne effect in experimental design.

References

Altheide, D., & Johnson, J. (1994). Criteria for assessing interpretive validity in qualitative research. In N. Denzin & Y. Lincoln (Eds.), *Handbook of qualitative research* (pp. 485–499). London: Sage Ltd.

Black, N. (1994). Why we need qualitative research. *Journal of Epidemiology and Community Health, 48*, 425–426.

Blumer, H. (1979). *Critiques of research, in the social sciences.* New Brunswick, NJ: Transaction Books.

Britten, N., & Fischer, B. (1993, July). Qualitative research and general practice. *British Journal of General Practice*, pp. 270–271.

Brown, P. (1992). Popular epidemiology and toxic waste contamination: Lay and professional ways of knowing. *Journal of Health and Social Behaviour, 33*, 267–281.

Denzin, N., & Lincoln, Y. (1994). *Handbook of qualitative research.* London: Sage Ltd.

Edwards, J., & Popay, J. (1994). Contradictions of support and self help: Views from providers of community health and social services to families with young children. *Health and Social Care in the Community, 2*, 31–40.

Fitzpatrick, R., & Boulton, M. (1994). Qualitative methods for assessing health care. *Quality in Health Care, 3*, 107–113.

Frankford, D. M. (1994). Scientism and economism in the regulation of health care. *Journal of Health Politics, Policy and Law, 19*(4), 773–799.

Fuchs, M. (1993). The reversal of the ethnological perspective: Attempts at objectifying one's own cultural horizon. Dumont, Foucalt, Bourdieu? *Thesis Eleven, 34*, 104–125.

Gabe, J., Kelleher, D., & Williams, G. (Eds.). (1994). *Challenging medicine.* London: Routledge.

Geertz, C. (1973). *The interpretation of cultures: Selected essays.* New York: Basic Books.

Graham, H. (1987). Women's smoking and family health. *Social Science and Medicine, 25,* 47–56.

Hammersley, M. (1987). *What's wrong with ethnography? Methodological explorations.* London: Routledge.

Marsh, C. (1982). *The survey method: The contribution of surveys to sociological explanation.* London: Allen and Unwin.

Maynard, A. (1991). The design of future cost-benefit studies. *American Heart Journal, 3*, 761–765.

Mulrow, C. (1994). Rationale for systematic reviews. *British Medical Journal, 309*, 597–599.

Plummer, K. (1983). *Documents of life: An introduction to the problems and literature of a humanistic method.* London: Allen and Unwin.

Popay, J., Rogers, A., & Williams, G. (1996). Qualitative research and the gingerbread man. *Health Education Journal, 55*, 1–3.

Popay, J., & Williams, G. (Eds.). (1994). *Researching the people's health.* London: Routledge.

Pope, C., & Mays, N. (1995). Reaching the parts other methods cannot reach: An introduction to qualitative methods in health and health services research. *British Medical Journal, 6996*(311), 42–45.

Rogers, A., & Pilgrim, D. (1995a). Experiencing psychiatry: An example of emancipatory research. In G. Wilson (Ed.), *Researching users views of community care services* (pp. 214–228). London: Chapman Hall.

Rogers, A., & Pilgrim, D. (1995b). The risk of resistance: Perspectives on the mass childhood immunization program. *Medicine health and risk: Sociological approaches* [Sociology of Health and Illness Monograph Series] L. J. Gabe (Ed.). Oxford, UK: Basil Blackwell.

Rosenberg, W., & Donald, A. (1995). Evidence based medicine: An approach to clinical problem-solving. *British Medical Journal, 310,* 1122–1126.

Secker, J., Wimbush, E., Watson, J., & Milburn, K. (1995). Qualitative methods in health promotion research: Some criteria for quality. *Health Education Journal, 54,* 1.

Stacey, M. (1994). The power of lay knowledge: A personal view. In J. Popay & G. Williams (Eds.), *Researching the people's health* (pp. 85–98). London: Routledge.

Stanley, L. (1990). Doing ethnography, writing ethnography: A comment on Hammersley. *Sociology, 24*(4), 617–627.

Tanenbaum, S. J. (1994). Knowing and acting in medical practice: The epistemological politics of outcomes research. *Journal of Health Politics, Policy and Law, 19,* 27–44.

Williams, G., & Popay, J. (1994). Lay knowledge and the privilege of experience. In J. Gabe, D. Kelleher, & G. Williams (Eds.), *Challenging medicine* (pp. 118–139). London: Routledge.

Williams, S., & Calnan, M. (1996). *Modern medicine: Lay perspectives and experiences.* London: UCL Press.

Woolfe, S., Battista, R., & Anderson, G. (1990). Assessing the clinical effectiveness of preventive maneuvers: Analytic principles and systematic methods in reviewing evidence and developing clinical practice recommendations. *Journal of Clinical Epidemiology, 43,* 891–905.

Zimmern, R L. (1995). *Challenging choices, complex decision-making.* Cambridge, UK: Colin Hollidge Design.

51

Sample Size in Qualitative Research

Margarete Sandelowski

A common misconception about sampling in qualitative research is that numbers are unimportant in ensuring the adequacy of a sampling strategy. The "logic and power" (Patton, 1990, p. 169) of the various kinds of purposeful sampling used in qualitative research lie primarily in the quality of information obtained per sampling unit, as opposed to their number per se. Moreover, an aesthetic thrust of sampling in qualitative research is that small is beautiful.[1] Yet, inadequate sample sizes can undermine the credibility of research findings. There are no computations or power analyses that can be done in qualitative research to determine a priori the minimum number and kinds of sampling units required, but there are factors, including the aim of sampling and the type of purposeful sampling and research method employed, which researchers can consider to help them decide whether they have collected enough data. These factors are the subject of this article.

Neither Small Nor Large, but Too Small or Too Large

Adequacy of sample size in qualitative research is relative, a matter of judging a sample neither small nor large per se, but rather too small or too large for the intended purposes of sampling and for the intended qualitative product. A sample size of 10 may be judged adequate for certain kinds of homogeneous or critical case sampling, too small to achieve maximum variation of a complex phenomenon or to develop theory, or too large for certain kinds of narrative analyses.

Source: *Research in Nursing & Health*, 18(2) (1995): 179–183.

Reported sample sizes are often too small to support claims of having achieved either informational redundancy (Lincoln & Guba, 1985) or theoretical saturation (Strauss & Corbin, 1990). Impatience, an a priori commitment to what will be seen, or a disinclination to see any more may incline researchers to stop sampling prematurely. Seeing nothing new in newly sampled units or feeling comfortable that a theoretical category has been saturated are functions involving the recognition of what is there and what can be made out of the data already collected, and then deciding whether it is sufficient to create an intended product. These functions are acquired through experience. For example, I have noticed in my own development and that of students with whom I have worked that beginning qualitative researchers often require more sampling units than more experienced researchers to "see" and to "make." One expert qualitative researcher (P. Stern, personal communication, 1989) intimated that we often have all the data we will need in the very first pieces of data we collect, but that we do not (or cannot) know that until we collect more. Ultimately, information can be deemed redundant or theoretical lines deemed saturated – only for now (Morse, 1989).

Conversely, sample sizes may be too large to support claims to having completed detailed analyses of data, especially the microanalysis demanded by certain kinds of narrative and observational studies. Even in qualitative projects aimed at explicating regularities across pieces of data, a high premium is still placed on discerning the particularities or idiosyncrasies presented by each piece of data. While qualitative studies may involve what are considered large sample sizes (over 50), qualitative analysis is generically about maximizing understanding of the one in all of its diversity; it is case-oriented, not variable-oriented (Ragin & Becker, 1989). Any sample size interfering with the case-oriented thrust of qualitative work can, accordingly, be judged too large.

Issues in Purposeful Sampling

One of the major differences between qualitative and quantitative research approaches is that qualitative approaches typically involve purposeful sampling, while quantitative approaches usually involve probability sampling (Kuzel, 1992; Morse, 1986, 1989; Patton, 1990). Patton (1990) described 14 different types of purposeful sampling, involving the selection for in-depth study of typical, atypical, or, in some way, exemplary "information-rich cases" (p. 169). Researchers in both domains of inquiry often have to resort to sampling they know is less than ideal for their purposes, but qualitative researchers value the deep understanding permitted by information rich cases and quantitative researchers value the generalizations to larger populations permitted by random and statistically representative samples. Although a sample of one will never be sufficient to permit generalization of findings to populations, it may be sufficient to permit the valuable kind of generalizations that can be made from and about cases, variously referred to as idiographic, holographic, naturalistic, or analyth generalizations (Firestone, 1993; Lincoln & Guba, 1985; Ragin & Becker, 1992; Simons, 1980; Stake & Trumbull, 1982).

In qualitative research, events, incidents, and experiences, not people per se, are typically the objects of purposeful sampling (Miles & Huberman, 1994; Strauss & Corbin, 1990). People, in addition to sites, artifacts, documents, and even data that have already been collected are sampled for the information they are likely to yield about a particular phenomenon. Sample size in qualitative research may refer to numbers of persons, but also to numbers of interviews and observations conducted or numbers of events sampled. People are certainly central in all kinds of inquiry approaches in the health sciences, but they enter qualitative studies primarily by virtue of having direct and personal knowledge of some event (e.g., illness, pregnancy, life transition) that they are able and willing to communicate to others and only secondarily by virtue of demographic characteristics (e.g., age, race, sex).

People versus Purpose

When qualitative researchers decide to seek people out because of their age or sex or race, it is because they consider them good sources of information that will advance them toward an analytic goal and not because they wish to generalize to other persons of similar age, sex, or race. That is, a demographic variable, such as sex, becomes an analytic variable; persons of one or the other sex are selected for a study because, by virtue of their sex, they can provide certain kinds of information. Accordingly, only as many persons of a particular sex are included in a study as is necessary to obtain that information. There is no mandate to have equivalent numbers of women or men or numbers of persons of each sex in the proportions in which they appear in a certain population.

Sampling on the basis of demographic characteristics presents something of a problem in achieving both informational and size adequacy in qualitative studies. There is currently a strong impulse (and federal mandate) to eliminate gender, race/ethnicity, and class bias in research by including members of minority or traditionally disempowered groups typically underrepresented in research, and by including women and men typically underrepresented in certain domains of research, such as men in family studies and women in studies of heart disease. Trost (1986) described a "statistically nonrepresentative stratified" sampling strategy whereby researchers can select persons varying in demographic characteristics to achieve representative coverage and inclusion. That is, while the sample is statistically nonrepresentative, it is informationally representative in that data will be obtained from persons who can stand for other persons with similar characteristics. In her illustration involving a study of families with teenagers, five sets of naturally and artificially dichotomized variables (one or two-parent family, one or two or more children, housed in an apartment or home, with a high or low income, and with a male or female teenager) were combined to yield 32 kinds of families to be sampled. A similar kind of sampling plan can be used to ensure inclusion of females and males, and persons varying in social class, race, cultural affiliation, religion, or other dimension.

Although this kind of sampling accommodates a new, laudable, and necessary moral consciousness concerning underrepresented and, therefore, often misrepresented groups by partially accommodating the logic of probability sampling, it may wholly contravene the logic of purposeful sampling. Strictly speaking, sampling for variation in race, class, gender, or other such background or person-related characteristics ought to be done in qualitative studies when they are deemed analytically important and where the failure to sample for such variation would impede understanding or invalidate findings (Cannon, Higginbotham, Leung, 1988). Deciding a priori that a sample will include a certain number or percentage of individuals in various demographic groups may meet federal and other mandates for inclusion of traditionally excluded persons, but it may also result in a sample with a kind of variation that has little analytic significance or detracts from analysis goals (Morse, 1989). More importantly, such a sample may be too small adequately to address the analytic importance of such factors as gender or race, or, alternatively, too large to favor the deep analysis that qualitative projects mandate.

One way to resolve this dilemma is to design studies in which a phenomenon is investigated in one group at a time (either simultaneously or sequentially). The design for such studies will include more than one purposeful sampling strategy: for example, homogeneous and maximum variation sampling, where person-related homogeneity is maintained while variation in the target phenomenon is sought. After a series of such studies has been completed, a larger synthesis of findings can be undertaken in which the researcher can more adequately address the question of whether and how a variable such as gender is important in understanding a phenomenon.

Sample Size in Different Kinds of Purposeful Sampling

Different kinds of purposeful sampling require different minimum sample sizes. For example, in deviant case sampling, where the intention is to understand a very unusual or atypical manifestation of some phenomenon, one case may be sufficient. Yet, even a sample of one requires within-case sampling (Miles & Huberman, 1994). The researcher must decide which of the varieties of data concerning the case to sample to explicate its a typicality. This is especially evident in cases involving aggregates of one, such as a family, community, or organization. Even when an individual is the focal one, the researcher must sample from the wealth of data obtainable from and about that individual.

In short, any one case offers a variety of data that must be sampled in sufficient quantity to make the case.

Maximum variation is one of the most frequently employed kinds of purposeful sampling in qualitative nursing research and typically requires the largest minimum sample size of any of the purposeful sampling strategies. As in any kind of sampling, the more variability there is within the confines of a qualitative project, the more numbers of sampling units the researcher will require to reach informational redundancy or theoretical saturation. Researchers wanting maximum variation in their sample must decide what kind(s) of variation they want to maximize and when to maximize each kind. One kind of variation already described is *demographic* variation, where variation is sought on generally people-related characteristics.

A second kind of variation is *phenomenal* variation, or variation on the target phenomenon under study. For example, the target phenomenon in a study of couples who have obtained positive fetal diagnoses is diagnosis, which varies on such dimensions as type and time of diagnosis, and the instrumentation used to make it. Like the decision to seek demographic variation, the decision to seek phenomenal variation is often made a priori in order to have representative coverage of variables likely to be important in understanding how diverse factors configure a whole. This kind of sampling is also referred to as selective or criterion sampling, where sampling decisions are made going into a study on "reasonable" grounds, rather than on analytic grounds after some data have already been collected (Glaser, 1978, p. 37; Schatzman & Strauss, 1973).

A third kind of variation is *theoretical* variation, or variation on a theoretical construct that is associated with theoretical sampling, or the sampling on analytic grounds characteristic of grounded theory studies. A theoretical sampling strategy is employed to fully elaborate and validate theoretically derived variations discerned in the data. Initial sampling for phenomenal variation permits these theoretical variations to be identified. A program of research employing grounded theory typically begins with a selective or criterion sampling strategy aimed at phenomenal variation and then proceeds to theoretical sampling (Sandelowski, Holditch-Davis, & Harris, 1992).

Researchers control the number of sampling units required to achieve informational redundancy or theoretical saturation by deciding which category of variation to maximize and minimize. This decision is a matter of fitting the sampling strategy to the purpose of and method chosen for a particular study and appraising the resources (including number of investigators and financial support) available to conduct the study. For example, purposeful sampling for demographic homogeneity and selected phenomenal variation is a way a researcher working alone with limited resources can reduce the minimum number of sampling units required within the confines of a single research project, but still produce credible and analytically and/or clinically significant findings.

Sample Sizes for Different Qualitative Methods

Just as different purposeful sampling strategies require different minimum sample sizes, different qualitative methods require different minimum sample sizes. Morse (1994) has recommended that phenomenologies directed toward discerning the essence of experiences include about six participants, ethnographies and grounded theory studies, about 30 to 50 interviews and/or observations, and qualitative ethological studies, about 100 to 200 units of observation.

Additional considerations in matching sample size to method are within-method diversity and the multiple uses of a method. Phenomenology offers a good illustration of how within-method diversity and the particular use to which a method is put can alter the requirements for sample size. In a phenomenological case study, one case can be sufficient to show something about an experience that a researcher deems significant for special display (e.g., Wertz, 1983). One case will not be sufficient, however, if the researcher's intention is to describe invariant or essential features of an experience. For example, a phenomenological study, as interpreted by Van Kaam (1959), will likely require 10 to 50 description of a target experience in order to discern its necessary and sufficient constituents. When phenomenological techniques are used in the service of a goal other than to produce a phenomenology, such as generating items for an instrument, at least 25 descriptions of an experience will likely be required.

Sample Sizes in Combined Qualitative and Quantitative Studies

Studies combining qualitative and quantitative approaches involve additional considerations in determining sufficient sample size. Indeed, so-called methodologically triangulated studies present researchers with many dilemmas (beyond the scope of this article), the resolution of which depend on the researcher's stance concerning the compatibility of the philosophies and practices of qualitative and quantitative inquiry.

With respect to sampling, the logics of probability and purposeful sampling are arguably sufficiently irreconcilable in most cases to preclude using the same subjects for both quantitative and qualitative purposes (Morse, 1991). Subjects selected for the purposes of statistical representativeness may not fulfill the informational needs of the study, while participants selected for information purposes do not meet the requirement of statistical representativeness. Accordingly, whether primarily quantitative or qualitative, or whether designed for purposes of completeness or confirmation (Breitmayer, Ayres, & Knafl, 1993), such combination studies would require two samples drawn simultaneously or sequentially according to the two logics of sampling.

Yet, it can also be argued that among persons chosen according to the logic of probability sampling, there will likely be articulate informants whose selection for the qualitative portion of a combined study can be justified as purposeful. The purposeful sample would have to be expanded only if the data obtainable from the participants already sampled was deemed informationally insufficient. Similarly, no additional sampling may be necessary in studies where further information obtainable from standardized instruments is desired about a purposefully drawn sample. The caveat here is that the researcher use the data from these instruments for purposes of fuller description, rather than to draw statistical inferences.

Conclusion

Determining an adequate sample size in qualitative research is ultimately a matter of judgment and experience in evaluating the quality of the information collected against the uses to which it will be put, the particular research method and sampling strategy employed, and the research product intended. Numbers have a place in ensuring that a sample is fully adequate to support particular qualitative enterprises. A good principle to follow is: An adequate sample size in qualitative research is one, that permits – by virtue of not being too large – the deep, case-oriented analysis that is a hallmark of all qualitative inquiry, and that results in – by virtue of not being too small – a new and richly textured understanding of experience.

Note

1. I am indebted to one of the anonymous reviewers of this article for the phrasing "small is beautiful."

References

Breitmayer, B. J., Ayres. L., & Knafl, K. A. (1993). Triangulation in qualitative research: Evaluation of completeness and confirmation purposes. *Image: Journal of Nursing Scholarship, 25,* 237–243.

Cannon, L. W., Higginbotham, E., & Liung, M. L. (1988). Race and class bias in qualitative research on women. *Gender & Society, 2,* 449–462.

Firestone, W. A. (1993). Alternative arguments for generalizing from data as applied to qualitative research. *Educational Researcher, 22,* 16–23.

Glaser, B. G. (1978). *Theoretical sensitivity: Advances in the methodology of grounded theory.* Mill Valley, CA: Sociology Press.

Kuzel, A. J. (1992). Sampling in qualitative inquiry. In B. F. Crabtree & W. L. Miller (Eds.), *Doing qualitative research* (pp. 31–44). Newbury Park, CA: Sage.

Lincoln, Y. S., & Guba, E. G. (1985). *Naturalistic inquiry.* Beverly Hills. CA: Sage.

Miles. M. B., & Huberman, A. M. (1994). *Qualitative data analysis: An expanded sourcebook* (2nd ed). Thousand Oaks, CA: Sage.

Morse, J. M. (1986). Quantitative and qualitative research: Issues in sampling. In P. L. Chinn (Ed.), *Nursing research methodology: Issues and implementation* (pp. 181–193). Rockville, MD: Aspen.

Morse, J. M. (1989). Strategies for sampling. In J. M. Morse (Ed.), *Qualitative nursing research: A contemporary dialogue* (pp. 117–131). Rockville. MD: Aspen.

Morse, J. (1991). Approaches to qualitative–quantitative methodological triangulation. *Nursing Research, 40,* 120–123.

Morse, J. M. (1994). Designing funded qualitative research. In N. K. Denzin & Y. S. Lincoln (Eds.). *Handbook of qualitative research* (pp 220–235). Thousand Oaks, CA: Sage.

Patton, M. Q. (1990). *Qualitative evaluation and research methods* (2nd ed). Newbury Park, CA: Sage.

Ragin, C. C., & Becker, H. S. (1989). How the micro computer is changing our analytic habits. In G. Blank, J. L. McCartney, & E. Brent (Eds.), *New technology in society: Practical applications in research and work* (pp. 47–55). New Brunswick, NJ: Transaction.

Ragin, C. C., & Becker, H. S. (1992). *What is a case? Exploring the foundations of social inquiry.* Cambridge: Cambridge University Press

Sandelowski, M., Holditch-Davis, D., & Harris, B. G. (1992). Using qualitative and quantitative methods: The transition to parenthood of infertile couples. In J. F. Gilgun, K. Daly, & G. Handel (Eds.), *Qualitative methods in family research* (pp. 301–322). Newbury Park, CA: Sage.

Schatzman, L., & Strauss, A. (1973). *Field research: Strategies for a natural sociology.* Englewood Cliffs. NJ: Prentice-Hall.

Simons, H. (Ed.). (1980). *Towards a science of the singular: Essays about case study in educational research and evaluation.* Norwich: University of East Anglia, Center for Applied Research in Education.

Stake, R. E., & Trumbull, D. J. (1982). Naturalistic generalizations. *Review Journal of Philosophy and Social Science, 7,* 1–12.

Strauss, A., & Corbin, J. (199). *Basics of qualitative research: Grounded theory procedures and techniques.* Newbury Park, CA: Sage.

Trost, J. E. (1986). Statistically nonrepresentative stratified sampling: A sampling technique for qualitative studies. *Qualitative Sociology, 9,* 54–57.

Van Kaam, A. L. (1959). Phenomenal analysis: Exemplified by a study of the experience of "really feeling understood." *Journal of Individual Psychology, 15,* 66–72.

Wertz, F. J. (1983). From everyday to psychological description: Analyzing the moments of a qualitative data analysis. *Journal of Phenomenological Psychology, 14,* 197–241.

52

Rigor or Rigor Mortis: The Problem of Rigor in Qualitative Research Revisited

Margarete Sandelowski

T he problem of rigor in qualitative research continues to arouse, beguile, and misdirect. As researchers, we have a much clearer understanding of the challenges involved in producing good qualitative work and of techniques that can be used to ensure its trustworthiness. Yet we also remain in danger of succumbing to the "illusion of technique"[1,2]: of making a fetish of it at the expense of perfecting a craft and of making rigor an unyielding end in itself, There is an inflexibility and an uncompromising harshness and rigidity implied in the term "rigor" that threaten to take us too far from the artfulness, versatility, and sensitivity to meaning and context that mark qualitative works of distinction. It is as if, in our quasi-militaristic zeal to neutralize bias and to defend our projects against threats to validity, we were more preoccupied with building fortifications against attack than with creating the evocative, true-to-life, and meaningful portraits, stories, and landscapes of human experience that constitute the best test of rigor in qualitative work.

In this article, I revisit the beguiling problem of rigor in qualitative research yet again.[3] What seems clearer to me now – after many years of reading and doing qualitative work – and what I hope to clarify here, is that rigor is less about adherence to the letter of rules and procedures than it is about fidelity to the spirit of qualitative work.[2]

Source: *Advances in Nursing Science*, 16(2) (1993): 1–8.

Reconceptualizing Validity

Scholars have increasingly disputed the conflation of validity with either truth or value (a scientifically valid work may be neither true nor valuable), and the reification, commodification, and reduction of validity to a set of procedures. They have also increasingly abandoned the storybook image of science to focus on what scientists actually do. As Elliot Mishler concluded, they have come to recognize that the work of science is, in part, defined by the social process of validation.[4]

According to Mishler, different communities of researchers differently warrant and evaluate claims to scientific worthiness. Because no general rules can be provided for appraising validity in particular studies or domains of inquiry, and because no standard procedure can be determined either for assigning weights to different threats to validity or for comparing different kinds of validity, validation is less a technical problem than a deeply theoretical one. For Mishler, the evaluation of the trustworthiness of any single project is inevitably a matter of judgment, whereby skilled researchers use their tacit understanding of actual, situated practices in their fields of inquiry to do their own work, to make claims for it, and to evaluate the work of others. Mishler emphasized the social world of scientists who strive to have their work accepted as good science. As social worlds are continually being made and remade, so are the practices that scientists use to support their claims-making. The social discourse on reliability, for example, is better understood as a particular way of warranting validity claims, rather than as a universal or abstract guarantor of truth. Indeed, as I discuss shortly, the effort to establish reliability (as it is conventionally portrayed in instructional literature) is often completely unwarranted in many qualitative projects and may, paradoxically, serve only to weaken claims to validity.

When validation is viewed as a culturally and historically situated social process, both experimentalist and interpretivist can be recognized as relying on contextually grounded linguistic and interpretive practices, rather than on rules assumed to be sufficiently abstract and universal for every project. Trustworthiness becomes a matter of persuasion whereby the scientist is viewed as having made those practices visible and, therefore, auditable; it is less a matter of claiming to be right about a phenomenon than of having practiced good science.

Reliability as a Threat to Validity

One of the most important threats to the phenomenological validity[5] (addressing the *true-to*) and, therefore, to the construct validity (addressing the *true about*) of qualitative projects is the assumption that validity rests on reliability. Investigators often claim that their findings are valid when, for example, they can show that research participants responded consistently over time and with each other concerning an experience, or that a panel of experts or persons other than the investigator coded information the same way. What is embedded in these examples is the notion of reality as external, consensual, corroboratory, and repeatable. What is being sought in these examples are coefficients of agreement or consensus on the nature of that reality.

What is forgotten is that in the naturalistic/interpretive paradigm, reality is assumed to be multiple and constructed rather than singular and tangible.[6] Moreover, what is ignored in the indiscriminate transfer to interpretive research of the assumption that a valid work must be a reliable one is that qualitative research is an art, or, at least, as much art as science, and that the nature of the narrative data that are the mainstay of qualitative work is inherently revisionist. To put it in phenomenological terms, repeatability is not an essential (or necessary or sufficient) property of the things themselves (whether the thing is qualitative research or the qualitative interview).

Qualitative Research as Art

As described in detail elsewhere,[7,8] there is a kinship between art and science, and qualitative research bridges these realms of meaning. Accordingly, any discussion of validity must occur in the context of the artfulness of qualitative inquiry. Renata Tesch elegantly summarized why the validity of an artful enterprise does not depend on replicable outcomes.[9] Indeed, according to Tesch, the result of a qualitative analysis should be viewed as

> a representation in the same sense that an artist can, with a few strokes of the pen, create an image of a face that we would recognize if we saw the original in a crowd. The details are lacking, but a good "reduction" not only selects and emphasizes the essential features, it retains the vividness of the personality in the rendition of the face.[9(p304)]

Similarly, a good qualitative data reduction grabs the "essence" of a phenomenon; it does not "flood (us) with so much detail (that we are) left with hardly a perception of the phenomenon at all."[9(p304)] Even when confronted with the same qualitative task, no two researchers will produce the same result; there will inevitably be differences in their philosophical and theoretical commitments and styles.

Tesch shows us not only why aiming for the so-called whole truth ("flooded with detail") may actually interfere with apprehending truth (the "essence"), but also why scientific notions of replicability are often completely at odds with the phenomenological validity sought by researchers working within the naturalistic/interpretive paradigm. Just as Dali's art is no less valid than Picasso's by virtue of differently re-presenting common phenomena, so too may different qualitative re-presentations of common phenomena all be valid ones. "There is no one correct way of drawing a face."[9](p305) The task for scholars in a practice-oriented discipline such as nursing is to find ways to apprehend and re-present these different representations to achieve the "fuller knowing" that advances knowledge and influences practice.

The Revisionist Nature of Narratives

A second critical factor invalidating the assumption that a valid work is always a conventionally reliable one is the inherently revisionist nature of the stories participants tell us in interviews. As described in more detail elsewhere,[10] these stories are remembrances about the past in a fleeting present moment soon to be past. Research participants often change their stories from one telling to the next as new experiences and the very act of telling itself cause them to see the nature and connection of the events in their lives differently. The idea of empirically validating the information in one story against the information in another for consistency is completely alien to the concept of narrative truth and to the temporality, liminality, and meaning-making function of stories.

The task for the researcher confronted with different versions of a life event is not to dismiss them as simply inconsistent with each other or to dismiss the storyteller as an unreliable informant. Rather, the researcher might, for example, consider whether the versions are truly inconsistent, or, if inconsistent, why discrepancies exist, or whether the two discrepant accounts even represent the same story. Although it may be a useful tool in some carefully selected instances, no reliability coefficient can ever adequately deal with the analytic challenges of narrative data.

Member Validation as a Threat to Validity

Member validation illustrates well not only the tenacity of the idea of reliability as the essential basis for validity, but also the complexity of all such techniques directed toward ensuring the rigor of qualitative research. Member validation, or the member check, is a technique scholars have proposed for establishing the validity of researchers' interpretations of data collected from research participants and for ensuring that these participants have access to what has been made of their experiences. The member check, accordingly, involves a professional obligation to do good science and a specifically ethical obligation to support members' right to know. As various scholars have described it,[6,11,12] member validation is an ongoing process throughout the life of a qualitative project. Researchers informally engage in member validation every time they seek clarification for or elaboration of meaning and intention from the people they interview or observe, or check out their evolving interpretations of the data they collect. Researchers formally engage in the process when they deliberately incorporate set procedures by which members can check the accuracy and adequacy of researchers' syntheses of data.

Member checking has been hailed as a way of enhancing the rigor of qualitative work by specifying a set of auditable practices and by virtue of its congruence with the qualitative goal of representing experience from the actor's point of view. Yet its potential to enhance qualitative work belies the deeply theoretical and ethical difficulties involved in this technique that may serve paradoxically to undermine the trustworthiness of a project. Indeed, what is often lost in the discourse on member checking is the recognition that both researchers and members are stakeholders in the research process, concerned with staking certain claims (to telling the truth, to being right), with maintaining certain personas (as good persons, subjects, scientists), and with frequently divergent interests, commitments, and goals. Even when members and researchers seem to have the same goals (such as to tell a good story or to promote an agenda), they may not. After all, there are different stories to tell and different agendas to promote.

For example, members will inevitably look for themselves and their own reality in researchers' accounts of their lives, but researchers strive to represent multiple realities in a way that still remains faithful to each member's reality. I have found in my own work that members are sometimes more interested in concrete descriptions of their own experiences than in abstract syntheses that incorporate them with other members' experiences. I recall in one of my studies one member's comment – on a synthesis I had given her to check – that certain incidents never happened to her or that she had never felt certain feelings. Such comments suggest the investment members have in their own experiences and the difficulty they may have in recognizing other peoples' concrete experiences as variants of their own, or as part of a larger abstraction. Scientific abstractions may appear to the member to be far removed from the "conventionalities and literalnesses"[13(p12)] of their own everyday lives. Indeed, "generalizations (of any kind) always tell a little lie in the service of a greater truth."[14(p205)]

Both members and researchers are interested in accounts that represent experience fairly, but they may have very different views concerning what a fair account is. Whereas members may be motivated to consent to participate in research to justify their actions or to defend the inevitability of certain outcomes, researchers may be motivated to conduct research to evaluate actions and to show the possibility of a variety of outcomes. Whereas members may strive to be accepted as good people, researchers typically strive to be accepted as good scholars; these goals may conflict.

The typically narrative nature of interview data makes the problem of determining accuracy of meaning and intention a deeply theoretical and moral one. As noted previously, the stories that members tell in interviews are themselves constantly changing. They represent members' efforts to order, find meaning in, and even live with the events in their lives at a particular moment in their lives. Stories previously told may elicit feelings members no longer have, regret, and/or have forgotten; a life event previously told as a tragedy may subsequently be told as a romance. Members may want such stories removed as data.

Again, the idea that information previously collected can be subsequently simply checked, corroborated, and/or corrected may be valid only for certain cases. Stories are not simply vehicles for the communication of information that can be easily categorized and counted for consistency; rather, they are time-bound interpretive, political, and moral acts. Researchers must account for both the informational contents in and the discursive features of interview data: for what is said and meant in the interview and for how the interview itself was made. Researchers employing the member-checking process are always obligated to ensure that any correction of contents or feeling tone is warranted as a correction and not as a new story that must be analyzed for its meaning and relation to other stories. Researchers may make serious analytic errors in attempting to find temporal, informational, or intentional consistency among stories. Moreover, analytic decisions become moral ones in the case of participants who wish to retract or alter information previously provided. Significantly, the information from any one interview "cannot be simply decontextualized to constitute a test of validity."[11(p164)]

Members may also simply not be in the best position to check the accuracy of an account. They may have forgotten the information they provided or the manner in which it was provided. A member in one of my studies insisted that a small portion of a transcript of an interview was incorrect. Yet, both the transcriptionist and I, while proofing the transcript against the audiotaped interview, heard her words as they appeared in the transcript. What the woman forgot was that she was crying during this portion of the interview and likely made statements she now sees as wrong. What I had to decide was whether the disputed information was analytically important; that is to say, did I have to resolve the problem of accuracy here? If I had to resolve it, how would I do it? For example, if I played the tape back to the woman, she would be forced to hear herself at a time when she was very distressed, and she would also be proven wrong about what she thought she had said. How would this implementation of the member-checking process affect her emotional health? These are only a few of the practical, theoretical, and ethical questions raised by this one incident alone. (As it turned out, the disputed lines were theoretically unimportant. I simply thanked her for correcting the lines and made a note of it on the transcript.)

Interestingly, a few participants have asked me for copies of their transcripts as remembrances for themselves. I provide these transcripts with the caveat that it may be difficult for them to relive the moment in time captured in those transcripts. For members, the effect of seeing in print what they once said or listening to themselves on tape may be similar to the effect of seeing oneself on videotape giving birth: somewhat bizarre and not wholly comfortable.[15] Importantly, whether shared with members as a remembrance or as part of a validation process, such play-by-play written or taped accounts of past events have effects that researchers have yet fully to explore.

Researchers engaged in member checking also have the problem of determining when to initiate a formal member-checking process and what synthesis of data to present to members to check. Because the member-checking process is itself a variable that may influence the findings, researchers have to make decisions about when during the research project to initiate formal procedures. The very act of reading a transcript for accuracy may not only lead the member to provide additional data that have to be analyzed, but it may itself also cause the member to revise his or her views and/or influence events still to be experienced in the course of the study.

Researchers may offer the member some lay rendition of the findings written or presented in everyday language accessible to the general public, or a scholarly synthesis that may be accessible only to other scholars. I recall one member who agreed to my everyday-English synthesis of a portion of her life, but who had difficulty understanding the scholarly synthesis prepared for a professional journal. The target audience for our work is often not a member group, but rather our own peers. Lay and scholarly syntheses are necessarily different from each other. Because they must adhere to different rules for representing data and often reflect different purposes, these syntheses may not be consistent with each other. Committed as many of us are to being accepted as good scholars and to telling scientific truths, we may say one thing in a report the member sees and another in a report the member does not even comprehend or may never see; neither of these versions will be lies nor will they constitute the whole truth. Importantly, the problem of member checking confronts researchers with all of the representational problems involved in trying to appeal to different audiences and in choosing the point of view and voice that will prevail in our reports of research. Indeed, we have yet to appreciate fully that decisions about how to present findings necessarily involve moral choices and that the conventional research report may be neither faithful to the letter or spirit of the phenomena addressed nor morally justified. In disseminating the findings of our research, we have yet to consider seriously the ethical implications of the choices we make or how artists (fiction writers, painters) resolve dilemmas involving differing voices and points of view.

Finally, member checking is itself socially constructed by the artifices and conventions of social interaction and research. Accordingly, members may participate in a formal checking process only to meet the expectations of researchers and to be good subjects; members may be uninterested in participating in such an exercise. In order to minimize conflict, members may be reluctant to disagree with researchers' interpretations. Moreover, different members may have very different views of the same interpretation.

Researchers have to address how the artifice of the research process itself may influence the validation process and whether the lack of convergence or consensus between researcher and member or among members themselves necessarily invalidates an interpretation.

As Bloor summarized it, members' responses are not "immaculately produced,"[11(p171)] but rather they are shaped and constrained by such factors as the: (1) nature of the interaction between researcher and member, member and member, and among researcher, member, and the audiences to which they desire to appeal; (2) social norms concerning politeness and consensus building; and, (3) frank conflicts of interest and need. Despite our claims to be "doing what comes naturally,"[6(p187)] the research process is inherently social and, therefore, itself subject to analysis as data in our studies.

Member checking exemplifies the practical and deeply theoretical, representational, and even moral problems involved in using such techniques. Indeed, practical problems are frequently theoretical, and representational problems are frequently both theoretical and moral. Although such techniques hold the promise of making the practices of qualitative researchers more visible and acceptable as science, they may cause as many problems as they resolve. Similar problems exist with such validation strategies as the expert panel, peer debriefing, and triangulation, where consensus or convergence may also be inappropriately sought, where the wrong expertise may be sought (for example, analytic expertise may be more relevant to a validation enterprise than clinical expertise), or where peers are also motivated by certain interactional constraints. We shall succeed in our efforts to ensure trustworthiness to the extent that we recognize the complexity of these strategies, analyze them critically, and select among them carefully. We shall succeed in our efforts to the extent that we are willing to consider also artistic resolutions to such problems as whose voices will be heard and what narrative stance to assume in reports of research.

Research is both a creative and a destructive process; we make things up and out of our data, but we often in-advertently kill the thing we want to understand in the process. Similarly, we can preserve or kill the spirit of qualitative work; we can soften our notion of rigor to include the playfulness, soulfulness, imagination, and technique we associate with more artistic endeavors, or we can further harden it by the uncritical application of rules. The choice is ours: rigor or rigor mortis.

References

1. Barrett W. *The Illusion of Technique*. New York, NY: Anchor Books; 1978.
2. Van Manen M. *Researching Lived Experience: Human Science For An Action Sensitive Pedagogy*. Albany, NY: State University of New York Press; 1990.
3. Sandelowski M. The problem of rigor in qualitative research. *ANS*. 1986;8:27–37.
4. Mishler EG. Validation in inquiry-guided research: the role of exemplars in narrative studies. *Harv Educ Rev*. 1990;60:415–442.

5. Bronfenbrenner U. The experimental ecology of education. *Teachers Call Rec.* 1976; 78:157–204.
6. Lincoln YS, Guba E. *Naturalistic Inquiry*. Beverly Hills, Calif: Sage; 1985.
7. Sandelowski M. The proof is in the pottery: toward a poetic for qualitative inquiry. In: Morse JM, ed. *Critical Issues in Qualitative Research*. Newbury Park, Calif: Sage; In press.
8. Sandelowski M. *Truth/Story-Telling in Nursing Inquiry*. Paper presented at Institute for Philosophical Nursing Research, Third Invitational Conference on Philosophy in the Nurse's World; May 4, 1993; University of Alberta, Banff, Alberta, Canada.
9. Tesch R. *Qualitative Research: Analysis Types and Software Tools*. New York, NY: Falmer Press; 1990.
10. Sandelowski M. Telling stories: narrative approaches in qualitative research. *Image J Nurs Sch.* 1991;23:161–166.
11. Bloor MJ. Notes on member validation. In: Emerson RM. ed. *Contemporary Field Research: A Collection of Readings*. Boston, Mass: Little, Brown; 1983.
12. Hoffart N. A member check procedure to enhance rigor in naturalistic research. *West J Nurs Res.* 1991;13:522–534.
13. Nisbet R. *Sociology As An Art Form*. New York, NY: Oxford University Press; 1976.
14. Barley N. *Not A Hazardous Sport*. New York, NY; Henry Holt; 1988.
15. McKay S, Barrows TL. Reliving birth: maternal responses to viewing videotape of their second stage labors. *Image J Nurs Sch.* 1992;24:27–32.

53

Establishing the Credibility of Qualitative Research Findings: The Plot Thickens

John R. Cutcliffe and Hugh P. McKenna

Introduction

Qualitative research is increasingly recognized and valued and its unique place in nursing research is highlighted by many (McKenna 1997, Benner & Wrubel 1989, Morse 1991, Denzin & Lincoln 1994). Despite this, some nurse researchers continue to raise epistemological issues about the problems of objectivity and validity of qualitative research findings (Altheide & Johnson 1994).

While much has been written about the psychometric-properties of qualitative research (Andrews *et al.* 1996) a review of the literature uncovered a great deal of conflict and confusion. It is reasonable to suggest that dilemmas do exist concerning the appropriateness of qualitative research approaches for the generation of useful theories. Therefore, this paper proposes to explore the issues relating to the representativeness or credibility of qualitative research findings. A critique will be undertaken of the commoner research methods and a rationale will be offered for the methods advocated by the authors.

The Principal Positions of Establishing the Credibility of Qualitative Research Findings

There exist distinct philosophical and methodological positions concerning the trustworthiness of qualitative research findings. Hammersley (1992) describes three such positions which can be summarized as follows:

Source: *Journal of Advanced Nursing*, 30(2) (1999): 374–380.

- Qualitative studies should be judged using the same criteria and terminology as quantitative studies.
- It is impossible, in a meaningful way, for any criteria to be used to judge qualitative studies.
- Qualitative studies should be judged using criteria that are developed for and fit the qualitative paradigm.

A fourth position suggests that the credibility of qualitative research findings could be established by testing out the emerging theory by means of conducting a deductive quantitative study (Moody 1990, Cutcliffe 1995, McKenna 1997).

Each of these positions warrants examination in more detail.

Qualitative Studies Should Be Judged Using the Same Criteria and Terminology as Quantitative Studies

Cavanagh (1997) suggests that qualitative researchers should strive to achieve reliable and valid results. Furthermore, he goes on to argue that qualitative researchers should give consideration to three different types of validity, content, hypothesis and predictive. Cavanagh (1997) also attempts to develop arguments for using measures of stability to determine the credibility of qualitative research findings. Here Cavanagh (1997) is recommending that the rigour of qualitative research findings can be judged using criteria and terminology that have been constructed in order to test the validity of results obtained from quantitative studies.

Jasper (1994) and Appleton (1995) construct similar arguments and submit that since qualitative research methods are often criticized for failing to address issues of reliability and validity clearly, researchers cannot ignore these parameters. They 'import' these quantitative terms and then 'translate' them into terms more often associated with qualitative studies such as 'truth value'. Therefore, by considering and addressing the 'truth value' of findings, researchers are addressing the inherent validity of their findings. Brink (1991) adopts a similar view when she argues that issues of validity are just as pertinent to qualitative research studies as they are to quantitative studies.

In considering these arguments, there is a need to examine the philosophical underpinnings of quantitative research approaches. A researcher who adopts a quantitative approach to the collection of data is viewing the world through a particular type of lens. The view suggests that the world can be explained and understood in terms of universal laws and objective truths (McKenna 1997). Its positivist and empiricist underpinnings suggest that there is only one reality and consequently a measure of the accuracy of this reality is its validity.

However, the qualitative researcher views the world through a very different lens. Key authorities on qualitative research point out that it is inappropriate to attempt to apply positivistic and empiricist views of the world to qualitative research (Benner & Wrubel 1989, Morse 1991, Denzin & Lincoln 1994). Qualitative research is based upon the belief that there is no one singular universal truth, the social world is multi-faceted, it is an outcome of the interaction of human agents, a world that has no unequivocal reality (Ashworth 1997b). It is concerned with describing, interpreting and understanding the meanings which people attribute to their existence and to their world.

Additionally, few would dispute that theory does not develop from empiricism alone (McKenna 1997). Carper (1978) described different ways of knowing: these were empirics, aesthetics, ethics and personal knowing. It is argued that these and the philosophical underpinnings of the research methods should influence the. way the resulting theory/findings are tested for accuracy. Chinn and Kramer (1995) assert that because there are different ways of knowing, the resultant theories should not be tested using only those methods advocated by empiricists. In other words a qualitative study is likely to lack credibility if it is critiqued using positivistic criteria. It matters little if this is carried out overtly or in a more covert form by importing and subsequently translating quantitative terms.

We would argue that qualitative research findings should be tested for credibility or accuracy using terms and criteria that have been developed exclusively for this very approach. Leinenger (1994 p. 97) makes this point most clearly when she states:

> We must develop and use criteria that fit the qualitative paradigm, rather than use quantitative criteria for qualitative studies It is awkward and inappropriate to re-language quantitative terms.

Accepting this, it is unfortunate that the research literature still proliferates with authors attempting to establish the credibility of qualitative studies using synonyms for quantitative approaches (Appleton 1995). There are also a number of authors who criticize the credibility of qualitative studies using criteria meant for quantitative studies (Cavanagh 1997). Such practices are likely to confuse and confound readers and undermine the very purposes and essence of qualitative research.

It is Impossible, in a Meaningful Way, for Any Criteria to Be Used to Judge Qualitative Studies

McKenna (1997) argues that some concepts within nursing are so abstract and nebulous that it is impossible to investigate these concepts using empirical measurements and consequently they lend themselves to qualitative enquiry.

Nursing theories produced by such methods may well be too abstract to apply in practice. Their strength lies in making practitioners think about their practice in creative and interesting ways. This implies that some theories produced by qualitative methods may not lend themselves to having their credibility established due to the extent of their inherent abstraction.

Some critics argue that the essential reflexive character and subjectivity of qualitative studies renders them incomplete, non-objective, and consequently impossible to check for complete authenticity of their findings (Altheide & Johnson 1994). Schutz's (1994) arguments follow a similar direction when she states that certain aspects of human experience cannot be accessed without the higher levels of awareness and consciousness that the researcher's subjectivity can bring. Furthermore, because the meanings uncovered in such investigations are only verifiable by subjective means, the application of any criteria, however defined, is inappropriate (Nolan & Behi 1995a). Despite her argument Schutz (1994) admits that nursing research needs to establish credibility and this necessitates a 'shared vision' with other informants.

Hammersley (1992) disagrees with the argument that no criteria can be produced which can help to establish the credibility of qualitative research findings. He suggests that all qualitative researchers should make some efforts towards this goal, otherwise researchers could be 'conjuring up' concepts, propositions and theories entirely from their imagination which do not reflect the phenomenon or situation under investigation. This sounds very similar to the process of writing fiction and thus shouldn't be described as research or science. Although, it should be noted that some qualitative researchers have compared qualitative research findings to stories or narrative tales (Clifford & Marcus 1985, Altheide & Johnson 1994). In essence, it is claimed that these researchers provide 'texts' which are in turn read and interpreted by the audience. The readers therefore construct their own meanings or readings from the text. However, Hammersley's (1992 p. 69) argument is cogent. He asserts:

> An account is valid or true if it represents accurately those features of the phenomena that it is intended to describe, explain or theorise.

McKenna (1997) supports this position, suggesting that whilst all ways of knowing should be respected, each must be subject to the rigour and analysis that knowledge requires. Altheide and Johnson (1994) adopt a similar position. They suggest that a critical question for qualitative researchers to consider is how should interpretative methodologies be judged by readers who share the same philosophical, epistemological and methodological underpinnings. They believe the answer to the question is that whilst qualitative researchers claim to interpret or make sense of social life, they must have a logic for assessing and communicating the interactive process through which the researcher acquired the information. They conclude (Altheide & Johnson 1994 p. 485):

> If we are to understand the detailed means through which human beings engage in meaningful action and create a world of their own or one that is shared with others we must acknowledge that insufficient attention has as yet been devoted to evolving criteria for assessing the general quality and rigour of interpretative research.

Qualitative Studies Should Be Judged Using Criteria that Are Developed for and Fit the Qualitative Paradigm

Qualitative researchers have identified a variety of approaches to judge the credibility of their findings. These warrant examination.

Burnard (1991) maintains that when researchers are generating patterns or themes from qualitative data, they can enhance the validity of the categorization method and guard against researcher bias by enlisting the assistance of a colleague. Both individuals then produce categories, independently of one another. Similarly other authors (Appleton 1995) suggest enlisting the assistance of an 'experienced' or 'expert' colleague to verify the data categorization, preferably one who is an expert in the area investigated.

This approach has several philosophical and epistemological difficulties. Firstly, since qualitative studies are normally indicated when there is an absence of theory pertaining to the specific phenomenon being studied, how likely is it that such 'experts' or 'experienced colleagues' will exist? Furthermore, what defines these individuals as 'experts' or 'experienced colleagues'? What criteria have they been subjected to in order to determine the extent of their expertise or experience? If such individuals do exist, this leads to the second difficulty. The process of theory induction and the production of categories/ themes depends upon the unique creative processes between the researcher and the data (Munhall & Boyd 1993, Schutz 1994). It is unlikely that two people will interpret the data in the same way, form the same categories/themes or concepts and produce the same theoretical framework. This is especially true if one researcher has been involved in every stage of the research process, including the data collection and data analysis stages, and the colleague has not. The main researcher's in-depth familiarity with the data and the subjects' world will undoubtedly affect the subsequent interpretation.

There is another potential problem with this approach. Enlisting the help of others to verify the categories/themes, somehow suggests that if more than one person thinks or agrees with the categorization, then this must be more accurate than one person's categorization. If this argument is expanded, it begins to support the positivistic philosophy that there is only one accurate interpretation, only one reality, and that the accuracy of an interpretation is increased as the number of people agreeing increases.

A positive outcome of qualitative researchers sharing their interpretation with colleagues would be the opportunity it provides for challenging the robustness of the emerging categories/themes. For instance, there may be issues or patterns the researcher has missed which the colleague may highlight. Furthermore through explaining the thinking behind choices made and the reasons for one line of enquiry and not another, the researcher can be assisted towards a more reasoned and complete interpretation.

Guba and Lincoln (1981, 1989) suggest another approach for establishing credibility for qualitative findings. They recommend that researchers leave an 'audit trail' so that the pathway of decisions made in the data analysis can be checked by another researcher. However, it is worth considering whether or not this method leaves any room for the 'hunches' or 'felt sense' of the emerging theory that can occur as the researcher becomes immersed in the data. Glaser and Strauss (1967) advocate the process of 'memoing', in that the researcher makes a note of key thoughts, hunches and lines of enquiry during data collection. It follows that these memos could serve as a form of audit trail. Yet there may be times when no rational explanation for such lines of enquiry may exist. Indeed Meleis (1991) maintains that theories evolve from ideas, which in turn are a product of amongst others, hunches, intuitions and inspirations. Perhaps, just as Benner (1984) describes how expert nurse practitioners make decisions based on intuitive knowing, it follows that experienced (or expert) qualitative researchers make decisions during their data collection based on similar intuitive knowing, leaving them unable to articulate why they made such a decision. They only audit trail this would leave would be, 'that it felt right to follow this line of enquiry'. This begs the question, do qualitative research findings uncovered as a result of following one's intuition or hunches, that leave a limited audit trail, have less credibility than those findings that do?

Guba and Lincoln (1981, 1989) also write of neutrality, where researchers can minimize their subjectivity and thus maximize the credibility of the findings. This is based upon the notion that the researchers' previous theoretical baggage would influence unduly the interpretations of the findings. When describing Husserlian phenomenological philosophy, Husserl (1964) describes a similar process. Husserlian philosophers and researchers using this form of phenomenology bracket their experience, judgement and beliefs out of their thinking and their studies to avoid these perceptions effecting the findings. Other authors (Rose *et al.* 1995, Jasper 1994) describe this process of bracketing, recognizing how one's intentionality can be addressed in Husserlian phenomenological research processes. Andrews et al. (1996) describe a process for making explicit the researcher's fore-understanding and Ashworth (1993, 1997b) holds the view that the credibility of the findings is increased if researchers first make explicit their pre-suppositions and acknowledge their subjective judgement. In essence good qualitative researchers account for themselves and show their hand in the research (Altheide & Johnson 1994).

Yet the value of such activities is not supported by all qualitative researchers. Researchers who base their beliefs on Heideggerian phenomenological philosophy (Heideggar 1962), such as Walters (1995), Benner (1984), Benner and Wrubel (1989), and Schutz (1994), each describe the creative interpretation that researchers bring to a study, and that this interpretation can be made richer by immersing themselves in the subject's world. As part of the subject's world the researcher is thus better equipped to gain a more complete understanding of it. As Altheide and Johnson (1994) suggest Heideggerian phenomenology always involves some part of the researcher in the induced theory.

According to Ashworth (1997a) the researcher's involvement in the world of the participants can be paradoxical. It may support the credibility in that the actual, multi-dimensional social world tends to impose its meanings on the research and counters the researcher's naive expectations. There is also the possibility that by interviewing and/or participant observation, the world and accordingly the lived experience of the researcher becomes more like that of the participants. This may reduce the possibility of the researcher constructing their own reality and not interpreting the participants' reality. Consequently any interpretation is more representative of the participants' reality. Alternatively, measures to increase objectivity, or maximize neutrality, may be thought necessary.

Therefore attempting to judge the credibility of qualitative research findings by means of examining the extent of researcher neutrality, or the extent of intentionality evident in the research, may be valuable for some qualitative approaches, but does not appear to be applicable to all approaches. What this does indicate is the need for clarity and precision regarding the specific qualitative approach being used. By being explicit the researcher then avoids further confusion with issues of credibility or authenticity of findings and as a result can add to the overall quality of the research (Cutcliffe 1997).

With many qualitative approaches, where the researcher endeavours to gain an insight into the social world of the participants, there appears to be an empathic process occurring between the researcher and the participants (Benner & Wrubel 1989, Bergum 1991, Schutz 1994, Walters 1995). The leads the authors to consider the following questions, does the extent or level of the researcher's empathy influence the authenticity of the findings? Would a more empathic researcher, one who is better equipped to enter into the participant's view of the world and the meaning they ascribe to their world, gain a more complete, comprehensive, authentic interpretation of the participant's world? Perhaps this is one reason why certain types of nurses gravitate towards these particular research methods. If so does this argument raise some training/educational implications for aspiring qualitative researchers? For example, should neophyte qualitative researchers receive training to develop their qualities and skills in being empathic and communicating empathy (Cassedy & Cutcliffe 1998)? If researchers with a greater empathic ability produce more truly representative interpretations, then it follows that a test of the credibility of the findings might include some assessment of the extent of empathy experienced by the participants.

Nolan and Behi (1995a p.589) identify another approach to establishing credibility in qualitative data. They maintain:

> All criteria developed for use in qualitative studies rely heavily on present-ing the results to those who were studied and asking them to verify whether or not they agree with them.

There is certainly evidence in the literature to support this statement with many authors advocating that the researcher return to the participants in order to verify the research findings (Guba & Lincoln 1981, Lincoln & Guba 1985, Turner 1981, Leininger 1994, Brink 1991, Ashworth 1993) However, even though few would dispute the value of this endeavour, there are still some issues worth exploring. An important question appears to centre around at what point in this process do the findings become credible? Should the researcher be concerned with each of the participants' verification or only a proportion of them? Should the researcher try to reach the point where a participant verifies all of the concepts, categories or theory, or only a proportion of these?

These questions also appear to be moving towards positivistic concerns, in that 'X%' of the participants verified 'Y%' of the theory and 'Z%' offered no verification. It is somewhat unlikely that each interviewee will recognize and thus verify the representativeness of the entirety of the emerging theory as each of them will have contributed only a portion of the data. Therefore it is quite possible that some participants will not recognize some of the emerging theory. This point illustrates the need for the opportunity for some explanation back to the interviewees in order that their verification may be more complete. If one participant agrees the theory is representative, then one could argue it has credibility, but at the same lime the researcher should make explicit where and how the respondents disagreed with the theory.

This difficulty can also be addressed by using the actual words of the par-ticipants (Glaser & Strauss 1967, Turner 1981, Melia 1982). If the emerging theory has captured the essence of the phenomenon or situation under investi-gation (representativeness) then the participants are likely to respond and recognize themselves in it, because it will have specific meaning for them. This is more likely to occur if the participants can recognize their own words.

In grounded theory data items are checked against one another repeatedly and compared and contrasted again and again. This provides a check on their representativeness (Munhall & Boyd 1993). A similar process can occur in phenomenology whereby the repeated reading of interview transcripts, and checking of one data item or theme against others can work as a check on their representativeness. By doing this distortions, inaccuracies and misinterpretations will be gradually discovered and resolved. Melia (1982) refers to the testing out/validation process that occurs in qualitative research where refining and checking the credibility of propositions, themes and categories that emerge in one interview can be verified in subsequent interviews. As a consequence, one of four responses can be obtained:

- The interviewee agrees with the authenticity of the data and the representativeness of the interpretation and adds nothing new (perhaps at this stage the categories have reached saturation) Glaser & Strauss 1967).
- The interviewee agrees with the authenticity of the data and the representativeness of the interpretation and adds further refinement and understanding to the category. A crucial component of category development.
- The interviewee disagrees with the authenticity of the data and the representativeness of the interpretation redirects the researcher's enquiry.
- The interviewee disagrees completely with the authenticity of the data and the representativeness of the interpretation and the researcher should completely rethink this line of enquiry.

Appleton (1995) argues that the process of triangulation increases the accuracy of qualitative research findings in that data from different sources can confirm the truth. Few would dispute that this is one of the principle benefits of triangulated methods (Redfern & Norman 1994, Begley 1996), However, if both sources of data provide inaccurate results, then all this method would do is confirm and support an inaccurate theory. If the triangulation of data produces inconsistent, conflicting or contradictory findings then this only adds to the researcher's confusion. Smith and Biley (1997) assert that establishing truth value or representativeness can be attained using three types of triangulation:

- Triangulation by means of constant comparative method. If a label appears repeatedly then the researcher can be satisfied with its existence.
- Triangulation regarding the variety of data collection methods. If each method produces the same, then the truth value is increased.
- Triangulation regarding the variety of participants – the more people assert the importance of an issue, the more they can be trusted.

However, the authors would disagree with the value of this third type as again it appears to be underpinned by positivistic thinking and so is inappropriate for qualitative studies. Given these arguments, it appears that some forms of triangulation can help establish the credibility of qualitative research findings, yet if used as the only method, data triangulation could be regarded as inappropriate. Nonetheless, it has to be accepted that if data triangulation or other triangulation methods are used in conjunction with other attempts to illustrate representativeness, then it should lend credibility to the findings.

Establishing the Credibility of Qualitative Research Findings by Conducting a Deductive Study, Testing Out the Emerging Theory

The process of triangulation as a method of establishing the credibility of qualitative research findings leads logically to the fourth distinct position. This entails carrying out a deductive study to test out the credibility of an induced theory. Because such an approach involves combining strategies from two research paradigms in one study it could well be described as across-method triangulation (Begley 1996). Redfern and Norman (1994) suggest that a specific advantage of using a triangulated study in nursing relates to the increased confidence in the results and a more complete understanding of the domain. More recently, Nolan and Behi (1995b) support this argument suggesting that triangulated studies help with the confirmation and completeness of the research findings. Confirmability is concerned with using different methods or approaches in the same study in order that one set of results confirms those of another. Completeness is concerned with using different methods within one study in order to get a more complete picture that might not be achieved if one method alone were used. The authors argue that if a triangulated approach is used in conjunction with other attempts to establish credibility outlined above, then the researcher has made a thorough attempt to address issues of representativeness and credibility of their qualitative research findings.

Conclusion

Guba and Lincoln (1981) maintain that qualitative data are credible when others can recognize experiences after having only read about them. Nonetheless, there is a strong case for undertaking more strenuous attempts to establish the credibility of qualitative research findings. This is essential if nursing wants to gain and maintain some credibility as a science (Schutz 1994). This paper argues that it is inappropriate to use quantitative terms as measures of credibility, either overtly or covertly by importing and translating such terms. Furthermore, since a blurred method can make establishing the credibility of the findings more difficult, it is in the researcher's interest to make explicit what qualitative approach they have used. The researcher should also make explicit what attempts/methods they have used to establish the credibility of their data interpretations.

Careful consideration should be given to selecting methods of credibility testing as some might be more worthwhile than others. Researchers are encouraged to return to the participants and attempt to gain verification. This process may benefit from using the words of the participants in the emerging theory. Any findings that were not recognized by the participants should be identified and, in particular, if disagreements existed these should be reported. The researcher might find it worthwhile to combine several methods of checking, including some form of triangulation.

Finally, perhaps the most useful indicator of the credibility of the findings produced is when the practitioners themselves and the readers of the theory view the study findings and regard them as meaningful and applicable in terms of their experience.

References

Altheide D.L. & Johnson J.M. (1994) Criteria for assessing interpretative validity in qualitative research. In *Handbook of Qualitative Research* (Denzin N. & Lincoln Y.S. eds). Sage London, pp. 485–499.

Appleton J.V. (1995) Analysing qualitative interview data: addressing issues of validity and reliability. *Journal of Advanced Nursing* **22**, 999–997.

Andrews M, Lyne P. & Riley E. (1996) Validity in qualitative healthcare research: an exploration of the impact of individual researcher perspectives within collaborative enquiry. *Journal of Advanced Nursing* **23**, 441–447.

Ashworth P.D. (1993) Participant agreement in the justification of qualitative findings. *Journal of Phenomenological Psychology* **24**, 3–16.

Ashworth P.D. (1997a) The variety of qualitative research: introduction to the problem. *Nurse Education Today* **17**, 215–218.

Ashworth P.D. (1997b) The variety of qualitative research: non-positivist approaches. *Nurse Education Today* **17**, 219–224.

Begley C.M. (1996) Using triangulation in nursing research. *Journal of Advanced Nursing* **24**, 122–128.

Benner P. (1984) *From Novice to Expert: Excellence and Power in Clinical Practice*. Addison-Wesley, New York.

Benner P. & Wrubel J. (1989) *The Primacy of Caring: Stress and Coping in Health and Illness*. Addison Wesley, New York.

Bergum V. (1991) Being a phenomenological researcher. In *Qualitative Nursing Research: A Contemporary Dialogue* (Morse J.M. ed.), Sage Newbury Park, California, pp. 55–71.

Brink P.J. (1991) Issues of reliability and validity. In *Qualitative Nursing Research: A Contemporary Dialogue* (Morse J.M. ed.), Sage Newbury Park California, pp. 164–186.

Burnard P. (1991) A method of analysing interview transcripts in qualitative research. *Nurse Education Today* **11**, 461–466.

Carper B.A. (1978) Fundamental patterns of knowing in nursing. *Advances in Nursing Science* **1**(1), 13–23.

Cassedy P. & Cutcliffe J.R. (1998) Empathy, students and the problems of genuineness: can we develop empathy on a short skills based counselling course? *Mental Health Practice* **1**(9), 28–33.

Cavanagh S. (1997) Content analysis: concepts, methods and applications. *Nurse Researcher* **4**(3), 5–16.

Chinn P. & Kramer M.K. (1995) *Theory and Nursing: A Systematic Approach* 4th edn. CV Mosby, St Louis.

Clifford J. & Marcus G. (1986) *Writing Culture: The Poetics and Politics of Ethnography*. University of California Press, Berkley.

Cutcliffe J.R. (1995) How do nurses inspire and instil hope in terminally ill HIV patients? *Journal of Advanced Nursing* **22**, 888–895.

Cutcliffe J.R. (1997) Qualitative nursing research: a quest for quality. *British Journal of Nursing* **6**(17), 969.

Denzin N. & Lincoln Y.S. (1994) Introduction: entering the field of qualitative enquiry. In *Handbook of Qualitative Research* (Denzin N. & Lincoln Y.S. eds), Sage London, pp. 1–18.

Glaser B. & Strauss A.L. (1967) *The Discovery of Grounded Theory: Strategies for Qualitative Research*. Aldine, Chicago.

Guba E.G. & Lincoln Y.S. (1981) *Effective Evaluation*. Jossey-Bass, San Francisco.

Guba E.G. & Lincoln Y.S. (1989) *Fourth Generation Evaluation*. Sage, Newbury Park, California.

Hammersley M. (1992) *What's Wrong with Ethnography?* Routledge, London.

Heidegger M. (1962) *Being and Time*. Harper Row, New York.

Husserl E. (1964) *The Idea of Phenomenology* (W. Alston & G. Nakhikan, trans.). Nijhoff, The Hague.

Jasper M.A. (1994) Issues in phenomenology for researchers of nursing. *Journal of Advanced Nursing* **19**, 309–314.

Lincoln Y.S. & Guba E.G. (1985) *Naturalistic Enquiry*. Sage, Newbury Park, California.

Leininger M. (1994) Evaluation criteria and critique of qualitative research studies. In *Critical Issues in Qualitative Research Methods* (Morse J. ed.), Sage, Thousand Oaks, California, pp. 95–115.

McKenna H. (1997) *Nursing Theories and Models*. Routledge, London.

Meleis A.I. (1991) *Theoretical Nursing: Development and Progress* 2nd edn. Lippincott, Philadelphia.

Melia K.M. (1982) 'Tell it as it is' – qualitative methodology and nursing research: understanding the student nurse's world. *Journal of Advanced Nursing* **7**, 327–335.

Moody L.E. (1990) *Advancing Nursing Science Through Research*. Volume 1. Sage, Newbury Park, California.

Morse J. (1991) Qualitative nursing research: a free for all? In *Qualitative Nursing Research: A Contemporary Dialogue* 2nd edn (Morse J. ed.), Sage, Newbury Park, California, pp. 14–22.

Munhall P.L. & Boyd C.O. (1993) *Nursing Research: A Qualitative Perspective* 2nd edn. National League for Nursing Press, New York.

Nolan M. & Behi R. (1995a) Alternative approaches to establishing reliability and validity. *British Journal of Nursing* **14**(10), 587–590.

Nolan M. & Behi R. (1995b) Triangulation: the best of all worlds? *British Journal of Nursing* **14**(14), 829–832.

Redfern S.J. & Norman I.J. (1994) validity through triangulation. *Nurse Researcher* **2**(2), 41–56.

Rose P., Beeby J. & Parker D. (1995) Academic rigour in the lived experience of researchers using phenomenological methods in nursing. *Journal of Advanced Nursing* **21**, 1123–1129.

Schutz S.E. (1994) Exploring the benefits of a subjective approach in qualitative nursing research. *Journal of Advanced Nursing* **20**, 412–417.

Smith K. & Biley F. (1997) Understanding grounded theory: principles and evaluation. *Nurse Researcher* **4**(3), 17–30.

Turner B. (1981) Some practical aspects of qualitative data analysis: one way of organising the cognitive processes associated with the generation of grounded theory. *Quality and Control* **15**, 225–245.

Walters A.J. (1995) The phenomenological movement: implications for nursing research. *Journal of Advanced Nursing* **22**, 791–799.

54

The Newfound Credibility of Qualitative Research? Tales of Technical Essentialism and Co-Option

Rosaline S. Barbour

A s qualitative researchers, we are fond of emphasizing the importance of context. We have, however, been curiously loath to examine the broader context in which we carry out our research (Barbour, 1998, 1999). We stand to learn much from cultivating a critical appreciation of the possibilities and constraints that we encounter as we go about generating data and analyzing, reporting, and disseminating our research; how we go about teaching and providing supervision; and how we approach collaboration. As qualitative researchers, we should extend our critical gaze to examine our own received wisdom and myth making, because this serves the same functions as does the storytelling of the people we typically study (Barbour & Huby, 1998).

A notable exception to this professional blind spot is Sally Hutchinson (2001), who has recently sought to take stock of the development of qualitative research. She has depicted the early stage in the progress of qualitative research from pariah paradigm to newfound respectability as having been characterized by what she terms "stopping." During this period, qualitative researchers constituted a dissenting voice, united by their shared experience of having manuscripts rejected by mainstream journals, which were seen as privileging reports written in the style and language of the positivist tradition. I would argue that although we have now reached another phase, where qualitative methods have achieved unprecedented acceptability, conflicts and tensions

Source: *Qualitative Health Research,* 13(7) (2003): 1019–1027.

continue to bubble under the surface and that these reflect divergent views concerning epistemology and, ultimately, the value of qualitative research.

In the current version of "commiserators' wisdom," tales of vigorously applied checklists have replaced those of uncomprehending or outright hostile editors and reviewers. Despite acting as a reviewer for several of the journals (such as the *British Medical Journal, British Journal of General Practice, The Lancet,* and *Social Science & Medicine*), which are frequently alleged to follow such an approach, I have found little evidence for this phenomenon, and I would suggest that researchers' fears are somewhat exaggerated. However, to paraphrase W. I. Thomas (1949), if those who seek to publish their qualitative research believe checklists to be real, then they are likely to be real in their consequences. Checklists are likely to have considerable appeal for those who might otherwise feel out of their depth in evaluating qualitative articles. Moreover, the situation will become more serious as an increasing number of qualitative articles are submitted to mainstream, journals and the identification of appropriate reviewers becomes ever more difficult – with the potential for co-option of those without direct experience of qualitative research.

Although the tick box approach that features in qualitative researchers' horror stories has yet to be enshrined in the journal-reviewing process, checklists (e.g., Hoddinott & Pill, 1979; Popay, Williams, & Rogers, 1998; Seale & Silverman, 1997) undoubtedly do circulate via journal clubs, critical appraisal sessions, and research methods training courses. Regardless of the intentions of their authors, who frequently have emphasized that checklists should be viewed as "indicative rather than constitutive of good practice" (Miller, 1997), checklists – with their bullet-point format – have a ready appeal. They appear to render manageable the complexities of the qualitative research process, offering an alternative to familiar templates developed for quantitative research. Thus, they frequently serve as a brief introduction to qualitative research both for those new to qualitative methods and to new audiences, such as practitioners, who find themselves under increasing pressure to become research active. Although specially tailored and packaged workshops and texts can make qualitative research more accessible to a wider constituency, there is a danger of dilution as an unintended consequence of such popularizing, as Krueger (1993) has pointed out in relation to the co-option of focus groups. A mechanistic overemphasis on fulfilling itemized checklists reduces qualitative research to what I have termed *technical essentialism.*

Although I have chosen to concentrate here on the negative potential of checklists, there is, undoubtedly, much to be said in their favor – depending on the spirit in which they are applied or invoked. They can be seen as a welcome development inasmuch as they have heralded the recognition that there is such a thing as bad qualitative research. They have also done much to perforate the unhelpful "preciousness" (Barbour, 1998) that has fre-quently character-ized the impassioned but, ultimately, obfuscating accounts of some qualitative acolytes. Seale (1999) advocates using checklists as an aide-mémoire, allowing the practicing researcher some time out in the "brain gymnasium" to critically examine his or her own research practice and to strive toward improvement. Using checklists in this way does not give rise to the problems associated with technical essentialism, however, and it is not with this approach that I wish to take issue.

Technical Essentialism

I have elsewhere (Barbour, 2001) enumerated some of the components of checklists (both published and the virtual checklists invoked by aspirant or rejected qualitative researchers). Most checklists include purposive sampling, respondent validation, multiple coding, triangulation, and, indeed, grounded theory (used as a means of linking data and resultant theory).

The growing reliance on purposive sampling reflects a welcome move away from convenience sampling to embrace the idea of selecting samples to reflect and examine the diversity present in the groups that we seek to study (Kuzel, 1992). However, when the term is cynically employed in a technical essentialist fashion, it frequently serves as little more than a legitimizing device for dressing up the details of the sample obtained rather than outlining the rationale and thinking behind a sampling frame constructed to provide a comparative focus for data analysis. Thus, purposive sampling is often employed as a retrospective justification rather than allowing for a detailed description of the processes engaged in as the research unfolded.

Likewise, the technical essentialist version of respondent validation, multiple coding, and triangulation also focus on outcomes rather than process. These checklist items are all concerned with demonstrating validity and implicitly rely on the notion of data as fixed and amenable to reanalysis and duplication of findings. Concordance between researcher and researched, between data sets, and between different coders is seen as strengthening the validity of the explanations advanced. This is perhaps clearest with reference to triangulation, which relies on the notion of a fixed point of reference and implies a hierarchy in terms of the value of data generated from different sources. If the technical essentialist construction of triangulation gains currency, however, and this is added to checklists (whether real or notional), then what will be the fate of well-designed single-method studies employing interviews, observational fieldwork, or focus groups?

The Co-Option of Grounded Theory

There is disturbing evidence that grounded theory, that bastion of the qualitative research process, has also been co-opted to serve as a component of technical essentialism. Bryman and Burgess (1994) had, of course, already alerted us to the prevalence of the somewhat cynical use of grounded theory as "an approving bumper sticker." Until relatively recently, however, the invoking of theory – in any shape or form – was the preserve of social scientists, some of whom have not been slow to realize that this was a powerful weapon in our boundary disputes with medical researchers eager to adopt qualitative methods (Chapple & Rogers, 1998).

A reading of recent journal articles, however, shows that the situation has changed markedly. Nowadays, it is commonplace to see grounded theory being used to justify the selection of (often spectacularly unremarkable) themes derived from qualitative data – often in the absence of any evidence of iterative refinement and revision of coding categories and gradual theory development. In their frequently cited chapter, Ritchie and Spencer (1994) did a sterling job in explaining clearly the complex process engaged in and previously reinvented afresh by generations of researchers as they searched for patterns in their data. The appeal of Ritchie and Spencer's "framework analysis" lies largely in its explication of steps that researchers can follow, including indexing, charting, and mapping, but they concede that some stages of analysis, "particularly those which involve inductive and interpretive thinking," are much more difficult to capture (p. 193). It is, therefore, not surprising that the most popular use of this citation relates to justifying researchers' choice of coding categories and themes in packaging and rendering manageable their data, documenting part of the process rather than illuminating the whole process involved in building up their interpretations and explanations. Again, this particular strategy (i.e., invoking "framework analysis" used in isolation) is consistent with the approach of technical essentialism.

Melia (1997) has argued that, in all probability, no one employs a grounded theory approach in its pure form. To portray data as speaking for itself (showing merely how data segments are coded without reference to other sources of inspiration) sidesteps some difficult problems and risks descending to the sort of uncritical romanticism that Atkinson (1997) has warned us against. As Miller (1997) pointed out, "Some of the most important interpretive possibilities of qualitative studies are established prior to data collection" (p. 6). We are unlikely to conceptualize a research question or to be able to formulate a research design that is fundable without explicit reference to existing bodies of knowledge and explicit or implicit reference to existing theoretical frameworks. Silverman (1993) commented, "Without an analytical basis, even detailed transcription can be merely an empty technique" (p. 16). We have some notion, even at the outset, of what our data are likely to look like and what we intend to do with it.

Melia (1997) has also talked of some "near mystical" passages in the original Glaser and Strauss (1967) text on grounded theory, and we can easily slip into reifying our data – refusing to be drawn on preliminary findings while we wait for transcription to be carried out, for example. Certainly, the welcome pause that this can afford after the rigors of generating data and negotiating relationships in the field goes some way toward explaining the popularity of this response. However, the reluctance shown by many qualitative researchers to use this time profitably to develop draft coding frameworks suggests an underlying belief in the sanctity of their data, with a corresponding underemphasis on the labor-intensive and creative tasks embodied in the process of analysis.

Originally advanced as a defense of empirical research against the criticisms of "grand theorists" (see Seale, 1999), grounded theory is also invoked as a distinct philosophical approach to qualitative research. This can, however, obscure or deemphasize its practical application. Used in this way, grounded theory allows for theory generation, and its strength lies precisely in its nonpartisan character, that is, it is amenable to very different and potentially contradictory theoretical paradigms. However, a technical essentialist approach overemphasizes the practicalities involved at the expense of the analytical.

Using grounded theory to link data and emergent theoretical explanations, however, does not absolve the researcher from engaging with existing bodies of theory. A technical essentialist version of grounded theory can appear to offer a refuge against the bewildering array of theoretical or philosophical positions in the current postmodern world. Although she is referring in this instance to inflated expectations of software analysis packages, Morse's (1997) comments serve to remind us of the researcher's agency: "Theories are actively constructed, not found . . . [and] they will continue to be constructed by human researchers" (p. 170). Technical essentialism thus affords a different view of the relationship between data and theory. It ultimately allows, at least in theory, for the contribution of sociological or anthropological literatures to be disregarded, because – if theory truly emerges from the data – the researcher is saved the burden of having to read extensively. Silverman (1992) observed wryly that many researchers are keen to adopt qualitative methods not so much for what these allow them to do as for what they allow them to avoid – that is, complex and taxing statistical calculations. In a technical essentialist application, grounded theory provides a justification for neglecting to embed qualitative research with reference to the existing literature or to use one's own data to interrogate, challenge, and develop previously formulated theoretical frameworks. It would be ironic if grounded theory were to be pressed into service in excusing researchers from juxtaposing local findings with universal (theoretical) explanations.

Qualitative researchers may bemoan the alleged application of checklists by unrelenting reviewers, but there is, nevertheless, some comfort to be derived from believing that we can thus make transparent the mechanics of the review process. The constraints on length of articles – especially when writing for clinical journals – can render us susceptible to the temptation of resorting to shorthand explanations of the process of qualitative research – "the awfulness of simplification" to which Morse (2001a) has referred. There is, then, an even more worrying and, perhaps, more invidious aspect to technical essentialism. It can be employed somewhat cynically, to advance a claim for credibility by demonstrating rigor through invoking the component parts enumerated in checklists. Thus, it can become a modus operandi for the aspirant journal contributor, becoming, as W. I. Thomas might have said, "real in its consequences," as checklist components are adopted as "technical fixes" (Barbour, 2001).

My argument is that technical essentialism has surfaced at this particular time because of the conjunction of several related developments. Some developments, such as the dual imperatives of publishing and securing research funding, have risen to the top of the academic agenda in this age of managerialism and research assessment exercises. However, qualitative researchers have also, at times, been instrumental in encouraging, albeit perhaps unwittingly, the growing reliance on technical essentialism.

The Legacy of Demystification

Alongside the growing respectability of qualitative research methods has come a demand for "experts" to provide training and supervision in previously uncharted waters, such as departments of primary care and other medical specialties. Qualitative researchers have been quick to embrace such opportunities, but – our considerable involvement in providing methods workshops notwithstanding – many share my own ambivalence with regard to this rush to embrace qualitative methods. Harding and Gantley (1998) were the first to raise doubts publicly about the advisability of reducing qualitative research training to a cookbook approach, in the way that many introductory courses do through providing a whistle-stop tour of different qualitative methods.

Although she is here reflecting on the consequences of providing a necessarily condensed account for the methods section of journal articles, Morse's (2001a) comments apply equally to the provision of research methods training. She argued that presenting qualitative research as involving a series of steps can "appear effortless and trite, concealing the conceptual struggles and skills essential in producing such research" (p. 435). Perhaps, then, this goes some way toward explaining both the enormous appeal of Ritchie and Spencer's (1994) chapter and the limitations of some of its subsequent applications.

Harding and Gantley's (1999) talk at the Association of University Departments of General Practice (AUDGP) Annual Conference held in London in 1999 was titled "You Only Want Me for My Methods." This presentation echoed the discomfort felt by many experienced but, often, somewhat isolated qualitative researchers in the face of a technical essentialist appreciation of their contribution to their respective departments, which emphasizes their skills in applying specific methods at the expense of their disciplinary grounding.

Charges of "sociological imperialism" (Chapple & Rogers, 1998) notwithstanding, the separation of method and theory can have very serious consequences. Technical essentialism also reifies data and relies on a notion of qualitative research methods as a means of collecting data, producing the same results in the hands of different researchers, provided that they employ the same tools, such as interviews or focus groups (Barbour, 1998). Such a view of the research process downplays the skills needed to elicit respondents' stories and also obscures the role and agency of the researcher and its impact on the nature of the data produced (in terms of form and content). Commenting on the teaching of undergraduate social scientists, Peter Collins (1998) has taken issue with a technical essentialist construction of the interview process. He argued,

> There is a tendency at the outset for students to see the interview as a kind of smash and grab opportunity in which they accost some innocent bystander and relieve them of whatever useful "data" they may have. They are aided and abetted in their assumptions by texts which imply a "model" interview in which objective interviewers extract objective facts from, presumably, objective subjects. (p. 1)

Paradoxically, some formulations of the research task, such as bearing witness in acting as a cipher for respondents to tell their stories, also collude with this view of research, downplaying the agency of the researcher and romanticizing interviewees' accounts (Atkinson, 1997). Recently, Hall and Callery (2001) argued that grounded theory has also overlooked the effect of interactions between researcher and participant on the construction of data. Following Mason (1996), I prefer to talk of generating data, thus acknowledging the important role of the researcher in creating the data via fieldwork relationships, the process of interpretation, and the particular personal and professional insights that he or she brings to bear on the research enterprise.

Many qualitative researchers employed within medical faculties find themselves occupying the position of "cuckoos in the nest," attempting to introduce a new approach within preexisting courses and formats (Harding & Gantley, 1999). We need to pay attention not just to the structural constraints under which we pursue our academic careers but also to those aspects of our workaday encounters, such as teaching and supervision, over which we retain a greater degree of control. These are most likely to provide the key to formulating a considered response to creeping technical essentialism.

Formulating a Considered Response

Through reexamining and developing our everyday approaches to carrying out research, teaching, and supervision, we can find ammunition for resisting the imperatives of technical essentialism. It is here, in our own backyard, that we can forge alternative responses that will strengthen and enhance the practice and rigor of qualitative research rather than letting it be subsumed to a set of overarching criteria or reduced to a checklist of procedures.

As Mauthner, Parry, and Backett-Milburn (1998) have shown, even the original researchers can draw out different themes from their data at different times, reflecting how their own interests have moved on. Journals such as the *British Medical Journal* now employ a procedure for quantitative articles whereby the version of the journal available on the World Wide Web contains more details of statistical analyses and results. Some online qualitative journals now employ a variant of the approach suggested by Hoddinott and Pill (1997), which allows the researcher to chart the many and varied influences that have impinged on the process of data generation, analysis, and writing up. Particularly for journals with strict word limits and restrictions on presenting of theoretical arguments (due to space constraints or a focus on practice), this enables the reader to both contextualize and evaluate the piece of research and the inferences drawn by the author. However, it is important that researchers continue to be encouraged to use such detail to analytic advantage in engaging with their data and interpretations; simply to deposit such information on the Web and leave readers to draw their own inferences would constitute a technical essentialist approach, complying with the letter rather than the spirit of such calls for contextual details.

Having asked six independent researchers to code the same focus group transcript, Armstrong, Gosling, Weinman, and Marteau (1997) reported that although their explanations and packaging of coding frameworks (including the language used) varied to an extent, there was significant agreement about issues worthy of comment. However, as Armstrong et al. acknowledged, this was a somewhat artificial situation. Normally a whole set of transcripts would have been available for analysis and for further discussion between coders. It would be interesting to speculate to as to whether analyses and packaging frameworks would converge or diverge as subsequent transcripts were analyzed. Crucial to such exercises is the background and level of experience of co-coders. To what extent are they steeped in or conversant with the central concerns of the research project in question? To what extent are they involved as the project unfolds? Morse (1997) pointed out that such secondary analysis by researchers removed from the project can "violate the process of induction," as their knowledge is necessarily limited to specific transcripts, which is likely to result in superficial analysis.

Barry, Britten, Barber, Bradley, and Stevenson (1998) have shown how the different knowledge bases and values of team members can influence the interpretation of data and thereby shape the process of analysis. I suspect that most experienced qualitative researchers already employ a pragmatic version of double-coding through supervision and team meetings. What is potentially valuable about this exercise is not the extent of agreement but the content and nature of any disagreements: the dialogue between supervisor and supervisee or coworker and how this feeds back into and informs the development of a coding frame. Such a session reproduces in microcosm the process of qualitative research itself, maximizing the analytic potential of exceptions or potential alternative explanations. It is incumbent on us to use such insights to advantage in attempting to unpick for others (i.e., students, new researchers, reviewers, and readers) the intricacies of the qualitative analysis process.

Conclusion

Given the important time and funding constraints under which most of us now carry out our research, collaborative exercises (such as those outlined here) might, indeed, provide a feasible alternative to the concept of data saturation and continuous returning to the field to check out and further develop emergent theories as originally advocated by Glaser and Strauss (1967). It is also important that we sidestep the possibility of developing a hierarchy of evidence and move to a consideration of parallel data and how this can be used to illuminate the phenomena we study. The materials are already at our disposal through our serial and even simultaneous involvement in different research projects, which can span a wide variety of topics. The challenge is to integrate this more explicitly into our teaching and supervision, drawing on the principles of the constant comparative method and analytic induction, allowing us to use exceptions to analytic advantage in continuously interrogating our data. (Such an approach might also ultimately help to avoid the theoretical congestion identified by Morse, 2000.) Although never far from the surface in the practice of qualitative research, these aspects of the analysis process have tended to have been treated as the "Cinderella" of grounded theory and have, as yet, escaped itemization in checklists. Green (1998) has reminded us, "Constant comparison does not stop within the researcher's own data set. Theoretical insight and comparative material comes from other research, perhaps outside the substantive field of interest" (p. 1065). It is constant comparison that provides the key also to contextualizing our research findings within the existing substantive and theoretical literature – a task that is often avoided (Morse, 2000). The constant comparative method also holds most promise as a basis for developing an appropriate and sympathetic approach to the ever-encroaching calls for meta-analysis of qualitative data (Morse, 2001b), an approach that could also reclaim grounded theory and provide a convincing alternative to technical essentialism.

Author's Note

An earlier version of this article was presented at the Sixth Qualitative Health Research Conference, held in Banff in 2000. I am grateful to those who attended for their helpful feedback. I would also like to thank the two anonymous reviewers for their constructive comments.

References

Armstrong, D., Gosling, A., Weinman, J., & Marteau, T. (1997). The place of inter-rater reliability in qualitative research: An empirical study. *Sociology, 31*(3), 597–606.

Atkinson, P. (1997). Narrative turn or blind alley? *Qualitative Health Research, 7,* 325–344.

Barbour, R. S. (1998). Mixing qualitative methods: Quality assurance or qualitative quagmire? *Qualitative Health Research, 8,* 352–361.

Barbour, R. S. (1999). The case for combining qualitative and quantitative approaches in health services research. *Journal of Health Services Research & Policy, 4,* 39–43.

Barbour, R. S. (2001). Checklists for improving rigor in qualitative research: A case of the tail wagging the dog? *British Medical Journal, 322,* 1115–1117.

Barbour, R. S., & Huby, G. (Eds.). (1998). *Meddling with mythology: AIDS and the social construction of knowledge.* London: Routledge.

Barry, C., Britten, N., Barber, N., Bradley, C., & Stevenson, F. (1999). Using reflexivity to optimize teamwork in qualitative research. *Qualitative Health Research, 9,* 26–44.

Bryman, A., & Burgess, R. G. (Eds.). (1994). *Analyzing qualitative data.* London: Routledge.

Chapple, A., & Rogers, A. (1998). Explicit guidelines for qualitative research: A step in the right direction, a defence of the "soft" option, or a form of sociological imperialism? *Family Practice, 15*(6), 556–561.

Collins, P. (1998). Negotiating selves: Reflections on "unstructured" interviewing. *Sociological Research Online, 3*(3). Retrieved February 13, 2003, from http://www.socresonline.org.Uk/3/3/2.html

Glaser, B., & Strauss, A. (1967). *The discovery of grounded theory.* Chicago: Aldine.

Green, J. (1998). Grounded theory and the constant comparative method [Commentary]. *British Medical Journal, 316,* 1064–1065.

Hall, W. A., & Callery, P. (2001). Enhancing the rigor of grounded theory: Incorporating reflexivity and relationality. *Qualitative Health Research, 11,* 257–272.

Harding, G., & Gantley, M. (1998). Qualitative methods: Beyond the cookbook. *Family Practice, 15,* 76–79.

Harding, G., & Gantley, M. (1999, July). *You only want me for my methods.* Paper presented at the Academic Departments of General Practice (AUDGP) Annual Conference, London.

Hoddinott, P., & Pill, R. (1997). A review of recently published qualitative research in general practice: More methodological questions than answers? *Family Practice, 14,* 313–320.

Hutchinson, S. A. (2001). The development of qualitative health research: Taking stock. *Qualitative Health Research, 11,* 505–521.

Krueger, R. A. (1993). Quality control in focus group research. In D. Morgan (Ed.), *Successful focus groups: Advancing the state of the art* (pp. 65–85). Newbury Park, CA: Sage.

Kuzel, A. J. (1992). Sampling in qualitative inquiry In B. F. Crabtree & W. L. Miller (Eds.), *Doing qualitative research* (pp. 31–44). Newbury Park, CA: Sage.

Mason, J. (1996). *Qualitative researching.* London: Sage.

Mauthner, N. S., Parry, O., & Backett-Milburn, K. (1998). The data are out there, or are they? Implications for archiving and revisiting qualitative data. *Sociology, 32*(4), 733–745.

Melia, K. M. (1997). Producing "plausible stories": Interviewing student nurses. In G. Miller & R. Dingwall (Eds.), *Context and method in qualitative research* (pp. 26–36). London: Sage.

Miller, G. (1997). Introduction: Context and method in qualitative research. In G. Miller & R. Dingwall (Eds.), *Context and method in qualitative research* (pp. 1–11). London: Sage.

Morse, J. M. (1997). Perfectly healthy, but dead: The myth of inter-rater reliability. *Qualitative Health Research, 7,* 445–447.

Morse, J. M. (2000). Theoretical congestion [Editorial], *Qualitative Health Research, 10,* 715–716.

Morse, J. M. (2001a). The awfulness of simplification [Editorial]. *Qualitative Health Research, 11,* 435.

Morse, J. M. (2001b). Steps and strategies [Editorial]. *Qualitative Health Research, 11,* 147–148.

Popay, J., Williams, G., & Rogers, A. (1998). Rationale and standards for the systematic review of qualitative literature in health services research. *Qualitative Health Research, 8,* 341–351.

Ritchie, J., & Spencer, L. (1994). Qualitative data analysis for applied policy research. In A. Bryman & R. G. Burgess (Eds.), *Analyzing qualitative data* (pp. 173–194). London: Routledge.

Seale, C. (1999). *The quality of qualitative research.* London: Sage.

Seale, C., & Silverman, D. (1997). Ensuring rigor in qualitative research. *European Journal of Public Health, 7,* 379–384.

Silverman, D. (1992). Applying the qualitative method to clinical care. In J. Daly, I. McDonald, & E. Willis (Eds.), *Researching health care: Designs, dilemmas, disciplines* (pp. 176–188). London: Routledge.

Silverman, D. (1993). *Interpreting qualitative data: Methods of analyzing talk, text and interaction.* London: Sage.

Thomas, W. I. (1949). *Social structure and social theory.* New York: Free Press.